SENSORY SUBSTITUTION AND AUGMENTATION

PROCEEDINGS OF THE BRITISH ACADEMY • 219

SENSORY SUBSTITUTION AND AUGMENTATION

Edited by
FIONA MACPHERSON

Published for THE BRITISH ACADEMY
by OXFORD UNIVERSITY PRESS

Oxford University Press, Great Clarendon Street, Oxford OX2 6DP

First edition published in 2018

British Library Cataloguing in Publication Data
Data available

Library of Congress Cataloging in Publication Data
Data available

Typeset by
Keystroke, Neville Lodge, Tettenhall, Wolverhampton

Printed in Great Britain by
Short Run Press Limited, Exeter, Devon

ISBN 978-0-19-726644-1

ISSN 0068-1202

A man may see how this world goes
with no eyes. Look with thine ears.

Might I but live to see thee in my touch,
I'd say I had eyes again!

William Shakespeare, *King Lear*

Contents

Illustrations

Figures

Tables

Notes on Contributors

Diana Acosta-Navas is a Graduate Fellow at the Edmond J. Safra Center for Ethics and a PhD candidate in the Philosophy Department at Harvard University. She completed her Master's degree at the National University of Colombia and her BA at Los Andes University. She has conducted research on the relation between visual perception and motor activity, as well as nativist theories of concepts. Her current research uses concepts from philosophy of language to assess efforts to empower vulnerable populations in post-conflict scenarios and situations of deep inequality.

Amir Amedi is the Director of The make SENSE Center for Brain imaging, Rehab and Augmentation of the SENSES. He is a Full Professor in the Department of Medical Neurobiology at the Hebrew University and the ELSC brain center. He holds a PhD in Computational Neuroscience from ICNC, Hebrew University, and was a Postdoctoral and Instructor of Neurology at Harvard Medical School. He is recipient of the Krill Prize for Excellence in Scientific Research, awarded by the Wolf Foundation (2011), the international Human Frontier Science Program Career Development Award (2004, 2009 respectively), and the JSMF Scholar Award in Understanding Human Cognition (2011). He has received two consecutive ERC grants (www.BrainVisionRehab.com 2013–2018; ExperieSENSE 2018–2023). He is an internationally acclaimed brain scientist with 15 years of experience in the field of brain plasticity and multisensory integration. He has a particular interest in visual rehabilitation and sensory substitution. In 2017 he co-founded www.ReNewSenses.com where his lab and his team are engaged in developing novel SSDs and topographic machine vision algorithms to help the visually impaired.

Malika Auvray is a CNRS researcher in cognitive sciences at the Institut des Systèmes Intelligents et de Robotique, Paris. Her main research interests are in sensory substitution and, more broadly, cross-modal interactions. She experimentally investigates learning the use of sensory substitution devices and the mechanisms involved in distal attribution. She challenges the distinction between the sensory modalities through the examples of these devices, and collaborates on the development of two visual-to-auditory conversion systems: the Vibe and Navig. She has published more than 40 articles or book chapters and has given 120 talks on sensory substitution, perception, and cross-modal interactions.

Umut Baysan is a Lecturer in Philosophy of Mind and Cognitive Science at the Faculty of Philosophy and St Anne's College, University of Oxford. Previously, he worked as a university teacher and a postdoctoral researcher at the University of

Glasgow, where he obtained his PhD in 2014. He works in philosophy of mind and metaphysics, specializing in the metaphysics of mind–body relations. His research has appeared in journals such as *Australasian Journal of Philosophy*, *Analysis*, *Philosophical Quarterly*, and *Minds and Machines*.

Robert Briscoe is Professor of Philosophy at Ohio University. His research takes an empirically oriented approach toward a range of topics in the philosophy of cognitive science, philosophy of perception, and philosophy of mind. He has published numerous papers on the role of action in perception, spatial representation, mental imagery, depiction, and pictorial experience. During the 2017–18 academic year, he was a Fulbright-Scotland Visiting Professor in the Department of Philosophy at the University of Glasgow.

David J. Brown is a Visiting Research Fellow in the Crossmodal Cognition Lab at the University of Bath and an Associate Lecturer in Psychology at Bath Spa University. He studied at the University of Sussex for his bachelor's and master's degrees before moving on to Queen Mary University of London for his PhD. His research interests primarily focus on visual-to-auditory and visual-to-tactile sensory substitution, as well as other more general cross-modal interactions.

Derek Brown is a Lecturer in the Centre for the Study of Perceptual Experience and Department of Philosophy at the University of Glasgow (though his chapter in this volume was written while he was a member of the Department of Philosophy at Brandon University). He works in philosophy of mind and perception, with particular interests in philosophy of colour and 'indirect' approaches to perception. He is co-editor of *Analysis and Interpretation in the Exact Sciences: Essays in Honour of William Demopoulos* (with M. Frappier and R. DiSalle, Springer, 2012) and *The Routledge Handbook of Philosophy of Colour* (with F. Macpherson, Routledge, forthcoming). He has held visiting appointments in philosophy at the University of Pittsburgh, the University of Glasgow, and the University of Cambridge.

Jonathan Cohen is Professor of Philosophy at the University of California, San Diego. He has published widely in philosophy of mind, philosophy of perception, and philosophy of language, and is the author of *The Red and the Real: An Essay on Color Ontology* (Oxford University Press, 2009), and co-editor of *Color Ontology and Color Science* (with Mohan Matthen, MIT Press, 2010) and *Contemporary Debates in the Philosophy of Mind* (with Brian McLaughlin, Blackwell, 2007).

Kevin Connolly is a philosopher and cognitive scientist who works on perception and learning. His research focuses especially on perception-based learning, as found in experts from wine tasters to radiologists to birdwatchers. He is the author of *Perceptual Learning: The Flexibility of the Senses*, forthcoming with Oxford

University Press. He is currently an Assistant Professor of Psychology at Minerva Schools at KGI, a new university founded on the principles of the science of learning. Prior to joining Minerva, he was an Andrew W. Mellon Postdoctoral Fellow at the University of Pennsylvania.

Jennifer Corns is Lecturer in Philosophy at the University of Glasgow. Her published research focuses on pain and affect. She aims to use philosophical tools and evaluate empirical research to make progress on topics that matter within and beyond the academy.

Ophelia Deroy holds the Chair of Philosophy of Mind at the Ludwig Maximilian University in Munich, as a joint appointment between the Faculty of Philosophy and the Munich Centre for Neuroscience. She is the former Deputy Director of the Institute of Philosophy at the School of Advanced Study, at the University of London, and an associate researcher at the Centre for the Study of the Senses in London. Her work focuses on how different kinds of information can be integrated across domains or agents, and has been published in many international journals in philosophy and cognitive science. In recent years, she has worked in close connection with cognitive neuroscientists, noticeably on the phenomenon of cross-modal correspondences, metacognition and the consequences of sensory deficits on multisensory perception. Her account of sensory substitution, developed with Malika Auvray, suggests it should be compared to other cases of non-natural 'cross-modal transfer', like the one occurring in reading.

Jérôme Dokic is Professor at the Ecole des Hautes Etudes en Sciences Sociales, Université PSL, and a member of the Institut Jean-Nicod in Paris. His research interests are perception, memory, imagination and, more recently, epistemic feelings and metacognition. He has published many articles on these topics, as well as the books *La philosophie du son* (with Roberto Casati, *Philosophy of sound*, Chambon, 1994), *L'esprit en mouvement. Essai sur la dynamique cognitive* (*Mind in motion. Essay on cognitive dynamics*, CSLI, Stanford, 2001), *Qu'est-ce que la perception?* (*What is perception?*, Vrin, 2nd edition, 2009) and *Ramsey: Truth and Success* (with Pascal Engel, Routledge, 2002).

Sarah Hillenbrand is a postdoctoral teaching fellow at Stanford University, with appointments in the Thinking Matters program and the Program in Writing and Rhetoric. She is also an adjunct professor of psychology at the University of San Francisco. The recipient of the National Science Foundation's Graduate Research Fellowship, she completed her doctoral research at the University of California, Berkeley, using brain scans to better understand the processes underlying human motor learning. More recently, her work has focused on writing, podcasting, and how rhetorical practices across multiple media shape the public understanding of science.

Katrine Iversen is a medical student in Brainlab, Department of Neuroscience and Pharmacology, University of Copenhagen.

Ron Kupers is Professor and Lab Coordinator of Brainlab in the Department of Neuroscience and Pharmacology, University of Copenhagen. He has worked on brain plasticity following sensory deprivation and in sensory substitution and the cerebral correlates of pain perception. With Maurice Ptito, he has investigated the cross-modal plastic processes involved in use of the Tongue Display Unit (TDU) which converts visual images into electrotactile pulses applied to the tongue via a grid made out of tiny electrodes.

Fiona Macpherson is Professor of Philosophy, and Director of the Centre of the Study of Perceptual Experience (www.gla.ac.uk/cspe), at the University of Glasgow, where she runs a Virtual and Augmented Reality Lab, and is editor of The Illusions Index (www.illusionsindex.com). She is a member of the Arts and Humanities Research Council and a trustee of the Kennedy Memorial Trust. She has been Visiting Professor at the universities of London, Umea, and Kentucky, as well as a Research Fellow at the Australian National University, a Rosamund Chambers Research Fellow at Girton College, Cambridge, and a Research Fellow at Harvard. She has published numerous papers on the mind and perception in philosophy and psychology journals, and many edited volumes, including *The Routledge Handbook of Philosophy of Colour* (with Derek Brown, Routledge, 2018), *Perceptual Imagination and Perceptual Memory* (with Fabian Dorsch, Oxford University Press, 2018), *Phenomenal Presence* (with Fabian Dorsch, Oxford University Press, 2018), *Hallucination* (with Dimitris Platchias, MIT Press, 2013), *The Senses* (Oxford University Press, 2009), *The Admissible Contents of Experience* (with Katherine Hawley, Wiley Blackwell, 2009), and *Disjunctivism* (with Adrian Haddock, Oxford University Press, 2008).

Paul Noordhof is Anniversary Professor of Philosophy at the University of York (having previously been Professor of Philosophy at the University of Nottingham). He has published work on causation and consciousness, self-deception and imagination. From 2006 to 2009 he held a Major Research Fellowship funded by the Leverhulme Trust for work on consciousness and representation.

J. Kevin O'Regan is ex-director of the Laboratoire Psychologie de la Perception, CNRS, Université Paris Descartes. After early work on eye movements in reading, he was led to question established notions of the nature of visual perception, and to predict, with collaborators, the phenomenon of 'change blindness'. His current work involves exploring his 'sensorimotor' approach to consciousness in relation to sensory substitution, sensory adaptation, pain, colour, space perception, and developmental psychology. He is interested in applying this work to robotics.

Kevin O'Regan has recently published a book, *Why Red Doesn't Sound Like a Bell: Understanding the Feel of Consciousness*, with Oxford University Press.

Achille Pasqualotto received his PhD in Psychology from Trinity College Dublin. Since then, he has worked as Post-doctoral Fellow at the University of Hong Kong and Collège de France, and as Assistant Professor at Sabanci University. In 2018, he joined Nanyang Technological University. His interests include: spatial memory, multisensory integration (esp. vision and haptics), sensory substitution, and brain stimulation.

Michael J. Proulx is Reader in Psychology at the University of Bath where he is Director of the Crossmodal Cognition Laboratory (www.bath.ac.uk/psychology/research/groups/crossmodal-cognition-lab) and Deputy Director of MARVEL (Mixed and Augmented Reality and Virtual Environments Lab, www.bath.ac.uk/comp-sci/research/marvel). His research focuses on several aspects of cross-modal cognition and multisensory processes, with a particular interest in the impact of blindness on cognition. He received his BS in Psychology from Arizona State University and his PhD in Psychological and Brain Sciences from Johns Hopkins University. He is a Fellow of the American Psychological Association and the recipient of a New Investigator Award in Experimental Psychology: Human Perception and Performance and a Science Showcase Award from the APA. He was also honoured as a torchbearer for the London 2012 Paralympic Games.

Maurice Ptito is Professor of Visual Neuroscience in the School of Optometry at the Université de Montréal. He is also an Adjunct Professor of Neurology and Neurosurgery at the Montreal Neurological Institute (McGill University) and Guest Professor in the Department of Neuroscience and Pharmacology at the University of Copenhagen. He currently holds the Harland Sanders Research Chair in Vision Science. He has authored more than 200 scientific publications and has received several awards and prizes, including the Sir John William Dawson Medal of the Royal Society of Canada and the Henry and Karla Hensen Prize (Denmark). He is a Fellow of the Royal Society of Canada, the Canadian Psychological Association, the American Academy of Optometry, and the Royal Danish Academy of Sciences and Letters. In 2013, he was made a Knight of the National Order of Quebec. The major goal of his research is understanding the mechanisms involved in visual plasticity in normal developing individuals, as well as those who were born without vision or lost their vision later in life. With Ron Kupers, he has investigated the cross-modal plastic processes involved in use of the Tongue Display Unit (TDU) which converts visual images into electrotactile pulses applied to the tongue via a grid made out of tiny electrodes. Using several brain imaging tools, they showed that the brains of blind individuals undergo extensive rewiring.

Dina Raveh is Professor (emerita) in the Department of Life Sciences, Ben Gurion University of the Negev, Beersheba, Israel. She studied for her BSc and MSc at the Hebrew University of Jerusalem, and for her PhD at the Weizmann Institute of Science, Israel; and did a post-doc at the Genetics Laboratory, Oxford University. She has been a Visiting Scientist at Yale University, the National Institute of Cancer (Frederick, MD), the Fred Hutchinson Cancer Center (Seattle, WA), the University of New South Wales (Sydney, Australia) and Auckland University (New Zealand). She has published research articles based on yeast as a model system for studying basic molecular cell genetics and how this knowledge is applied in medicine, in journals such as *Proceedings of the National Academy of Sciences USA*, *Molecular Cell Biology*, *PLoS Genetics*, etc. Her current interest in brain research was stimulated by a project on tinnitus research with Professor Grant Searchfield at Auckland University and by her association with the Amedi research group.

Laurent Renier is a Scientific Collaborator at the Université Catholique de Louvain (UCL, Belgium) and the Director of the Visual Impairment Department and the Archipel Center at the Royal Institute for the Deaf and Blind in Brussels (Institut Royal pour Sourds et Aveugles, IRSA, Belgium). He is a specialist in brain plasticity and has published several scientific papers on blindness, human perception and sensory substitution.

Barry C. Smith is a professor of philosophy and director of the Institute of Philosophy at the University of London's School of Advanced Study. He is also the founding director of the Centre for the Study of the Senses, which pioneers collaborative research between philosophers, psychologists and neuroscientists. From 2013 to 2019 he was the Arts and Humanities Research Council's Leadership Fellow for the Science in Culture Theme, and he has held visiting professorships at the University of California at Berkeley, Simon Fraser University, British Columbia and the École Normale Supérieure in Paris. A philosopher of language and mind, his principal research is on the multisensory nature of perceptual experience, focusing on taste, smell and flavour. He has written theoretical and experimental papers, publishing in *Nature*, *Food Quality and Preference*, and *Chemical Senses and Flavour*. In 2007, he edited *Questions of Taste: The Philosophy of Wine* (Oxford University Press); in 2008, he edited *The Oxford Handbook of Philosophy of Language* (with Ernest Lepore, Oxford University Press); and in 1998, *Knowing Our Own Minds* (with Crispin Wright and Cynthia Macdonald, Oxford University Press). In 2010 he wrote and presented a four-part series for the BBC World Service called *The Mysteries of the Brain*, and in 2017, he wrote and presented a ten-part series for BBC Radio 4 called *The Uncommon Senses*.

Charles Spence received his PhD in experimental psychology from the Department of Psychology at the University of Cambridge in 1994. He is a university professor in the Department of Experimental Psychology at Oxford University. Professor Spence heads the Crossmodal Research Laboratory in the Department of Experimental Psychology, Oxford University (http://psy.medsci.ox.ac.uk/research/crossmodal-research-laboratory). He has published over 800 articles in top-flight scientific journals over the last couple of decades. Professor Spence has been awarded the 10th Experimental Psychology Society Prize, the British Psychology Society: Cognitive Section Award, the Paul Bertelson Award, recognizing him as the young European Cognitive Psychologist of the Year, and the Friedrich Wilhelm Bessel Research Award from the Alexander von Humboldt Foundation in Germany. He has published a number of edited volumes, and has published: *In Touch with the Future: The Sense of Touch from Cognitive Neuroscience to Virtual Reality* (with A. Gallace, Oxford University Press, 2014); *The Perfect Meal* (with B. Piqueras-Fiszman, Wiley-Blackwell, 2014); and *Gastrophysics: The New Science of Eating* (Viking Penguin, 2017).

David Suarez is Lecturer in the Department of Philosophy at the University of California, Berkeley. He has published on phenomenology, cognitive science, and the philosophy of mind. In his work on 'phenomenological naturalism' he argues that in order to understand how the world becomes available to us in experience we must reconceive nature along the lines explored by phenomenologists.

Jamie Ward is Professor of Cognitive Neuroscience at the University of Sussex. He is best known for his research on synaesthesia, but has wider research interests in multisensory perception, embodied cognition, and sensory substitution. In addition to publishing extensively in journals, he is the author of leading textbooks (*The Student's Guide to Cognitive Neuroscience*; *The Student's Guide to Social Neuroscience*) and Editor-in-Chief of *Cognitive Neuroscience*.

Thomas D. Wright has a BSc and PhD from the University of Sussex. His thesis was entitled 'Towards a better understanding of sensory substitution: the theory and practice of developing visual-to-auditory sensory substitution devices' and was funded by the EPSRC. His research integrates software development with experimental methods from cognitive psychology, and also draws on evidence from the neurosciences.

Preface and Acknowledgements

The conference, where the vast majority of these papers were delivered, took place from 26 to 28 March 2013 at the British Academy in London. It was generously funded by the British Academy, and a grant from the Social Science and Humanities Research Council of Canada awarded to The Network for Sensory Research, which is directed by Professor Mohan Matthen at the University of Toronto, and which involves four other partners: Susanna Siegel (Harvard), Alex Byrne (MIT), Barry Smith and the CENSES: Centre for the Study of the Senses (London), and myself and the Centre for the Study of Perceptual Experience (Glasgow). It was also funded by a grant from the Chancellor's Fund of the University of Glasgow. I am very grateful to the generosity of these funders without whom the conference could not have taken place.

There are many people who deserve my thanks for helping me in organizing the conference. Malika Auvray (Institut des Systèmes Intelligents et de Robotique, Paris) provided advice about the work of many psychologists on the topic. Angela Pusey and staff at the British Academy made many of the practical arrangements and advised me on practical matters. I would also like to thank the speakers and all those who attended for their excellent contributions throughout the conference.

The conference was followed by a public event where many of the speakers and attendees put on practical demonstrations of the sensory substitution and augmentation devices that we had been discussing during the conference. This was a historic moment when, for the first time ever, these devices were gathered together in one location. I would like to thank Jon Bird (City University, London) for his advice and enormous practical help in setting up this event.

The papers delivered at the conference, together with a video of the practical demonstration events, can be found on the Centre for the Study of Perceptual Experience's website at: www.gla.ac.uk/cspe.

This volume is the first on the topic of sensory substitution and augmentation. It shows that there is a growing amount of current research on the subject. What the volume makes clear is that this research is still in its infancy. There is much disagreement among researchers as to the nature of the devices, how they work, the nature of the mental states that they cause in people using them, and about their practical value. This volume is required precisely because it makes these disagreements perspicuous, and I hope that it will spur further work towards exploring and resolving these issues. That surely will add to our understanding of perception and make progress in helping those who would like their senses enhanced. Philosophers, psychologists, and neuroscientists all contribute to the discussions on these topics in this volume, and I hope that the value of interdisciplinary work on this topic becomes manifest, and people come to see that many disciplines have an important contribution to make to the debates about sensory substitution and augmentation.

I would like to thank the contributors to this volume for their thoughtful contributions, and for their patience as this volume was brought to press. I would also like to thank Brigid Hamilton-Jones of the British Academy for her help in compiling this volume. And, finally, I would like to thank the British Academy for publishing this volume in their Proceedings of the British Academy series.

Fiona Macpherson
March 2018

1

Sensory Substitution and Augmentation: An Introduction

FIONA MACPHERSON

Abstract In this essay I outline the main questions and the debates about sensory substitution and augmentation devices. I describe the two most studied modern sensory substitution devices (TVSS and the vOICe) and one sensory augmentation device (the feelSpace belt). I discuss whether use of these devices gives rise to new sensory experiences of objects or just new perceptual judgements about objects. Then, on the assumption that new sensory experiences are being had, I consider what sensory modality is operative—the substituted or the substituting one, or another altogether. I examine the evidence concerning whether the experiences had in sensory substitution are of a two- or a three-dimensional world. And I also examine the evidence about the nature of those experiences with respect to whether colour is represented in them. I consider whether there are any limits to what information or what experiences can be given via sensory substitution. And I discuss whether the results from sensory substitution experiments can be used to support certain theories of perception at the expense of rivals, and to provide illuminating examples of distinctions that some people want to make in articulating a theory of perception. Furthermore, the practical use of sensory substitution and augmentation devices is considered. Finally, I will provide a brief overview of the rest of the essays that this volume contains and the host of further interesting issues that the authors consider and address.

1.1 What Are Sensory Substitution and Sensory Augmentation?

THE SENSES ARE OUR windows on the world. They constitute the various ways that we have of perceiving the world. Vision, hearing, touch, taste, smell, proprioception,

Proceedings of the British Academy, **219**, 1–42.

and balance, among others, are the ways that we humans, and other creatures, have of gaining empirical knowledge about the world.

Losing a sense is a terrifying prospect. Becoming blind or deaf, losing the sense of touch or taste, or any of the other senses, would cut oneself off from important and valuable features of the world. The loss of certain experiences would itself be hard to come to terms with and, practically speaking, many important activities would become more difficult: negotiating one's way around the world, communicating with other people, and avoiding danger. Even the prospect of losing one's sense of smell, the sense that most people might choose to lose, if forced to choose to lose one of them, has been shown often to have dire consequences. Unlike the loss of other senses, which typically lead to temporary depression followed by a period of readjustment, the loss of smell can often lead to lasting depression.[1] Lack of enjoyment of food, inability to monitor one's body odour, increased social anxiety, impaired sex-life, and the loss of the strong connection between smell and the emotions, are among the effects of losing this sense. The prospect, therefore, of being able to replace vision, hearing, smell, or any other sense, in full or in part, by exploiting another sense or senses, is an immensely attractive prospect for some—a prospect that potentially could transform for the better the lives of those who have lost a sense. This is the prospect of sensory substitution.

For those who have been born without a sense, or lost a sense very early in life, rather than late in life, the issue of whether one should provide, or try to provide, the missing sense is a complicated one. For example, some people in the Deaf community see themselves as being differently abled compared to those people born with hearing, and not as people who are impoverished and need to be 'cured'. While people who are deaf lack access to sound, they have access to something that hearing people typically do not: the rich and distinctive Deaf language and culture. They are keen to preserve this and they would not want this to be lost by giving a sense of hearing to all deaf people.[2] Nonetheless, some people who have been born without a sense, or who have lost one very early in life, would like to be able to have that sense—or at least the possibility of discovering whether they would prefer a life that included having that sense. In the case of blind people, for example, the potential to be less reliant on other people sometimes provides a large motivating factor to gain sight. And so, at least for some people born without one of the human senses, or who lost one early, the possibility of gaining such a sense is a highly attractive prospect, in addition to it being so for those who lose a sense later in life.

While the prospect of being able to replace a sense is potentially transformative for those who have lost a sense, it also gives rise to new and rather exciting ideas. If replacing a sense is possible, then could we extend our existing senses, or could

[1] See Deems et al. (1991), Gudziol et al. (2009), and Seo et al. (2009).

[2] See Hyde and Power (2006).

we give ourselves whole new senses? Who hasn't thought that it would be interesting to be able to hear or smell the range of stimuli that we know that dogs can and that humans, at least without augmentation, cannot? What schoolchild hasn't thought that having X-ray vision might be fun? Perhaps having an extended sense or having a new sense could be useful in some circumstances. When one hears about the senses that some nonhuman animals have—such as electric senses or magnetic senses, senses that open up whole new possibilities for finding out about the world, navigating through it, and acting upon it—who wouldn't want to acquire such senses, even if only on a temporary basis? Sensory augmentation devices try to deliver these possibilities.[3]

We can state more formally what sensory substitution and sensory augmentation amount to. In sensory substitution, one tries to replace a missing sense by delivering some or all of the information usually gathered by one sense to another sense. What counts as a missing sense in a person in this context is determined by considering the normal sensory capacities of humans. More generally, what counts as a missing sense in a creature is determined by considering the normal sensory capacities of the species of which the creature is a member. Sensory substitution has been attempted using modern technology since the 1960s, although, arguably, other more low-tech means have been around for a lot longer. For example, the use of Braille is a way to get information about words on a page to those who are blind by exploiting their sense of touch. Likewise, the use of a cane by blind people is a way of using touch to get information about obstacles in the world—obstacles that would typically be detected by sight by those that have it. Bach-y-Rita and Kercel (2003) suggest that writing itself may be considered the first sensory substitution device as it is a way of presenting information about words to vision—information that before the invention of writing was gained through hearing the spoken word. The promise of modern technology is to provide powerful tools to replace missing senses—ideally, to replace a missing sense *in toto*, although whether that is possible is as yet unknown. The goal that falls short of the ideal is to provide as much useful information as possible—information that one normally gets through a missing sense—by means of another sense.

An extension of this idea yields sensory augmentation. Rather than replace a missing sense with another, one tries to create a novel sense or enhance an existing sense. To do this, one has to do that which one does in sensory substitution: deliver information to a subject via a sense that does not usually deliver that information. This is why sensory substitution and augmentation are closely related. As we increasingly learn of the senses of nonhuman animals, so the intriguing possibilities of senses we can imagine giving people grow.[4] Among others, we can

[3] Some philosophers, such as Nudds (2004) and Richardson (2013), have, in line with Aristotle, argued that there are only five senses. I reject this view and argue against it in Macpherson (2011a) and (2013).
[4] See, for example, Hughes (2001).

imagine having a magnetic sense that allows us to detect magnetic fields and their properties, as pigeons do and use to navigate long distances; and we can envisage having an electric sense enabling us to detect electric fields, as many fish have; or we can contemplate having echolocation, as, for example, bats have. It might also be possible to make our senses more sensitive and thus, for example, responsive to higher or lower sounds, more and more diffuse smells, larger and smaller frequencies of electromagnetic radiation, and so on. Possessing such senses might allow us to help ourselves, and each other, in ways that we could not before. For example, having the ability to detect objects in front of us in the dark—an ability that echolocation confers—might help us in various rescue situations, as might a keener sense of hearing or smell than that which we typically have.

In addition to their potential to increase the sensory abilities of people, sensory substitution and augmentation devices might also deliver enriched experiences to people in virtual-reality computer-simulated worlds—and in a way that could be delivered over the internet. It is very easy to transmit images and sounds to people via screens and speakers using the internet, giving them visual and auditory experiences of a virtual world. By using vibromotors placed on a person's body we can also give them experiences of touch corresponding to a virtual world. But what about experiences in other sensory modalities? That is not so easy. But sensory substitution and augmentation might be able to help. Sensory substitution might allow us to get information to a person that they would normally get from modalities other than sight, hearing and touch via those modalities—modalities that it is easy to send information to over the internet. If that is right then we might be able to enrich people's online virtual experience. For example, devices have been created that use tactile stimulation on the tongue to give people information about their position with respect to gravity—in other words information about their balance—that they would normally get through their vestibular sense.[5] Using such a device, one could send information about a person's orientation to gravity corresponding to the position that a person is in in a virtual world. This is just one example of many possibilities that sensory substitution and augmentation may open up.

In conclusion, it is hoped that modern sensory substitution and augmentation devices will be able to replace or expand our senses. But to what extent has this been achieved to date? To what extent are the experiences created by sensory substitution devices like the sensory experiences that we are trying to replace? To what extent can we augment people's senses, providing them with new information and new experiences? The first aim of this introduction is to delve deeply into this question to discover the usefulness of these devices, to outline the different sorts of experience that might be created, and what the evidence tells us about

[5] See Tyler et al. (2003).

these experiences. While there are some reasons to be hopeful about the powers of sensory substitution devices, there are also reasons to wonder whether they will ever really have the practical applications that we hope they might have. The second aim is to look to see whether the study of modern sensory substitution and augmentation devices can shed light on the nature of our senses and perception in general. Much of the philosophical, psychological, and neuroscientific work that takes place concerning sensory substitution and augmentation is keenly aware of the possibility that it might help our understanding and it seeks to comprehend many different aspects of perception.

In the sections that follow, I outline the main questions and the debates about sensory substitution and augmentation devices that have arisen in the literature to date. In section 1.2, I will describe the two most studied modern sensory substitution devices and one sensory augmentation device. This is vital to allow the reader to have a clear idea of what sensory substitution and augmentation devices are, how subjects' behaviour changes when they use them, and what subjects say about their experience. This forms part of the evidence that is used to assess how these devices work. In section 1.3, I will discuss whether use of these devices gives rise to new sensory experiences of objects or just new judgements about objects. In section 1.4, on the assumption that new sensory experiences are being had, I will consider what sensory modality is operative—the substituted or the substituting one, or another altogether. I will examine the evidence concerning whether the experiences had in sensory substitution are of a two- or a three-dimensional world. And I will also examine the evidence about the nature of those experiences with respect to whether colour is represented in them. In section 1.5, I will consider whether there are any limits to what information or what experiences can be given via sensory substitution. In section 1.6, I will discuss whether the results from sensory substitution experiments can be used to support certain theories of perception at the expense of rivals, and to provide illuminating examples of distinctions that some people want to make in articulating a theory of perception. In section 1.7, the practical use of sensory substitution and augmentation devices will be considered. Finally, in section 1.8, I will provide a brief overview of the rest of the essays that this volume contains and the host of further interesting issues that the authors consider and address.

1.2 Sensory Substitution and Augmentation Devices

The most famous sensory substitution device is the Tactile Visual Sensory Substitution (TVSS) device, which was developed by Paul Bach-y-Rita, initially with the help of Carter Collins (Bach-y-Rita et al. 1969). The device tries to replace vision by exploiting the sense of touch. Subjects who use the TVSS are either blind people or sighted people who are blindfolded. The original equipment consisted of a dentist's chair adapted so that on the back of the chair was a grid of solenoid vibrators—in other words a grid of metal pins each of which is able to vibrate. A camera was mounted on the side of the dentist's chair that produced a black and white image. This image determined which of the solenoids vibrated. If one imagines the black and white image overlaid on top of the grid of solenoids, those solenoids that would vibrate would be those whose locus was within a white region of the image. For example, if the image consisted of black on the left-hand side and white on the right-hand side then the solenoids on the right-hand side of the grid would vibrate and those on the left would not. If the image consisted of a white circular area in the middle of a black background, then a circle of solenoids in the middle of the grid would vibrate and the rest would not. More complicated patterns could be produced, limited only by the resolution of the camera image, the resolution of the grid of solenoids, and the resolution of the skin in being able to detect them.

Later, portable versions of the device were created in which a grid of vibrating pins was strapped to a subject's back or stomach, and the camera was mounted on the subject's forehead. Later still, a version was created that, instead of using vibrating solenoids on the skin, used a grid of electrodes that could carry an electrical charge (rather than vibrate) and which were placed into the mouth to rest against the tongue (Bach-y-Rita et al. 2003). This device is called a tongue display unit (TDU).

One reason for using the TDU is that the tongue is very sensitive to touch. Different parts of the body are more or less sensitive to touch. One way that this is measured is by a two-point discrimination test, in which a series of either one or two pinpoints is placed on the subject's skin and the subject has to report whether they felt one or two pinpoints pressing against them. (The test is carried out with the eyes closed.) The smallest distance between two pinpoints that a subject can reliably identify through touch as being two pinpoints, rather than one, is the subject's two-point threshold. In normal subjects, the two-point threshold of the back and the stomach is rather large. For example, on the back it is between 36 and 75 mm. The fingertips are very sensitive and have a two-point threshold of 2–4 mm. The tongue is even more sensitive at around 1 mm.[6] Given that we normally want the hands to be free to carry out tasks, one can appreciate why the tongue is used. It allows for a higher resolution of image to be given to a subject, compared to the back or stomach, without limiting a subject's ability to engage with the world using their hands.

In order to practise using the device, subjects were told what was in front of them, or felt what was in front of them, when they were wearing the device. The idea was to learn what tactile stimulation corresponded to what objects and properties

[6] See Campbell (2006: 453).

being in front of them. The goal was to be able to subsequently identify things using only the device.

After wearing such devices and practising with them for a few hours, subjects could:

- recognize a range of common objects in front of them at a distance from their body, such as a cup, a telephone, and a toy horse;
- point accurately to objects in space; and
- judge objects' distance and absolute size (that is their size independent of distance from the subject/camera).

In order for the practice to be successful, thereby allowing the subjects to subsequently identify things using only the device, it is often reported that the subjects had to be able to move the camera. It is certainly true that if the camera was stationary then subjects could not learn to use the device. However, it is an interesting question to what extent *self-movement* is necessary. For example, if the camera is moved by another person but subjects know how it is being moved—either because they are told, or because they can feel the camera so they know how it is being moved—would that be sufficient to allow subjects to learn to use the device? Current evidence does not settle this question.

Subjects are also asked to report what it is like for them when they are training using the device. They say that initially they are only aware of the tactile stimulus and tactile experience that they have. However, after a great deal of practice, they report experiencing objects out in the world in front of them. This is often called 'externalizing' objects and properties. They do not report the tactile stimulus or a tactile experience (although they can pay attention to the tactile stimulation if they want to and come to report on a tactile experience). Moreover, subjects report their experience in quasi-visual terms, that is, using some of the language that people normally use to report their visual experience. (I will discuss this point in more detail below.)

After around thirty hours of practice with the TVSS, subjects:

- could make complex pattern discriminations;
- could recognize the faces of members of laboratory staff; and
- displayed a looming response when the camera lens was unexpectedly zoomed.

The second point is illustrated nicely by the following report that a subject gave when identifying what was in front of her while using a TVSS device: 'That is Betty; she is wearing her hair down today and does not have her glasses on; her mouth is open, and she is moving her right hand from her left side to the back of her head.'[7]

[7] Bach-y-Rita (1972: 6).

Let me explain the third point in more detail. When a camera lens is zoomed, the image it captures changes so that things in the distance appear to move forward and expand their apparent size—that is they increase the area of the image that they occupy. This makes it look as if things in the distance are rushing toward the camera. In response to this unexpected event, the subjects automatically moved their head and body backwards— and did so even if the tactile sensation that they were receiving was on their back—seemingly supporting the subjects' reports that they localized the objects that they were detecting as being in front of them in the external world, and not where the tactile sensation was.

Another sensory substitution device that has received much attention, study, and use is the vOICe, which was developed by Peter Meijer.[8] The aim is to give people vision by using the sense of hearing, and so, like the TVSS, the device is used by either blind people or sighted people who are blindfolded. This device uses a camera mounted on a subject's forehead or glasses and converts the camera image into a 'soundscape'. This is a sound stimulus that lasts one second that begins with a click to indicate the start of the period. Consider the X-axis and Y-axis of a camera image. The X-axis is represented by the duration of the sound over the one second. The Y-axis is represented by the pitch of the sound. And the volume of the sound corresponds to the brightness of each pixel. This means that unlike the TVSS, which can signal only black and white, the vOICe can signal black and white and shades of grey in between.

Consider the image of a sloping line in Figure 1.1. This would be represented by the vOICe by a click to indicate the start of the image, and then a brief silence followed by a note of rising pitch, followed by a brief silence. And consider the image of three dots in Figure 1.2. This would be represented by a click, a brief silence, and then a brief low-pitched sound followed by a brief silence, then a brief high-pitched sound followed by a brief silence, and then a brief medium-pitched sound again followed by a brief silence. After the one-second duration of the soundscape, it repeats again, starting with a click. More complex images elicit more complex sounds, with highly complex sound yielding very highly complex soundscapes. However, as with the TVSS, with practice, subjects can come to recognize objects using the device, and they report vision-like experiences: reports of a stable world appearing to be in front of them.

Now that I have described two of the most used and studied sensory substitution devices, I turn to describe one sensory augmentation device: the feelSpace belt. Recall that in sensory augmentation, one sense is used to try to create a new sense or enhance an existing one. The feelSpace belt, developed by Peter König, tries to give people a sense of magnetic north. The device consists of thirty vibrating actuators fitted on the inside of a belt that is worn round the waist. A compass

[8] See Meijer (1992). The capitalization of 'OIC' brings to mind the phrase, 'Oh, I see'.

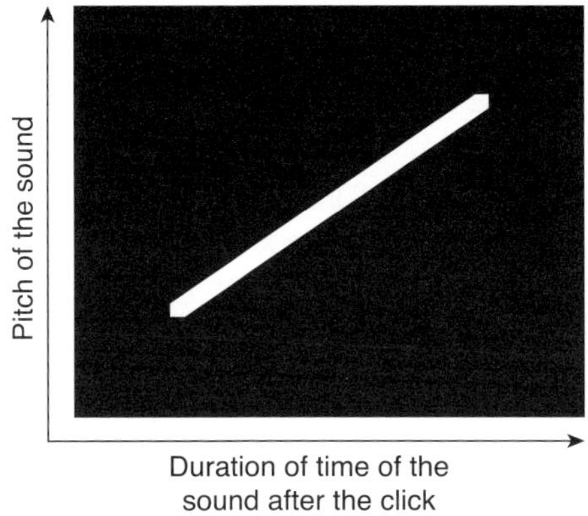

Figure 1.1 How a sloping line is represented by the vOICe.

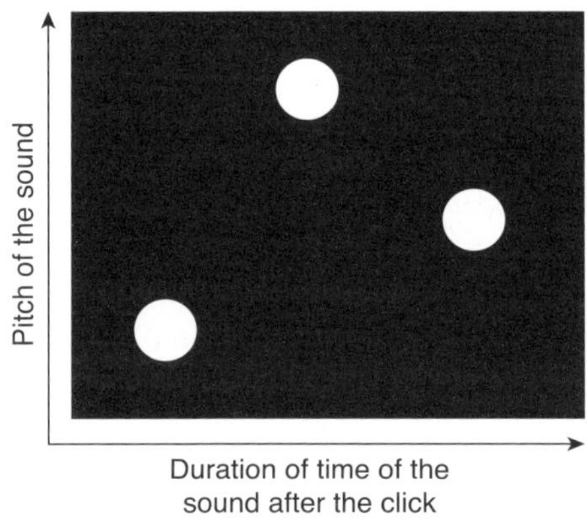

Figure 1.2 How three dots is represented by the vOICe.

detects magnetic north, and makes the actuator that is facing north vibrate. As the wearer moves around, the actuator that vibrates changes as the wearer's orientation towards magnetic north alters. After six weeks' training consisting of wearing the belt constantly, subjects who wore the belt were better than controls at certain navigation tasks. Nagel et al. (2005) report that two out of four subjects who were trained to use the belt reported changes in their perceptual experience. They said that it was hard to describe the new experience, but that it was a sense of space different from that which they had before. They were more aware of the direction of their home or office when they were at various different locations. One subject said, 'reference points are intuitively present and help a lot in navigating around and understanding relations between places' (Nagel et al. 2005: R22). This awareness was clearly distinguished from the additional tactile stimulation that the belt provided. Surprisingly, the additional spatial awareness was relative to landmarks, not to magnetic north, as the experimenters had expected.

I have now explained what sensory substitution and augmentation are, and I have explained the workings of three devices. The devices allowed discriminations of objects or directions in new ways, and in the two sensory substitution cases, subjects often reported having new experiences described in quasi-visual terms. In the sensory augmentation case two subjects reported having new experiences. In the next section, I will examine the evidence concerning whether new experiences are had and, in the section following that, I will consider whether those alleged experiences are in a new modality. Subsequently, I will examine other properties of those alleged experiences.

1.3 Do Subjects Have a New Sensory Experience?

In this section I will focus on what is reported to be the new 'quasi-visual' experience that subjects come to have after practice with the TVSS and the vOICe. Do subjects come to have a new sensory experience, as they often report? Recall that many subjects reported a new experience of stable objects in space external to, and in front of, them. What is clear is that new information is getting to the subjects that allows them to do things they couldn't do before: identify and discriminate objects. But are subjects doing this because they have a new experience in addition to or instead of that experience which they had at the start of their training—an experience in addition to or instead of the tactile experience in the case of the TVSS, or the auditory experience in the case of the vOICe? The alternative to the idea that they did have a new experience is the idea that subjects just come to make new judgements or come to form new beliefs about objects that are in front of them—judgements or beliefs that are inferred from the tactile or auditory experiences that they have at the start of their training with the sensory substitution devices and that they continue to have throughout the training.

It is very difficult, *in general*, to tell when a subject is having a sensory experience about something as opposed to making a judgement or having a belief about that thing.[9] So even in cases of perception that do not involve sensory substitution or augmentation there are often disputes about what is, say, visually experienced, and what is simply believed in response to that visual experience. One reason is that philosophers are not agreed on what objects and properties visual experience can represent, and thus on what sorts of visual experiences there are. Some philosophers think that only low-level properties such as size, shape and colour can be represented in visual experience, while others think that many other properties

[9] See Macpherson (2012) for detailed discussion.

besides can be represented, such as natural-kind properties, like being a pine-tree, or artificial-kind properties, such as being a table.[10] Moreover, some philosophers think that experience is simply belief or the acquisition of belief. For example, David Armstrong held that 'perception is *nothing but* the acquiring of knowledge of, or, on occasions, the acquiring of an inclination to believe in, particular facts about the physical world, by means of our senses' (1961: 105). Along similar lines, more recently, Katherin Glüer-Pagin (2009) has argued that experiences are beliefs with contents of the form *x looks F*.

In what follows, I will assume that sensory experiences are *not* to be equated with judgements or belief on the grounds that sensory experiences have a distinctive sort of phenomenology (by which I mean subjective character, or way that it is like, for the subject of the experience) that judging or believing lacks, and on the grounds that perceptual experiences play a different rational role, and have a different structure, from that of belief and judgement.[11] And, for ease of exposition, I will talk as if sensory experiences can have high-level content. (Nothing turns on this. Those people who believe that experiences do not have high-level contents can simply take my descriptions of experiences with high-level contents as specifying, in an informal manner, experiences with the sort of low-level contents that they would suppose such specifications to suggest.)

So, how can we tell whether the subjects who use the TVSS and the vOICe have new experiences about objects in the world in front of them or whether they simply make judgements about such objects based on their tactile or auditory experience? What evidence is there that can help us decide whether subjects are having new experiences?

One piece of evidence is the looming response—the automatic moving backwards away from the direction in which the camera is pointed—that TVSS subjects exhibit when the camera lens is, unbeknown to them, zoomed in, which I mentioned in the previous section. People have been impressed with this fact, pointing out, particularly, that this effect occurs even when the tactile stimulation is on a subject's back. Subjects don't try to move away from the location of the tactile stimulation, but from the direction in which the camera is pointing, suggesting that they are experiencing objects in front of them in the direction that the camera is pointed. It is argued that the fast automatic looming response could only be driven by sensory experience of objects in front of the subject, and could not be driven by judgement, which does not occur quickly enough to drive the response. It is argued that perceptual experience occurs more quickly than judgement, which occurs as a response to, and hence at a later time than, such experience.

However, one might question the premises of this argument. Might there not be fast automatic judgement formation once subjects have practised sufficiently using a device? Do we have really good evidence that judgement could not occur on the

[10] This debate is summarized in Macpherson (2011b).
[11] See Crane (1992) on these latter two points.

sort of timescale that could drive the looming response? I believe that this issue has not been investigated enough. Another concern stems from the performance of subjects in identifying objects using sensory substitution: it does not seem to be a fast automatic process at all. Most subjects have to pay great attention and be fully engaged with the task of identifying the objects in front of them in order to succeed at it. Moreover, recognition of an object in around ten seconds would be considered a good performance using a sensory substitution device. This is clearly far longer than one would take to recognize an object if one had a normal visual experience of it. One thought is that the experiences or judgements of objects' identity may take some time to have, but there may be a basic experience, an experience simply as of something being out in the world in front of them, that subjects have that precedes the experience or judgement that subjects have of objects' identity. Another thought is that subjects can make a fast automatic judgement that something is out in the world in front of them, which precedes the identification of which objects are in front of them. It is very hard to determine which is the correct account.

Another fact that some people think tells in favour of the hypothesis that subjects are having a new sensory experience is that congenitally blind people who use sensory substitution devices report that they come to have perceptual concepts that they did not have before—concepts such as parallax, perspective, shadow, and interposition of objects. One could try to argue that the best explanation of this new concept formation is that the congenitally blind people are having new experiences, which allow them to grasp the perceptual concepts that they did not previously.

However, one might question this conclusion on the ground that there is a good alternative explanation of what is going on that has not been ruled out. That explanation is that the congenitally blind subjects can simply form new beliefs about what is in front of them, and the relationship that those objects bear to them in egocentric space, and that it is coming to have these new beliefs that explains why they gain the new perceptual concepts. This explanation gains further support from the detailed observations of Kennedy (1993) that congenitally blind people can make and use raised-line drawings using touch, and, in virtue of doing so, come to have concepts, such as perspective, that previously it was thought they could not have. This suggests that there are many ways that blind people could come to have these concepts and new visual experiences are not required.

A third piece of evidence that people have used to argue for the conclusion that subjects are having new experiences is that one can create correlates of visual illusions using sensory substitution devices. For example, Renier et al. (2005) created a version of the Ponzo illusion using an auditory-visual sensory substitution device. In the Ponzo illusion, two lines of equal length appear unequal when they are placed at different positions on converging lines.[12] And Bach-y-Rita (1984)

[12] The Ponzo illusion can be seen and is discussed in this online article: Donaldson and Macpherson (2017).

reports creating the waterfall illusion using the TVSS. The waterfall illusion is one in which stationary objects appear to be moving. It is caused by looking first at a constantly moving stimulus for some time before looking at stationary objects.[13] How can this piece of evidence be used to argue that subjects are having new experiences? Importantly, one can get these illusions to persist, even when the subject knows conclusively that they are illusions. This is crucial because the persistence of a state that represents the world to be some way, in the face of conclusive counter-evidence that the world is not that way, is one of the standard tests used to identify that a state is a perceptual experience rather than a judgement. The reason is that if one judged something to be the case, and then conclusive counter-evidence was brought against that judgement, then one would expect one's judgement to change—at least it ought to change, on pain of irrationality. However, this is not the case for perceptual experiences. Illusory perceptual experiences can, and do, persist in the face of conclusive counter-evidence, without one being irrational. Thus, the creation of representational states that persist despite the subject knowing that they are not veridical, and without evidence to think that they are being irrational, provides some evidence in favour of the thought that the states created are perceptual experiences and not judgements.

Unfortunately, however, that evidence is not conclusive. One can defend the view that a judgement rather than a perceptual experience is being created by the use of sensory substitution devices by claiming that the judgement formed is not one that represents, say, that there *are* lines of unequal length in front of one—a judgement that would have to be overturned by the conclusive counter-evidence that the lines were of equal length, on pain of irrationality—but a judgement, say, to the effect that there are lines that *appear* to be of unequal length in front of one. That judgement need not vanish in the face of conclusive counter-evidence because how things *are* does not strictly determine how things *appear*. Thus, unfortunately, this alleged test for perceptual experience is not as conclusive as one would hope. Further debate on this topic would have to consider whether the notion of appearance that this defence uses can be cashed out in a way that does not make reference to perceptual experience.

One might think that one could settle the issue by scanning the brains of subjects who are using sensory substitution devices to find out whether they are having a perceptual experience—and if so in which sensory modality—or whether they are making a judgement. However doing that would have to rely on having clearly established correlations between experiences in certain modalities and their absence. But when creating experience in unusual ways, such as through substitution, it is far from clear that we know enough about such correlations to determine through scanning what is going on. For example, while people used

[13] The waterfall illusion can be seen online and is discussed in Macpherson and Baysan (2017).

to think that each sensory modality was associated with a different area of the cortex, increasingly, people are now doubtful whether there are any areas of the cortex that are solely correlated with one modality.[14] In particular, what is called the 'visual' cortex may be active whenever any *spatial* experience is had, rather than whenever any *visual* experience is had. Moreover, one also has to bear in mind that when people lose, or have never had, a particular sense, then their brain develops in a nonstandard way and areas of the cortex that would otherwise have been used to process information from a particular sense may be co-opted to do other tasks, making it difficult to draw conclusions about what sort of mental state is occurring from the area of the brain that is active. For example, stimulating the 'visual' cortex of early blind subjects using transcranial magnetic stimulation (TMS) during Braille reading produced *tactile* experiences in early blind subjects, which were reported as the existence of extra dots, missing dots, or dots that did not make sense.[15]

One might think that the way forward is to study the detailed reports of the subjects' experience. Can we not rely on subjects' reports of their own mental states to determine whether they are having a new experience?

As I discussed earlier, many users of sensory substitution report having a distinctive new experience. But how reliable are such reports? There is no objective test to see whether a subject's report of having an experience is correct, or whether, in general, a subject is reliable in reporting his or her mental life. And even if we take the case of ordinary mundane experience that many of us regularly have, such as our common or garden visual experience of objects in front of us had through using our eyes, there is disagreement as to what that experience is like. I have already mentioned above that there is disagreement on whether natural or artificial kinds can be represented by experience. But there are also debates about whether visual experience is of a three-dimensional world, or of a two-dimensional world with an accompanying judgement representing the third dimension—a debate that has persisted for hundreds of years.[16] Another case in point is whether our visual experience is as rich as we normally take it to be. Some people think that our experience is not as detailed and highly precise as we typically take it to be, and that we do not represent colour in the periphery of our visual field. If they are right, then most of us misreport our visual experience a lot of the time. I am not here endorsing the view that experience is not as rich as we take it to be, but using the disagreement about this issue to show that there are a variety of considerations—this one being a rather radical one—that may lead us not to trust subjects' reports about their experience.

[14] For example, Vetter et al. (2014) have found that they can read off 'visual' cortex what auditory stimulus a subject has heard.
[15] See Cohen et al. (1997).
[16] See Smith (2000).

Moreover, when it comes to the experiences that are reported when subjects are using sensory substitution and augmentation devices, there is actually quite some disagreement about the nature of the experience. Recall that two out of four of the subjects who trained with the feelSpace belt said that they had new experiences of the space around them. But two of the subjects did not report that they had such new experiences. What is going on? Are two of the participants correct and two wrong? How could we tell? Or are both right: two correctly reporting that they had no new experience and two correctly reporting that they did have a new experience? Likewise, among those who report quasi-visual experience when using the TVSS or the vOICe, some report that they have two-dimensional experience, and some report that they have three-dimensional experience.[17] Are some of those people misreporting their experience, and if so which? Or are people just different and some have two-dimensional experience and some have three-dimensional experience?

There are numerous reasons to think that some people have a new experience and some do not—and therefore that there are simply interpersonal differences among those who use sensory substitution and augmentation devices. If that is true, there is reason to think that the different reports by the subjects reflect this fact. In other words, disparate reports do not necessarily indicate that we should not trust the reports because some are not accurate. I will now explain what reasons there are to think that there could be interpersonal differences among sensory substitution users—reasons that I think not enough people who are thinking about this issue take suitable account of, and so overlook the idea that some people may be having new experiences while other people may only be making new judgements.

The first reason is that people who use sensory substitution devices have different sorts of ability. While some people using these devices have no disability and are normally sighted (typically wearing a blindfold when using the sensory substitution device), some people are late blind, some early blind, and some are congenitally blind. There is reason to think that different kinds of subjects using these devices will have different responses because their brains have developed in different ways. Second, we need to bear in mind that sensory substitution devices are different from one another. Perhaps some sensory substitution devices are more likely to give new sensory experiences than others; or some more likely to give two-dimensional experience, and some more likely to give three-dimensional experience. Third, it is also important to note the different training regimes that people have undergone when they are making their reports about their experience. Sometimes people have undergone tens of hours of practice with a device. Sometimes people have undergone hundreds of hours of practice. And in one case, a subject used a device for four years, and during two of those years they used the

[17] See Ward and Meijer (2010).

device constantly. Fourth, is the different level of motivation of subjects using a device. Some people are exceptionally keen to use a device and to find out what information they can get about the world using it. Some subjects become very quickly demotivated when using a device. They are disappointed that the use of the device doesn't give instant results. They are put off on account of how it feels to use the device—sometimes by how frustrating it is to learn to use it, sometimes by the lack of affect that they feel while using the device—and they therefore don't like to use it. Not surprisingly, this motivational factor might affect what happens to a subject when they use the device. For example, it may be that sustained attention and effort are required in order to come to have a new experience and that is unlikely to occur in people who are not highly motivated to practise with the device. Finally, fifth, there may just be innate differences between people that determine whether or not they have a new experience after practice with a sensory substitution or augmentation device. In short, there are many complex factors that may affect what it is like for people to use these devices, and thus what they report. Researchers should be very careful not to over-generalize and draw conclusions about what is happening in all instances of sensory substitution and augmentation use, when their evidence base consists in just a limited range of instances of that use.

To sum up this section, showing that subjects do have a new experience, rather than come to make new judgements about the world, is a real challenge. There are no straightforward decisive practical tests for determining whether a mental state is a perceptual experience or a judgement. And most likely there are complex interpersonal differences that mean that we have to look carefully at the precise details of each case to try to decide what is going on in that case. We will have to weigh the evidence carefully in each case and decide where the balance of probability lies.

In the next section, I will suppose that (at least some) subjects using sensory substitution devices are having new experiences and I will investigate what we should think the nature of those experiences is.

1.4 What is the Nature of the Experience Produced by Sensory Substitution?

Let us suppose that (at least some) subjects who use sensory substitution devices for some reasonable period of time come to have new experiences. What are those experiences like? I will first investigate what the modality of the experience is. Second, I will investigate whether the experiences are of a two-dimensional world or of a three-dimensional world. Third, I will consider whether the experiences represent colour, and if not, what that means these experiences are like.

1.4.1 The Modality Issue

Consider TVSS use. Are people using vision to perceive the world (that is, the substituted modality) or are they using touch (that is, the substituting modality)? And are the new experiences that some people have visual ones or tactile ones? And consider the vOICe. Are people using vision to perceive the world (that is, the substituted modality) or are they using hearing (that is, the substituting modality)? And are the new experiences visual ones or auditory ones? Or are none of these descriptions correct? In order to think about these questions we need to step back a little and consider the factors that differentiate the sensory modalities.

There are four traditional competing views about how one should individuate the senses. One view is that what determines the type of a sensory modality is the nature of the sensory organ: an eye in the case of vision; an ear in the case of hearing; skin in the case of touch; and so on.[18] A second view is that what determines the identity of a sensory modality is the nature of the proximal stimulus that impacts on the sensory organ. So, for example, light in the case of vision; sound waves in a medium in the case of hearing; pressure and temperature in the case of touch; and so on. A third view is that what is important is what the experiences in a modality represent. So, for example, the shape, size, and colour of objects at a distance from the body in the case of vision; sounds or objects producing sounds, including pitch, volume, and timbre properties, in the case of hearing; and the shape, size, surface texture, and temperature of objects pressing up against the body, including the pressure with which they press, in the case of touch; and likewise for the other senses. The fourth traditional view is that what is important is the conscious nature of the experiences that the modality produces—which is determined by what it is like to have them (or their 'phenomenal character'). The idea here is that visual experiences, auditory experiences, tactile experiences, and so on, each have a unique feel to them that determines the modality that is operative.

Many people think that the phenomenal character of an experience is to a large extent determined by what an experience represents. This is because when we describe the phenomenal character of our experience we typically do so by describing what objects and properties the experience represents. These people would consider the third and fourth criteria to be the same or to yield the same results.

[18] For the purposes of this essay, I will assume that touch is one modality. However, that fact has been questioned. Plato thought that what is commonly thought of as touch is really three distinct senses: a pressure, a temperature, and a pain sense, partly on the grounds that there are three very different sorts of phenomenal experience associated with each of these. Some modern scientists also believe that touch is actually three modalities but for different reasons. They have found that there are distinctive receptors that detect temperature, pressure, and painful stimuli, and that there are separate spots in the skin receptive to pressure, warmth, cold, and painful stimuli. And so on these grounds they posit there are three distinct senses. See Macpherson (2011a).

While these accounts of the individuation of the senses all agree on the fact that vision, audition, touch, taste, and smell—the five Aristotelian senses—operating normally and in normal conditions are all different from each other, they are competing theories because they yield different answers in other cases about what type a particular sense is. To explain this, I will consider what each theory says about the sense that is being used when someone uses a TVSS.

The first theory says that what is important is the nature of the sensory organ. In the TVSS, what is the sensory organ? It is tempting to think that the sensory organ is the camera that is detecting the scene in front of the subject. And it might be tempting to think that the camera is a type of eye. With those assumptions in place, this theory would yield the result that the sense being used is vision. However, one could deny that a camera is an eye—it is just a man-made camera. In that case, this theory would yield the result that the sense is a new one—one that has a camera for an organ. Alternatively, one could argue that the sensory organ is the skin, for it is the skin that is the organ of the subject that receives a stimulus. With that assumption in place, this theory would say that the sensory modality is touch. Another option would be to think of the whole TVSS system as being the sensory organ—the camera plus the vibrating pins and the subject's skin. This would mean that the sense was a new one—neither vision nor touch.

It is interesting to note that this theory does not tell us how to determine which physical object is the sensory organ, and it does not tell us how to identify what type of organ something is. The theory needs supplementing by accounts of those things in order to yield a verdict.

The second theory says that what is important is the nature of the proximal stimulus. But what is that? When considering the previous theory we noted that we could take the sensory organ to be either the camera or the skin. In using this second theory, we face a similar choice. We could take the proximal stimulus to be the light that hits the camera, or we could take it to be the pressure of the pins that touch the subject's skin. The former would yield the verdict that the sense in operation was sight. The latter would yield the verdict that the sense in operation was touch.

Again note that this theory does not tell us how to determine what the proximal stimulus is in unusual cases. And it also does not specify what the proximal stimuli are for the normal operation of the Aristotelian senses in normal conditions. For example, is visible light—light of roughly 400–750 nanometres—the proximal stimulus of vision, or is the proximal stimulus any form of electromagnetic radiation, so that a sense that detected gamma rays, or X-rays or microwaves or radio waves would count as vision?

The third theory tells us to look to what the experiences produced by a sensory modality represent. Here one might think that we can discern a clearer result. Haven't we determined that the new experiences had in sensory substitution represent objects in front of the body of the subject? Do they therefore not represent that which visual experiences represent? The experiences using TVSS seem to represent more closely that which vision does, compared to any other sensory modality, and so one might conclude that the modality in operation here is vision.[19] However, as I will spell out in more detail later, it is plausible to think that some or all of these experiences do not represent colour. For many people, including Aristotle, that is a defining feature of visual experience, and so they hold that if an experience does not represent colour then it cannot be visual. (I, myself, see no reason to think that colour must be represented by visual experiences, as I will explain below.) What type of experiences are such experiences then? They don't seem like tactile experiences, as, unlike tactile experiences, they represent objects at a distance from the body, and they don't represent pressure or temperature. So perhaps they are a novel type of experience.

However, one might try to make a case that those experiences are tactile. Some psychologists have postulated that practice using a sensory substitution device gives one a novel experience but one that is in the substituting modality. They have suggested that learning to use a sensory substitution device is a bit like learning certain language skills, such as learning to read or learning a new language. For example, Bach-y-Rita said:

> The learning process may be similar to that which takes place in children with normal sensory and motor systems, or in adults learning a foreign language or Morse code, or in deaf persons learning manual communication.
>
> (1984: 153)

And Jones (2004) says:

> Meijer likens the process of learning to recognize sounds as shapes to acquiring a foreign language. Novices begin by mastering an elementary visual alphabet: a circle, a rectangle, a triangle, an oval. Since, generally speaking, all other shapes can be said to be combinations of these, the wearer of such a device begins to gain 'fluency' that makes recognizing whether a door is open or closed, or whether a chair is occupied, almost second nature.

[19] In section 1.3, I mentioned that there may be interpersonal differences between people with regard to whether they come to have new sensory experiences or whether they come to be able to make new judgements about the world. Of course it could be the case that the phenomenal character of new experiences produced by sensory substitution devices is different from subject to subject. For example, Auvray et al. (2007) asked sighted participants what it felt like to perceive with the vOICe. Some participants said that their experience was close to vision, others that it was closer to audition. And one of the participants said that her experience was visual when she was locating an object in space, and auditory when she was recognizing the shape of the object. In the text above, I focus on the reports of the subjects in the TVSS case, which seem less variable. Again, note that the device used, and the amount of practice subjects have, and which task they are performing, are three among many factors (the others of which I outlined in section 1.3) that might affect the nature of subjects' mental states when using a sensory substitution device. Therefore, there may again be large interpersonal differences between people when using sensory substitution devices.

When one learns to read, one learns to recognize words, which one could not do before. Recognizing words becomes fast and automatic, but we don't think that people are having non-visual experiences when they are reading. It seems that they come to have a new type of visual experience that allows them to recognize new things. Perhaps this is a good analogy for what goes on in those who practise a lot with the TVSS. They are having new tactile experiences that allow them to recognize objects at a distance from their body, which they could not do before.

Another option is to think that the new experiences are amodal or meta-modal experiences in the sense that they represent that which one might think all sensory modalities can represent: objects occupying certain portions of space. However, it is not entirely certain that every modality can represent that. Can smell, for example? Exactly what smell experiences represent is highly disputed. (See Batty (2013) for discussion of this modality.) Perhaps then they are amodal or meta-modal in the sense that at least two sensory modalities can represent those objects and properties and spatial relations. Another option is that they are experiences in a novel modality—neither vision nor touch. I favour this last option, as I will explain below.

According to the fourth theory we need to think about the phenomenal character of the experiences that are being had. Are they visual or are they tactile or neither? The same considerations as were adduced for the third theory would carry over and apply to this theory also.

Elsewhere (Macpherson 2011a), I have argued that we do not need to choose between the four theories of how to individuate the senses. I believe that people have felt compelled to do so because they subscribe to a sparse model of the senses. That is a model according to which there are relatively few types of senses—perhaps the Aristotelian five, or perhaps those plus a few others—and those senses are relatively discrete, that is, distinctive from each other. I hold that consideration of cases such as sensory substitution, but also cases of animal senses, some of which are to some degree like ours and some of which are very unlike ours, and consideration of possible but non-actual senses, show that the senses cannot be clearly divided up into a limited number of discrete kinds. The differences between the senses amount more to a difference of degree, rather than a difference of kind. Rather than try to pigeonhole all the senses into a small number of discrete categories, we should simply note what each sense is like in respect of each of the criteria that the four theories ask us to consider. For each of the properties that these theories claim individuate the senses, we can note, if we like, how different or similar each sense is to one of the five Aristotelian senses with respect to that property, but that is relatively unimportant. One advantage of this view is that one does not have to decide on many factors that were left unspecified by the four theories. For example, one does not need to say what an eye is, or whether the camera or the skin is the proximal stimulus. One does not need to determine whether the proximal stimulus is light or electromagnetic waves more generally, or whether it is pressure on the skin. One simply needs to record all the facts about these features of a sensory modality, and where one records different facts, there one records different types of perceptual system. Thus, on my account, perception using TVSS is somewhat like normal human vision, somewhat like normal human touch, and somewhat unique, and thus it should count as its own distinctive sensory modality—a TVSS modality.

1.4.2 The Two- or Three-Dimension Issue

Another question that we can raise about new experiences that people might have when using sensory substitution devices is whether they represent two- or three-dimensional objects and space. In other words, when people using these devices make depth judgements are they doing so because they experience the third dimension or is it inferred from an experience of two dimensions?

An interesting source of evidence comes from Guarniero, a congenitally blind PhD student of Bach-y-Rita, who studied the TVSS in his doctoral thesis. He also used the TVSS for three weeks himself and wrote about his experience. He said:

> Very soon . . . the sensations no longer felt as if they were located on my back . . . By this time objects had come to have a top and bottom; a right side and a left; but no depth—they existed in an ordered two-dimensional space, the precise location of which has not yet been determined . . . In order to judge distance I had to master some of the cues of monocular vision, namely familiar size and interposition. I also made use of the fact that, when things are viewed from above, those farther away appear higher in the visual field. Even when interposition was the only cue I used, the objects still appeared two-dimensional and I had to infer that one was behind the other.
>
> (1974: 101–104)

This is very clearly a report in favour of the two-dimensional view.

However, recounting their studies with the vOICe, Ward and Meijer report on two of their subjects:

> Both CC and PF report being able to perceive depth. However, both of them report that this ability occurred after having 'flat' visual experiences of edges and shading . . . PF . . . reports her sense of depth perception arising in a kind of Eureka moment: 'I was washing dishes . . . and looked down into the sink to make sure that the water had got out and I realised "Oh! I can see down. I can see depth." And I stepped back from that sink and looked down again to make sure that I wasn't fooling myself, and I walked slowly through my house looking into the rooms and it was like incredible. I could see into the room. That flat drawing now has depth to it. I can sense it.'
>
> (2010: 496)

PF was late blind and had been using the vOICe for four years, and during two of those years she had been using it immersively.

What these results again point to is that there are probably a whole host of factors (that I outlined in section 1.3) that may affect subjects' experience. Different subjects probably experience different things, and, indeed, the same subject may experience different things at different times. Nonetheless, the clear and well-documented reports of CC and PF, which attest to gaining three-dimensional perceptual experience after having had only two-dimensional perceptual experience, are rather compelling evidence that three-dimensional perception can be experienced.

1.4.3 The Colour Issue

What does the evidence say about the experience of colour in the new experiences in those who use sensory substitution devices, supposing, as we did above, that they do have new experiences?

To be clear, we have to distinguish between chromatic and achromatic colour. The achromatic colours are black, white, and all the shades of grey in between. The chromatic colours are all the rest, that is, all the colours that have some hue value, such as red, green, blue, yellow, and so on. Do those who use the TVSS and the vOICe have chromatic or achromatic colour experience or no colour experience? Clearly no chromatic colour information is captured about the world or relayed to subjects using those devices. However, one might think that black and white information is given to TVSS subjects. (Recall that pins either press against the subject or they do not, with white areas in the image driving the pins to vibrate and press against the subject and black areas causing the absence of the pin press.) And one might think that black and white and grey-scale information is being given to subjects who use the vOICe. (Recall that the volume of the sound captured the lightness/darkness dimension of the components of the image.) And one might suppose that this means that subjects using a TVSS will have experience of black and white, and subjects using the vOICe will have experience of black and white and shades of grey in between. However, that supposition is too quick.

Consider that one might tell the subjects how the devices work, and which stimuli correspond to white, black, and degrees of lightness. However, one needn't do that. If one did not, then subjects would not know whether pressure corresponds to white or black and whether increasing volume means increasing or decreasing lightness. In such a case, what would subjects' experience be like?

It is wise here to consider the early blind, the late blind, and the sighted separately from the congenitally blind. One might imagine that the early blind, the late blind, and the sighted might have experiences of black and white and lightness because their visual system simply assigns blackness, whiteness, and different degrees of lightness to the pressure or volume stimuli, drawing on its stored representations of those colours. Perhaps it would make little practical difference which way round the visual system assigned those colours with respect to the ability of the subjects to identify which objects were in front of them. After all, we could have built the devices differently so that pressure signalled blackness and increasing volume signalled increasing darkness, rather than the other way around. Either way, subjects would have experiences of white and black and degrees of lightness, and whether they corresponded to the image that was driving the device, or were inverted with respect to that image, need not concern us with respect to the question of whether achromatic colour is represented.

Evidence for this hypothesis comes from Ward and Meijer who report PF, a late blind subject with some residual vision, using the vOICe saying:

> Just sound? . . . No, it is by far more, it is sight! There IS true light perception generated by The vOICe. When I am not wearing The vOICe the light I perceive from a small slit in my left eye is a grey fog. When wearing The vOICe the image is light with all the little greys and blacks . . . The light generated is very white and clear then it erodes down the scale of color to the dark black.
>
> (2010: 495)

However, although only achromatic colour information is delivered to subjects, this might not limit the nature of the experiences that subjects have. For example, later in her life, in a dialogue between PF and JW (one of the experimenters), PF said that colours had started to appear in her experience:

> PF: . . . Over time my brain seems to have . . . used my memory to color everything.
>
> JW: But if you look at someone's sweater or pants you wouldn't necessarily know the color? It could be blue or red.
>
> PF: My brain would probably take a guess at that time. It would be greyish black. Something I know such as grass, tree bark, leaves, my mind just colors it in.
>
> (2010: 497)

This suggests that the visual systems of people who have previously had sight can fill in colours—be they achromatic or chromatic—based on the memory of colours, or based on pure guess work. If that is right, then it is tempting to think that a congenitally blind person, who must lack such memories, would not experience this. This supposition is backed up to some degree by a study by Kupers et al. (2006) that found that blind subjects trained with a TDU reported only tactile sensations on the tongue when TMS was applied to their visual cortex, while similarly trained sighted subjects reported only phosphenes (that is, hallucinatory visual experiences of lights). This suggests that the congenitally blind do not have experiences of lightness or darkness (nor of achromatic colour) when they use the TDU. It does, however, raise an interesting question about what the experience of the congenitally blind is like when they use a sensory substitution device. Do they have vision-like experiences of objects at a distance from the body that don't involve experience of chromatic or achromatic colour?

As mentioned previously, Aristotle, and almost all philosophers since then, have said that there can be no visual experience of form without colour.[20] They think that we experience distal form in virtue of experiencing differences in colour. If that is right, then there is a worry that if congenitally blind people are not experiencing colour then perhaps they are not experiencing distal form. Perhaps this would give us a reason to think that they are merely judging what the distal form of the objects in front of them is. While it is true that humans typically experience distal form in virtue of experiencing differences in colour, must it be the case? Is another sort of experience of distal form possible?

An interesting case to consider with respect to this question is bat echolocation. Bats send out a high-frequency 'chirrup' sound and listen for how long it takes the sound to return (if indeed it does) in the form of an echo, because it bounces off objects in front of them. This allows bats to determine what objects are in front of them and how far away they are. It allows them to negotiate through their environment skilfully and quickly, dodging obstacles such as tree branches, and catching moths in the dark. Clearly, using echolocation, bats can detect three-dimensional objects at a distance from their body. But notice that in so doing—in detecting distal form—they don't detect colour. They don't use a form of perception that is able to pick up information about colour. So what is the bats' experience like?[21]

One idea is that bats experience distal form by experiencing sound reflectance. If that is right, then perhaps one needn't experience colour to experience distal form, but perhaps one needs to detect some quality or other. If one must experience distal form by experiencing some quality or other, what quality do congenitally blind people using the TVSS or vOICe experience?

One suggestion is that they experience distal form in virtue of experiencing light reflectance, for that is what drives the camera on the TVSS and the vOICe. However, as stated before, subjects needn't know whether a substitution device signals white or black with pressure, or increasing lightness or darkness with volume. But more than that, they needn't know what is driving the TVSS at all. For example, we could have built a device that was not driven by light reflectance but which was driven by something else that was capable of informing subjects about what was in front of them. We could, for instance, have built a device that worked by converting sound-reflectance information into tactile or auditory stimuli. Therefore, based just on the information that they receive through the sensory substitution device, it is not clear how blind subjects could be experiencing distal form in virtue of experiencing light reflectance for they, or their brains, may have no idea about what is driving the system that they are interacting with.

[20] See Macpherson (2015: 115) for further details.

[21] Of course this question was famously asked by Nagel (1974) who thought that in principle one cannot know everything about what it is like to be a bat. However, even if that were true, it does not stop one knowing many things about what it is like to be a bat, as Akins (1993) cleverly shows.

Are there any other properties in virtue of which the congenitally blind might be experiencing distal form? The only other suggestion that I can think of is that they are experiencing distal form in virtue of experiencing the pressure that they feel on their skin in the case of the TVSS or in virtue of the sound properties that they hear in the case of the vOICe. However, it is very hard to imagine how they can experience a property—form—that they experience as being some distance in front of them, in virtue of experiencing another property—pressure or sound—that they experience as being on their skin or coming through headphones. Of course, in a causal sense of 'in virtue of', the subjects are experiencing distal form in virtue of experiencing the pressure on their skin or the sound from the headphones. But that is not what is at issue here. Such a causal claim is not disputed by anyone in these cases. What is at issue is whether the subjects *experience* the distal form as being constituted by a pressure/nonpressure boundary on their skin or a sound/nonsound or sound with a different volume coming from the headphones.

To understand what I mean here, consider a device which was such that whenever you saw a green triangle, it caused you to simultaneously have an experience of a purple square. In a causal sense of 'in virtue of', you experience the square in virtue of experiencing the green triangle. But in another sense of 'in virtue of' you do not experience the square in virtue of experiencing the green triangle. You do not experience the square/nonsquare boundary as being constituted by the green/nongreen boundary, or the triangle/nontriangle boundary. You experience the square as being constituted by the purple/nonpurple boundary. I call the sense of 'in virtue of' in which one sees the square in virtue of the purpleness, and not in virtue of the greenness or the triangularity, the 'phenomenal sense' of in virtue of. I have argued elsewhere that when one experiences one property in virtue of experiencing another in the phenomenal sense, then one must experience those properties as being at the same location.[22] This is not what is experienced by congenitally blind subjects using the TVSS or the vOICe. The pressure or the sound is not experienced as being at the same location as the distal objects. Therefore, I believe that they are not experiencing the distal form in virtue of, in the phenomenal sense, the pressure or the sound. Thus, as there are no good candidates for being the property in virtue of which, in the phenomenal sense, subjects experience the distal form, I suggest that they experience pure distal form—that is they experience distal form without experiencing it in virtue of, in the phenomenal sense, any other property.

In Macpherson (2015), I argue that there are other interesting mental phenomena, unrelated to sensory substitution, that back up the idea that one could experience distal form without experiencing it in virtue of, in the phenomenal sense, any other property. Such cases include a special case of achromatopsia, experiences of phantom contours, experiences of amodal completion, and certain

[22] See Macpherson (2015).

forms of type two blindsight. Spelling out the details of all of these cases would take me too far from my present purposes, but the interested reader can pursue my arguments in that paper. Moreover, in that paper, I argue that even though subjects in certain cases are not having experiences of colour, there is reason to still think that their experience is visual—or at least more like visual experience than experience in any other of our sensory modalities. This is because their experience is of distal objects, it is caused by the proximal stimulus of visible light, and it is caused by the operation of the eyes. Thus, unlike Aristotle and many other philosophers, I don't think that visual experiences have to be experiences of chromatic or achromatic colour. However, as I outlined in section 1.4.1, because I hold a very fine-grained taxonomy of the senses that takes them to differ in degree and not kind, I think that TVSS perception and vOICe perception are different from any of our senses and so count as *sui generis* ways of perceiving the world, and hence as being senses distinct from vision, hearing, or any of the senses that humans have without technological intervention.

However, in whichever modality one believes the experiences of congenitally blind subjects using the TVSS or the vOICe to be in, I see no good reason to think that the fact that they do not experience colour justifies thinking that they cannot be having perceptual experience at all and must, instead, be simply making judgements about the objects in the world in front of them.

1.5 What Are the Limits of Sensory Substitution?

Thus far, I have discussed the TVSS and the vOICe. These are sensory substitution systems that convey the shape, size and location of objects in space. There are variants of these devices that substitute for these properties too. I have also discussed the feelSpace belt—a device that has been used to try to give people a sense of spatial direction: magnetic north. Other kinds of sensory substitution system exist that I have not yet mentioned. One kind of device tries to substitute for the orientation of a person with respect to gravity, in other words substitute for the vestibular sense. Various forms of these devices exist. Some exploit electrical stimulation on the tongue as the substituting modality (see Tyler et al. 2003), others exploit audition (see Dozza et al. 2004), and others still vibrotactile stimulation on the body (see Goebel et al. 2009). It is interesting to note that in all of the devices just mentioned, all of the properties that are being substituted are 'common sensibles'.

Aristotle divided up properties into proper sensibles and common sensibles. Proper sensibles are properties that are only detected through one sensory modality. For example, Aristotle thought colour is only detected through vision and so is a proper sensible of vision. Pressure is only detected through touch and so it is a proper sensible of that modality. Sweetness is only detected through taste and so it is a proper sensible of taste. In contrast to this, Aristotle thought that shape is a common sensible as it can be detected by more than one sense: both vision and touch. Size, position in space, and direction are also common sensibles for they are all perceivable by more than one sense.

All the properties that I have so far spoken about substituting or providing through augmentation are common sensibles. Size, shape, and location relative to the body are clearly common sensibles. When it comes to magnetic north, we don't get the direction of magnetic north *as such* given to us through any sense without augmentation, but all egocentric directions are available through many different senses to us, for example through hearing and touch, and many egocentric directions are available through vision. It is easy to see how one could provide information through each of those modalities about which direction was magnetic north. Thus, all the properties that we have been considering are properties that can be detected by more than one sensory modality. Given this, one might wonder whether one can only substitute for, or augment to provide, properties that are common sensibles. Or, in addition, can one substitute for proper sensibles such as taste, smell, or pitch properties?

When we substitute for spatial properties we map each spatial dimension that is being substituted onto a separate dimension created out of a set of qualities in the substituting modality. For example, in TVSS the two-dimensional camera image is mapped onto a two-dimensional patch of skin. And in the vOICe the two-dimensional camera image is mapped onto the dimensions of pitch and time of occurrence after a click. In the case of the feelSpace belt, information about the direction of magnetic north is mapped onto positions on the belt.

One might think therefore that to substitute for a proper sensible, such as taste, one has to create a mapping from dimensions of taste qualities to dimensions in another modality. One problem with this approach is that it is not clear whether each of the sensory modalities has dimensions along which we can plot each experience in that modality. For example, Wilson and Stevenson (2006) suggest that, behind the difficulties of modelling olfactory quality space, is a false assumption about olfactory experience. This is the assumption that olfactory experience is analytic—that it has various, basic distinguishable components. Instead, they argue, olfactory experience is largely synthetic; that is, the various properties of the odorant stimulus produce a largely irreducible experience. As a result, Wilson and Stevenson suggest abandoning classification schemes that attempt to model olfactory properties by means of a quality space. If they are right, then this would present a great problem for creating a way of substituting for the sense of smell.

Nonetheless, let us focus on a case in which we think that there are dimensions along which one can map the experiences in the modality. One could imagine the taste dimensions consisting of degrees of intensity of the basic tastes: salty, sweet, sour, bitter, umami. And one could imagine mapping these dimensions onto other sensory dimensions. For example, a degree of pressure of a stimulus on the little finger might indicate a degree of saltiness; a degree of pressure on the ring finger might indicate a degree of sweetness; and so on for each finger, and each dimension of taste. But if one hooked up a subject to such a substitution system how would they know which qualities the pressure on the fingers referred to? If a subject had never experienced those qualities before, how could experiencing pressure on their fingers give them experiences as of taste qualities?[23]

When subjects use the TVSS and the vOICe, we tell them what the tactile and auditory stimulation corresponds to, namely shape, size and location information, and subjects can often find out what it corresponds to by feeling the objects in front of them—thereby using an existing sense to calibrate the substituted sense. Moreover, subjects know what shape, size and location are, for, even if they have never had sight, those are properties that one can come to be aware of through other modalities.

Now consider again the hypothetical tactile-taste substitution system that I described above. While we could tell subjects using the system that pressure on their fingers referred to different levels of basic tastes, one might think that subjects who have never had a taste sensory modality would not know what the basic tastes were, for they haven't had any awareness of them. They have only had such properties described to them, and reasonably we could question whether such descriptions gave them knowledge of what such properties are really like.[24] So one might have a strong intuition that such a system would not cause experiences of taste in subjects using it. Rather, it seems more likely that subjects would just form judgements about what tastes were being indicated to be present by the system. Moreover, even if a subject had taste memory and taste imagination, and could come to remember or imagine taste automatically in response to the pressure on the fingers, an experience of the memory or imagination of taste would seem to be a very impoverished experience compared to really tasting things. It is this fact that leads many diets to come to an end!

The intuition articulated in the last paragraph was that pressure on the fingers, caused by a device that could detect tastes, together with subjects being told what the pressure on their fingers referred to, would not cause subjects to have perceptual experiences of taste. However, this view is challenged by those who hold the sensorimotor theory of perception. Hurley and Noë (2003) hold such a view and they claim that what determines whether subjects come to have experiences in the substituted modality depends on whether they can acquire and use the common laws of sensorimotor contingency that the substituted modality shares

[23] The astute reader will notice that the same question arose when I considered whether we could substitute for colour—a property almost universally taken to be a proper sensible: the proper sensible of vision. In that case, I noted that memory might provide one with a means to know which property the sensory substitution device was signalling. It is of some interest to note that on my view, according to which there is a *sui generis* TVSS modality, colour can no longer be thought of as a proper sensible because one can experience it in the TVSS modality as well as the visual modality.
[24] See Jackson (1986) for further articulation of this point.

with the perception that takes place by means of the sensory substitution device. (Sensorimotor laws are the laws that describe how one's perceptual experience changes in response to the way one acts on the world.) In the case of TVSS they think that this would happen:

> as you move around an object, hidden portions of its surface come into tactile-visual view, just as they would if you were seeing them. As you move closer to an object, its apparent tactile-visual size increases, just as it would if you were seeing it. As you turn to the left, objects in 'view' swing to the right in your tactile-visual field, just as they would if you were seeing them. What it is like to see is similar to what it is like to perceive by TVSS because seeing and TVSS-perception are similar ways of exploring the environment: they are governed by similar sensorimotor constraints, draw on similar sensorimotor skills, and are directed toward similar visual properties, including perspectivally available occlusion properties such as apparent size and shape.
> (Hurley and Noë 2003: 144–145)

This is an interesting suggestion about when and why one comes to have visual-like experiences when using a TVSS. Suppose that it is true. Does this mean that one could substitute for proper sensibles such as taste and smell? The question will turn on whether there could be enough sensorimotor contingencies in common between our ordinary perception of taste and a sensory substitution system for taste, such as the one I have described. I am not convinced that there could be, nor am I convinced that there could be enough sensorimotor contingencies in common between ordinary taste and a sensory substitution system for taste that would differentiate the sensorimotor contingencies from those involved in the detection of other proper sensibles such as smell. And even if that could be guaranteed, the question of whether we should accept the sensorimotor theory of perception has not been settled, and requires further investigation.

In short, there are intuitions on both sides concerning whether sensory substitution or augmentation of proper sensibles is possible. To my mind there is not enough evidence supporting the intuition that it is possible, hence I would hedge my bets on the conclusion that sensory substitution or augmentation of proper sensibles is not possible. An exception to this might be cases where memory is able to give one experiences of the properties that are being substituted, but whether memory is capable of producing the same sort of experience as perception is highly debatable.

If only the common sensibles can be substituted or augmented, at least in people who have no memory of the properties that we are trying to substitute, then this restricts sensory substitution and augmentation to, roughly, properties of the shape and location of objects. Perhaps this makes the possibilities of the types of sensory substitution and augmentation more limited than one might have hoped for. And perhaps one might feel rather disappointed at such a conclusion. However, knowledge of spatial properties is crucial for getting around the world and so they are particularly useful ones to be able to substitute in people who lack them, or to augment in cases where we wish to extend the range of our sensory powers.

1.6 Sensory Substitution and Theories of Perception

There are many different theories of perception in philosophy and psychology. One reason that theorists have been interested in sensory substitution is that many hoped that the results from sensory substitution experiments could be used to support certain theories at the expense of rivals, and to provide illuminating examples of distinctions that some people want to make in articulating a theory of perception.

One such case is the sensorimotor theory that I have just discussed above. Hurley and Noe (2003) claim that what determines the conscious nature of an experience is the sensorimotor constraints that govern that experience. Thus they claim that if one uses a sensory substitution system, say one that substitutes for vision using touch, then if the experiences one has obey the sensorimotor constraints of vision, rather than touch, one will have experiences with visual, and not tactile, phenomenal character. And they claim that this is so even if the part of the brain that processes the incoming perceptual signals is the tactile cortex, rather than the visual cortex. The way that they express this last point is that in these cases there is 'cortical deference', rather than 'cortical dominance'. The phenomenal character of the experience is not determined by where in the cortex the perceptual signal is processed or by what phenomenal character activation of that part of the cortex has produced in the past.

Many factors make it unclear whether sensory substitution experiments support the sensorimotor theory. Several of these have been discussed above about the nature and limits of the experiences that can be produced using sensory substitution. As we have seen, the evidence about what experience is produced in which circumstances is extremely messy. Different experiences are produced in different circumstances. So the evidence does not clearly tell for or against the theory. Second, the sensorimotor contingencies that are produced by sensory substitution are, at best, a sub-set of those produced by the normal operation of the substituted sense, so one would expect any experience to be only partially like that produced normally in the substituted modality. Further, the substituting modality still seems to be operative, and one can attend to experiences had in that modality, while using sensory substitution. So again, the phenomenal character of the experience or experiences that are had is going to be more complex than that of those had while using the substituted modality in normal conditions. Thus, weighing up the phenomenal character of those experiences and determining whether it coincides with the relevant sensorimotor contingencies is exceptionally difficult, and, to my mind, inconclusive. Finally, even if we could clearly show that sensory substitution yields experiences that are phenomenally like those had in the substituted modality, that alone does not show that the sensorimotor theory is correct. Other factors besides sensorimotor contingencies could be the cause of those experiences. For example, part of the within-the-head functional role of the experience—specifically the effects of the state leading to the subject holding certain beliefs about the way the world is—might be responsible. In short, evidence from sensory substitution does not settle whether the sensorimotor theory is true or false.

Another debate about the nature of perception that people hoped sensory substitution might help to settle is the debate about whether perception (broadly understood) involves two distinct elements: sensation and perception (narrowly understood); and if so, what the relationship is between them.

In fact, comprehending what this distinction amounts to is difficult. Contemporary accounts of the distinction vary widely—often without the explicit realization that there is such disparity. Matters are not helped by the fact that many philosophers and psychologists reject the distinction—in part because the distinction is unclear, in part because there are such different understandings of it, but most importantly, because many contemporary theorists think that it is impossible to identify two separate elements answering to the descriptions given of them. Goldstein and Brockmole (2017), writing in their classic textbook, *Sensation and Perception*, do not use the term 'sensation' except in brief discussions of the history of the subject, or to explain why they do not use it! They say that the book's title reflects the fact that:

> [s]ensation was discussed in the early history of perceptual psychology, and courses and textbooks followed suit including *sensation* in their titles. But . . . researchers eventually stopped using the term sensation . . . [and] as far as we are concerned, everything that involves understanding how we experience the world through our senses comes under the heading of perception.[25]

Bearing in mind the caveats just mentioned, let me nonetheless attempt to give an account of the distinction between sensation and perception (narrowly understood). In the most general of terms, sensation is most usually taken to refer to some basic element involved in the use of the senses or, equivalently, in perception (broadly understood), while perception (narrowly understood) refers to a more complex element. Often sensation is spoken of occurring earlier than perception (narrowly understood), and often it is claimed that perception (narrowly understood) is based on sensation, with sensation coming earlier in a causal process that leads to perception (narrowly understood). However, importantly, that is not always so. Thomas Reid, who gives an early and very influential account of sensation, is most often interpreted as holding that sensation and perception involve parallel processes and that perception is immediate and not formed on the basis of sensation.[26] Looking to a prominent contemporary advocate of the distinction,

[25] Goldstein and Brockmole (2017: 6).

[26] There is some dispute among scholars over this point which is nicely summarized in Nichols (2007: ch. 5). Nichols himself concludes that Reid does not think sensation is required for perception (narrowly understood). Nichols notes, as do many other scholars, that Reid was the first person to make the distinction between sensation and perception clear. Hamlyn (1961), in his excellent book-length account of the history of sensation and perception, argues that Reid was the first to make it clear since

Nicholas Humphrey is quite explicit in holding a similar view. For him, sensation and perception (narrowly understood) are parallel processes and perception (narrowly understood) is not based on sensation. A third account is that sensation and perception are held to occur simultaneously with sensation taken to be a pure core and hence a part of perception (narrowly understood). For example, Dretske (1969: 75, quoted in Ben-Zeev 1984) maintains:

> if one systematically strips away from a given perceptual act all the accretions due to past experience, all the collateral information, anticipations, interpretive and inferential elements, all the habitual or conditional associations, then one will be left with a 'pure sensory core'—the given of sense experience.

Sometimes, particularly on this latter view, it is held that we are not normally aware of our sensations but that, with training, we can become so.[27]

What kind of things are sensations and perception taken to be and how have various people distinguished them? Answers to these questions give rise to the different accounts of the distinction between sensation and perception (narrowly understood).

Philosophers since Aristotle's time have discussed sensation and perception.[28] And they have taken sensation to be a conscious mental state, and perception (narrowly understood) either to be or to (typically) involve a different conscious mental state—a perceptual experience—or further elements of a conscious state beyond that given by sensation that together with sensation form a perceptual experience (broadly understood). In contrast to this, some psychologists take sensation and perception (narrowly understood) to be different types of physiological processing. I think that it is important to be very clear which of these one means when talking about sensation and perception.

Of course, one might think that physiological processing and mental states will line up nicely, and one might even have hopes of one day identifying them. With that in mind, one might thereby attribute to the more primitive mental states sometimes called 'sensations' some of the properties that one attributes to the more primitive physiological processing sometimes called 'sensations'. And one might thereby attribute to the more sophisticated mental states sometimes called 'perceptual experience' some of the properties of the more sophisticated physiological processing sometimes called 'perception'. This is precisely what Boring (1942: ch. 1) states happened in the late nineteenth century. Sensation and perception conceived of as mental states by philosophers were synthesized with and conjoined to a conception of sensation and perception as physiological processes

Aristotle. However, readers should note that, as I indicated earlier in the text, Reid's account is far from universally adopted by scholars.

[27] See Clark (2007).

[28] See Hamlyn (1961).

by psychologists. This yielded a conception of sensation and perception in which sensations and perceptions were mental states that corresponded to two different levels of processing.

However, it is clear that such an approach is controversial. Whether such identification can be made is open to debate. Moreover, such identification will not always be feasible, given that some of the accounts of the basic physiological processing said to constitute sensation are so primitive, such as the registering of light on the retina, that it would simply not be plausible to identify it with any conscious mental state. However, other accounts of the properties of sensation, considered as a physiological process, are more amenable to identification with conscious mental states, and one could apply them to both physiological processing and to mental states, as we shall see.

One important account of the distinction between sensation and perception (narrowly understood) is that sensation involves the passive reception of sensory input in the sense that it is devoid of active mental contributions such as memory, past experience, expectation, interpretation, judgement and thought.[29] In the case of physiological processing, the idea is that when we see an object, such as a table—which is called the 'distal stimulus'—light bounces off the table and enters our eyes. The light is called the 'proximal stimulus' as it is that, rather than the table, which has a direct causal impact on our body. The registering of the light and the turning of it into an electrical signal in the nerves, carried out by the transducers in the eye, is a process which some claim is such that the signal does not 'display any degree of independence from the [proximal] stimulus' (Ben-Zeev 1984: 328). And this process, together with some nerve firings slightly further down the causal chain that are all also thought not to display any independence from the proximal stimulus, is sometimes called sensation.[30] In contrast, perception (narrowly understood) is a process that uses active mental contributions such as memory, past experience, expectation, interpretation, judgement and thought, so as to produce something that doesn't just correspond with the proximal stimulus—in our example, the light that impacts on the retina—but, hopefully, something that corresponds to the distal object that the light bounced off—the table. We know that many different distal stimuli are compatible with the same proximal stimulus and hence, if it exists, the same sensation. On this view, the role of perception is therefore to recover the most likely distal stimulus given the sensation and background knowledge and assumptions either built into the visual system and the mind or learned by them.

One can apply this sort of idea to sensation and perception (narrowly understood) conceived of as being or involving conscious mental states. Sensation would be a mental state that is passive and devoid of active mental contributions such

[29] See Hamlyn (1961) and Ben-Zeev (1984).
[30] See Clark (2007).

as memory, past experience, expectation, interpretation, judgement and thought. Perception (narrowly understood) would be, or involve, a perceptual experience that was active in the sense that it did involve such contribution. (And one may hold that perception is in some sense based on sensation, or one may adopt an alternative account as detailed above.)

Some people will disavow this idea of sensation, as they may disavow the idea that there is any such purely passive processing or mental states. However, denying this need not lead one to deny *tout court* that there is sensation, because this is not the only account of the distinction between sensation and perception.

One alternative idea is that sensation is a feeling of what is going on in me—of how I am being affected by various stimuli—whereas perception is consciousness of objects and properties external to one. It is this reading that yields the conception of sensation as including pains, itches, and tickles. It is associated with the having of subjective feelings and affect. According to Hamlyn (1961: 189), 'while sensations may be caused by stimuli affecting our body, to have a sensation is not necessarily, or even generally, to know anything about its cause'. In contrast, perception is, or involves, a mental state that represents what is happening in the world around me. The idea is that when we perceive (broadly understood), we are aware of how we are being impacted on by the world—which is to be identified with sensation—and we are aware of what the world is like—which is to be identified with perception (narrowly understood). Humphrey (1992) advocates this elucidation of the sensation/perception distinction and endorses it as the correct account of perception (broadly understood).

A third idea is that sensations have no representational content—they have no meaning or they are not about anything.[31] Meaning and representation only get a grip in perception (narrowly understood). This idea of the distinction between sensation and perception (narrowly understood) is that which Thomas Reid advocated. He claimed, sensation 'hath no object distinct from the act itself'. In contrast, he held that perception (narrowly understood) involved a 'conception or notion of the object perceived', and a 'strong and irreducible conviction and belief of its present existence'.[32]

What is the relationship between these last two conceptions of the distinction between sensation and perception? Are they distinct? Yes. This is because it is possible to hold the latter without the former. One can hold the view that sensations represent my body and what is happening to it—for example that the skin on my hand is being deformed or heated—and thus they are not totally lacking a representational nature.

Sometimes researchers endorse one of these three accounts of sensation and perception, sometimes they hold more than one of these to be true. Often, they

[31] See Ben-Zeeve (1984) for a summary of the positions of those who have held this view.

[32] Reid (1785/1941), Essays 1 & 2, quoted in Hamlyn (1961: 460).

are not clear enough about which account they hold. The keen reader can find an elaboration on these conceptions of sensation and perception, and a detailed account of their historical development, in Hamlyn (1961) and Ben-Zeeve (1984).

How has sensory substitution been thought to help in deciding whether perception (broadly understood) involves both sensation and perception (narrowly understood)? Humphrey (1992) argues that in normal vision we have both visual sensations of the light at our eye, plus visual perception (narrowly understood) of distal objects such as tables and chairs. In TVSS use, he claims that we have a tactile sensation, caused by the vibrating pins on our body, plus visual perception (narrowly understood) of distal objects. This, he claims, shows us that the same visual perception (narrowly understood) can be accompanied by different sensations, as well as it being the case, as is widely agreed, that, if there are sensations, the same sensation can be accompanied by different perceptions (narrowly understood). Thus, he argues that sensory substitution helps to establish that there are doubly dissociable sensational and perceptual aspects to using our senses.

In a similar vein, Ned Block (1996) argues that sensory substitution supports the idea that there is a non-representational element to perceptual experience—that he calls qualia, and that he might easily have called sensation given the third definition of sensation articulated above—that is distinct from the representational aspects of perceptual experience. As we have already noted, people using TVSS report that they can attend to the tactile stimulation on their back, although they usually do not do so; they usually attend to the objects apparently in front of them. Block says that in attending to the tactile stimulations the subjects are attending to the sensation that accompanies their visual perception of external objects. In like manner, he says that during normal perception people usually just attend to the objects and properties given to them in perception, and don't normally attend to the non-representational elements of their experience—the qualia or sensational elements—but he claims it is possible for them to do so, and that therefore they exist, with sensory substitution providing a clear example of the different introspectible elements of perception (broadly understood).

Both of these arguments rely on the thought that the tactile element of TVSS use should be considered as being sensation, in one way or another, and the only sensational element occurring during the use of the TVSS, while the visual element should be considered to be the only perceptual (narrowly understood) element occurring during it. However, these thoughts are highly questionable. One might think that there is both tactile and visual perception taking place (which may or may not involve both sensation and perception (narrowly understood)). Why think that the tactile element involves only sensation? Why not think that it involves both tactile sensation of how the pins affect my body and tactile perception of those pins, in addition to the visual perception taking place? Or why think that the tactile element isn't just perception (broadly construed) that is not composed of sensation and perception (narrowly understood)? Why think that the visual element does not involve a sensational element? Or does not involve perception (broadly understood) that is not composed of sensation and perception (narrowly understood)? Without answers to these questions—thus without independent arguments backing up the existence of sensation and perception (narrowly understood), and how those terms apply to what occurs in sensory substitution—the case of sensory substitution should do nothing to boost our credence in the existence of a distinction between sensation and perception (narrowly understood). The evidence from sensory substitution does not alone provide evidence for the distinction, unless already seen through the lens of a theory that endorses those notions and their appropriate application to the case of sensory substitution.

In addition, as I have taken pains to show earlier in this essay, it is not straightforward at all to conclude that there are perceptual visual experiences occurring in TVSS use, or experiences in the substituted modality in sensory substitution more generally. Indeed, why think that that TVSS involves either tactile elements or visual elements at all? One might argue, as I explored in section 1.4, that its use constitutes a new sensory modality that is neither tactile nor visual. Or one might hold that it is purely tactile, perceptually speaking, and only involves judgements that are visual-like. And, moreover, what the experiences involved are like is a matter of great dispute and may be highly variable. Thus, the messiness of the evidence concerning the conscious mental states occurring in sensory substitution also foils its use as a clear demonstration of the existence of and distinction between sensation and perception (narrowly understood).

1.7 Practical Use

As we have seen above, there appears to be some potential for sensory substitution devices to help those who have lost a sense, and for augmentation devices to provide us with more information than we already obtain through the ordinary use of our senses. However, we have also seen some of the limitations of these devices. Many substitution devices do not give perceptual experiences that are identical to those that are missing. They perhaps give aspects of those experiences, and perhaps only in some people, and in particular conditions, and perhaps after a great deal of practice with the devices. Perhaps in some cases they do not give new experiences at all, only the ability to make judgements about the world. I also noted that many people who suffer from sensory loss (although not all) do not like using these devices and do not adopt them into their lives.

One reason that this may be so is a point that one should be clear about—clearer about than I have been thus far. It is that the TVSS, and the vOICe, and similar devices are rather limited with respect to the types of situation in which they work. Lighting has to be bright, and the stimuli have to be clearly differentiable from their background. So test stimuli are often used that consist of very dark objects on a white background or vice versa. In other words, in many instances the devices only work well in very artificial situations. Moreover, the resolution of the devices is fairly limited. The visual acuity of users of a TVSS device is very low. Sampaio et al. (2001) claim that blind users averaged an acuity of only 40/860 using it. In short, people cannot use TVSS and TDU devices in everyday perceptual situations effectively.[33] So, despite the high hopes that Bach-y-Rita had in the 1960s and 1970s that sensory substitution devices would transform the lives of those who had lost senses, sensory substitution devices are not in common use.

It remains to be seen if advances in technology will allow people to make more useful devices in the future—and at an affordable price. What I hope to have shown in this introduction is that if these practical problems can be overcome—and that is a big if—there is reason to be hopeful that some people may be able to come to have new perceptual experiences using these devices: experiences that represent some features of the world that are of practical importance to us.

1.8 The Essays in This Volume

The essays in this volume represent the latest psychological and philosophical thinking about the many different aspects of sensory substitution and augmentation that I have discussed above.

Renier gives a comprehensive overview of the nature of sensory substitution from a psychologist's point of view, arguing that sensory substitution devices can give people experiences in the substituted modality. Smith responds to Renier, arguing that sensory substitution does not give someone an experience that has the phenomenal character of an experience in the substituted modality. He claims that the substituting modality takes on some of the functions of the substituted modality, making the perceptual experiences they each produce somewhat more like each other than they would otherwise have been.

Corns' essay looks in detail at claims about the perceptual nature of sensory substitution. She differentiates the claims that sensory substitution comprises a natural modality, that it comprises a unique modality, and that it comprises a perceptual process, and she investigates closely the evidence for each claim.

Noordhof argues that in sensory substitution the substituting sense plus the sensory substitution device is not always appropriately classified as the substituted sense. He gives an alternative account according to which properties putatively proprietary to a sense modality can be presented in another modality in cases of substitution. He draws lessons for the development of any kind of representationalist or relationalist theory of phenomenal properties.

[33] See Collins (1985).

Hillenbrand et al. discuss the work of Amir Amedi's lab and investigate the nature of brain plasticity and cross-modal connections in sensory substitution, focusing on the vOICe. Brown's essay provides commentary on work from Amedi's lab. In particular he discusses the idea that sensory substitution devices may facilitate behavioural transference of skills across sense modalities and that these skills are therefore amodally represented. He argues that this conclusion is not warranted from the evidence that the Amedi lab present.

Ptito et al. investigate the nature of brain plasticity and cross-modal connections in sensory substitution focusing on what occurs with use of a TDU.

The essay by Proulx et al. focuses on what we can learn about spatial navigation from sensory substitution. This allows us to compare sensory substitution systems for their practical usefulness, together with their effects on the brain, and their implications for theories of cognition and cross-modal correspondences.

O'Regan defends the sensorimotor theory of perception and its account of sensory substitution. He argues that it is not plasticity which gives rise to the change of experience observed after practice with sensory substitution, but changes in the modes of interaction with the world which plasticity allows.

Briscoe is interested in whether active control of the camera is necessary for the emergence of distal attribution in TVSS. He thinks that it is but he gives an account of this that is at odds with that given by supporters of the sensorimotor theory of perception. He holds that the information gained by moving the camera helps to solve the causal inference problem faced by subjects' perceptual systems, namely the problem of working out what the most probable source of stimulation in the substituting modality is.

Wright and Ward define a very broad range of sensory tools, among which sensory substitution devices are just one kind. They distinguish this group of tools as ones that provide 'raw' sensory information. They differentiate these from other sensory devices that operate at a higher symbolic or conceptual level, thus providing a new taxonomy of sensory tools, and a new definition of sensory substitution.

Cohen's essay also distinguishes between sensory substitution devices that provide 'raw' sensory information—the basic form of energy to which visual receptors are normally responsive—and those that provide information about higher-level emergent features whose nature is not determined by the basic form of energy. He suggests that one could build better sensory substitution devices by building devices that provide information about such emergent features, in addition to the basic forms of energy. Cohen lays out a programmatic vision of how the design of useful sensory substitution devices should proceed.

Connolly explores ways in which the extensive literature on perceptual learning can be applied to help improve sensory substitution devices. He then uses these findings to answer the question of whether the sensory experience had when using sensory substitution devices should be classified in the substituted modality, in the substituting modality, or in a new sense modality.

In contrast to Cohen and Connolly, Spence lays out a negative picture of the prospects of sensory substitution devices being able to help those with sensory loss in a practical manner. He sets out fundamental and technological limitations of substitution devices. He also examines the negative hedonic tone that use of these devices frequently engenders.

The essay by Suarez et al. picks up on the theme established in Spence's essay about the lack of positive emotional experiences that users of sensory substitution devices often report. Suarez et al. suggest a practical way of overcoming this problem.

Lastly, Dokic also considers the emotional and hedonic experiences associated with sensory substitution. He argues that they are constituted by noetic feelings such as familiarity and presence. He explicates a view according to which neither familiarity nor presence can be reproduced in sensory substitution. However, he argues against this view, drawing on the idea that such feelings can arise at the post-perceptual level, as well as at the perceptual level. He also draws on the psychological literature on metacognition, which leads him to a more optimistic view about whether positive feelings can be enjoyed by trained users of sensory substitution devices.

The depth and breadth of these essays attests to the enormous importance of sensory substitution and augmentation in thinking about the nature of perception, perceptual experience, and brain plasticity and organization, particularly cross-modal plasticity and organization. It also attests to the interaction between perception and emotion, and the importance of the feelings that people have when using sensory substitution and augmentation devices. The potential for these devices to alter the skills and abilities that we may have through their use is as yet uncertain, yet these essays push forward our understanding of why this is so. In the end, our own ability to affect our perception through technology may prove to be the key to fully understanding its nature.

References

Akins, K. (1993) What is it like to be boring and myopic? In B. Dahlbom (ed.) *Daniel Dennett and His Critics*. Oxford: Oxford University Press, 124–160.

Armstrong, D. M. (1961) *Perception and the Physical World*. New York: Humanities Press.

Auvray, M., Hanneton, S. and O'Regan, J. K. (2007) Learning to perceive with a visuo-auditory substitution system: localization and object recognition with the Voice. *Perception* 36: 416–430.

Bach-y-Rita, P. (1972) *Brain Mechanisms in Sensory Substitution*. New York: Academic Press.

Bach-y-Rita, P. (1984) The relationship between motor processes and cognition in tactile vision substitution. In W. Prinz and A. F. Sanders (eds) *Cognition and Motor Processes*. Berlin-Heidelberg: Springer-Verlag, 150–159.

Bach-y-Rita, P. and Kercel, S. W. (2003) Sensory substitution and the human–machine interface. *Trends in Cognitive Sciences* 7(12): 541–546.

Bach-y-Rita, P., Collins, C. C., Saunders, F. A., White, B. and Scadden, L. (1969) Vision substitution by tactile image projection. *Nature* 221: 963–964.

Bach-y-Rita, P., Kaczmarek, K. A. and Tyler, M. E. (2003) A tongue-based tactile display for portrayal of environmental characteristics. In L. Hettlinger and M. Haas (eds) *Psychological Issues in the Design and Use of Virtual and Adaptive Environments*. Mahwah, NJ: Lawrence Erlbaum Associates.

Batty, C. (2013) Smell, philosophical perspectives. In H. Pashler (ed.) *Encyclopedia of the Mind*. Thousand Oaks, CA: Sage.

Ben-Zeev, A. (1984) The passivity assumption of the sensation-perception distinction. *British Journal for the Philosophy of Science* 35: 327–343.

Block, N. (1996) Mental paint and mental latex. In E. Villanueva (ed.) *Perception* (Philosophical Issues 7). Atascadero, CA: Ridgeview Publishing Co.

Boring, E. G. (1942) *Sensation and Perception in the History of Experimental Psychology*. Oxford: Appleton-Century.

Campbell, W. W. (2006) *DeJong's The Neurologic Examination*, 6th edn. Philadelphia: Lippincott Williams & Wilkins.

Clark, A. (2007) Sensory and perceptual consciousness. In M. Velmans and S. Schneider (eds) *The Blackwell Companion to Consciousness*, 445–455.

Cohen, L. G., Celnik, P., Pascual-Leone, A., Corwell, B., Faiz, L., Dambrosia, J., Honda, M., Sadato, N., Gerloff, C., Catala, M. D. and Hallett, M. (1997) Functional relevance of cross-modal plasticity in blind humans. *Nature* 389: 180–183.

Collins, C. C. (1985) On mobility aids for the blind. In D. Warren and E. R. Strelow (eds) *Electronic Spatial Sensing for the Blind: Contributions from Perception, Rehabilitation, and Computer Vision*. Dordrecht: Martinus Nijhoff Publications, 35–64.

Crane, T. (1992) The nonconceptual content of experience. In T. Crane (ed.) *The Contents of Experience*. Cambridge: Cambridge University Press.

Deems, D. A., Doty, R. L., Settle, R. G., Moore-Gillon, V., Shaman, P., Mester, A. F. et al. (1991) Smell and taste disorders: a study of 750 patients from the University of Pennsylvania Smell and Taste Center. *Archives of Otorhinolaryngology: Head and Neck Surgery* 117: 519–528.

Donaldson, J. and Macpherson, F. (2017) Ponzo illusion. In F. Macpherson (ed.) *The Illusions Index*. www.illusionsindex.org/i/ponzo-illusion.

Dozza, M., Chiari, L. and Horak, F. B. (2004) A portable audio-biofeedback system to improve postural control. *Conference Proceedings of the IEEE Engineering in Medicine and Biology Society* 7: 4799–4802.

Glüer-Pagin, K. (2009) In defence of a doxastic account of experience. *Mind and Language* 24: 297–373.

Goebel, J. A., Sinks, B. C., Parker, B. E., Richardson, N. T., Olowin, A. B. and Cholewiak, R. W. (2009) Effectiveness of head-mounted vibrotactile stimulation in subjects with bilateral vestibular loss: a phase 1 clinical trial. *Otology and Neurotology* 30(2): 210–216.

Goldstein, B. and Brockmole, J. R. (2017) *Sensation and Perception*, 10th edn. Boston, MA: Cengage Learning.

Guarniero, G. (1974) Experience of tactile vision. *Perception 3*(1): 101–104.

Gudziol, V., Wolff-Stephan, S., Aschenbrenner, K., Joraschky, P. and Hummel, T. (2009) Depression resulting from olfactory dysfunction is associated with reduced sexual appetite—a cross-sectional cohort study. *Journal of Sexual Medicine* 6(7): 1924–1929.

Hamlyn, D. W. (1961) *Sensation and Perception: A History of the Philosophy of Perception*. London: Routledge & Kegan Paul.

Hughes, H. C. (2001) *Sensory Exotica: A World beyond Human Experience*. Cambridge, MA: MIT Press.

Humphrey, N. (1992) *The History of the Mind*. New York: Simon and Schuster.

Hurley, S. and Noë, A. (2003) Neural plasticity and consciousness. *Biology and Philosophy* 18: 131–168.

Hyde, M. and Power, D. (2006) Some ethical dimensions of cochlear implantation for deaf children and their families. *Journal of Deaf Studies and Deaf Education* 11(1): 102–111.

Jackson, F. (1986) What Mary didn't know. *Journal of Philosophy* 83: 291–295.

Jones, W. D. (2004) Sight for sore ears: Dutchman develops auditory imager for the blind. *IEEE Spectrum*, 1 February. http://spectrum.ieee.org/biomedical/devices/sight-for-sore-ears.

Kennedy, J. M. (1993) *Drawing and the Blind: Pictures to Touch*. New Haven, CT: Yale University Press.

Kupers, R., Fumal, A., de Noordhout, A. M., Gjedde, A., Schoenen, J. and Ptito, M. (2006) Transcranial magnetic stimulation of the visual cortex induces somatotopically organized qualia in blind subjects. *Proceedings of the National Academy of Sciences USA* 103(35): 13256–13260.

Macpherson, F. (2011a) Individuating the senses. In F. Macpherson (ed.) *The Senses: Classical and Contemporary Readings. Oxford:* Oxford University Press.

Macpherson, F. (2011b) The admissible contents of experience. In K. Hawley and F. Macpherson (eds) *The Admissible Contents of Experience.* Oxford: Wiley-Blackwell.

Macpherson, F. (2012) Cognitive penetration of colour experience: rethinking the issue in light of an indirect mechanism. *Philosophy and Phenomenological Research* 84(1): 24–62.

Macpherson, F. (2013) Can science tell us that we smell? *Mind and Language* online symposium on the Brains Blog on Louise Richardson's 'Flavour, taste, and smell' (*Mind and Language* 28(3): 322–341). http://philosophyofbrains.com/2013/06/06/louise-richardson-synpo.aspx.

Macpherson, F. (2015) The structure of experience, the nature of the visual, and type 2 blindsight. *Consciousness and Cognition* 32: 104–128.

Macpherson, F. and Baysan, U. (2017) Waterfall illusion. In F. Macpherson (ed.) *The Illusions Index*. www.illusionsindex.org/ir/waterfall-illusion.

Meijer, P. B. L. (1992) An experimental system for auditory image representations. *IEEE Transactions on Biomedical Engineering* 39: 112–121.

Nagel, S. K., Carl, C., Kringe, T., Märtin, R. and König, P. (2005) Beyond sensory substitution—learning the sixth sense. *Journal of Neural Engineering* 2: R13–R26.

Nagel, T. (1974) What is it like to be a bat? *Philosophical Review* 83: 435–450.

Nichols, R. (2007) *Thomas Reid's Theory of Perception*. Oxford: Oxford University Press.

Nudds, M. (2004) The significance of the senses. *Proceedings of the Aristotelian Society* 104(1): 31–51.

Reid, T. (1785/1941) *Essays on the Intellectual Powers of Man*, ed. A. D. Woozely. London: Macmillan.

Renier, L., Laloyaux, C., Collignon, O., Tranduy, D., Vanlierde, A., Bruyer, R. and De Volder, A. G. (2005) The Ponzo illusion using auditory substitution of vision in sighted and early blind subjects. *Perception* 34: 857–867.

Richardson, L. (2013) Flavour, taste, and smell. *Mind and Language* 28(3): 322–341.

Sampaio, E., Maris, S. and Bach-y-Rita, P. (2001) Brain plasticity: 'visual' acuity of blind persons via the tongue. *Brain Research* 908(2): 204–207.

Seo, H. S., Jeon, K. J., Hummel, T. and Min, B. C. (2009) Influences of olfactory impairment on depression, cognitive performance, and quality of life in Korean elderly. *European Archives of Otorhinolaryngology* 266(11): 1739–1745.

Smith, A. D. (2000) Space and sight. *Mind* 109(435): 481–518.

Tyler, M., Danilov, Y. and Bach-y-Rita, P. (2003) Closing an open-loop control system: vestibular substitution through the tongue. *Journal of Integrative Neuroscience* 2: 159.

Vetter, P., Smith, F. W. and Muckli, L. (2014) Decoding sound and imagery content in early visual cortex. *Current Biology* 24(11): 1256–1262.

Ward, J. and Meijer, P. (2010) Visual experiences in the blind induced by an auditory sensory substitution device. *Consciousness and Cognition* 19: 492–500.

Wilson, D. A. and Stevenson, R. J. (2006) *Learning to Smell: Olfactory Perception from Neurobiology to Behavior*. Baltimore, MD: Johns Hopkins University Press.

2

Sensory Substitution: From Sensations to Phenomenology

LAURENT RENIER

Abstract Sensory substitution refers to the use of one sensory modality (e.g. hearing) to supply environmental information normally gathered by another sense (e.g. vision) while still preserving some of the key functions of the original sense. For example, the use of auditory signals might give information about visual scenes. The development of sensory substitution devices has profoundly changed the classical definition of sensory modalities and contributed to the emergence of a new form of perception. In the last decade, our knowledge about cognitive and brain mechanisms involved in sensory substitution has grown considerably, bringing new insights into human perception. The phenomenological experience of perceiving via a sensory substitution device can now be discussed in the light of current scientific knowledge. Thanks to technological advances and scientific achievements, sensory substitution has become a real alternative for restoring some functions of a defective sensory organ (e.g. sight in the case of blindness or hearing in the case of deafness). This essay addresses some of the major questions raised by sensory substitution, including discussions regarding the nature of perception arising from the use of such devices, demonstrates how the study of sensory substitution enhances our understanding of human perception and brain plasticity, and provides a short overview of rehabilitation potentialities.

2.1 Introduction

THE TERM 'SENSORY SUBSTITUTION' was introduced at the end of the 1960s to indicate the use of one sensory modality to supply environmental information normally gathered by another sense (e.g. the use of sound to provide information about visual scenes; Bach-y-Rita et al. 1969). Following the first attempts to create tools to compensate for the loss of sight (e.g. the long cane to assist blind people in their

Proceedings of the British Academy, **219**, 43–59.

movements), Paul Bach-y-Rita and his collaborators developed the first sensory substitution device that was specifically dedicated to the scientific investigation of brain plasticity in early blind people (Bach-y-Rita et al. 1969; Bach-y-Rita and Kercel 2003). Since this pioneering work, the increasing interest in sensory substitution has given rise both to the development of various sensory substitution devices and to numerous studies in the cognitive neuroscience sphere (Renier and De Volder 2005). Sensory substitution has now become a vast field of study and constitutes both a research topic and a means to investigate other domains such as human perception (including what we might think of as 'synthetic' or 'artificial synaesthesia') and brain plasticity. The purpose of this chapter is to provide an overview of some sensory substitution devices, to summarize the main questions explored over the last decades in this research area, to demonstrate how sensory substitution contributes to the study of brain function and human cognition, and to evaluate the rehabilitation potentialities of available systems.

2.2 Sensory Substitution Devices

While virtually every sense can be replaced by another one using human–machine interfaces, most sensory substitution devices were developed for vision substitution and there have been very few attempts to develop devices to substitute the olfactory and gustatory modalities. Vision is the predominant sense in sighted humans (Rock et al. 1999) and the most investigated one. The visual sense plays a central role in how we represent and interact with the world around us. The primacy of vision is structurally embedded in cortical organization since about one-third of the cortical surface in primates is involved in visual processes (Kupers et al. 2011). Therefore, it is not surprising that the visual sense is also the most frequently substituted via sensory substitution devices (either via auditory or tactile modalities). Besides vision, however, there have been some attempts to replace hearing and the vestibular function by the tactile modality.

2.2.1 Vision substitution

Historically, the first efficient sensory substitution instrument developed to replace vision was the long cane. This very simple instrument was used to assist blind people in their displacements (Hoover 1950). At the beginning of the nineteenth century, Louis Braille, who suffered blindness himself at the age of 3, invented one of the first sensory substitution systems which used an arbitrary code (Mellor 2008; but for previous systems see also the Ecriture Nocturne of Charles Barbier de la Serre and the Embossed Alphabet of Valentin Haüy, e.g. Monnier 1989). Braille was further developed into a successful reading and writing system using a tactile code. The cane and Braille are still used today all around the world by blind people in their everyday lives.

Following these first successful steps, electronic versions of the long cane (e.g. laser cane and other obstacle detectors) were intended to improve orientation and mobility by providing spatial information (Kay 1961; Farmer 1978). Later, these sonar aids evolved into head-mounted versions, such as the well-known Sonicguide (Kay 1974; see also www.batforblind.co.nz/index.php) which used pitch and binaural balance, i.e. difference in the stimulation intensity between the ears. Those devices provided the user with information about obstacle location and distance. Other approaches such as the 'SeeHear' chip from Caltech (Nielson et al. 1989) use binaural directional cues, much as natural human echolocation does. Human echolocation, initially described as 'facial vision' (Supa et al. 1944), is the ability of humans to detect objects in their environment by actively creating sounds (e.g. by tapping their canes, stomping their foot or making clicking noises with their mouths) and sensing echoes from those objects (Thaler et al. 2011).

In the same period as that of the Sonicguide, Bach-y-Rita and his collaborators (1969) developed the Tactile Vision Substitution System (TVSS), offering the possibility of both localizing *and* recognizing objects. Currently, two main classes of vision sensory substitution devices exist, tactile and auditory. In other words, what would usually be visual information is fed to the senses in the form of touch or sound. These 'modern' vision sensory substitution systems consist of a video camera coupled with a human–machine interface. The human–machine interface transmits the information to the brain either through tactile sense or the auditory modality, the so-called 'sensory substitution channel' (Bach-y-Rita and Kercel 2003).

The TVSS and visual-to-tactile substitution devices

The original TVSS mapped black-and-white images from a video camera to a vibrotactile belt worn on the abdomen at a resolution of 20 × 20 pixels in the tactile array. This 'new generation' of devices opened the way to the scientific study of sensory substitution. The TVSS in its pneumatic, electric or vibrotactile variants (Kaczmarek et al. 1991; Zappe et al. 2004) uses various skin areas of the body as the peripheral sense organ for input: the abdomen, the back, the thigh or the forehead, as well as the tongue, may be used for this purpose. Of these, the tongue, which is a very sensitive organ, seems more suitable than other body parts, as demonstrated by studies using a substitution device known as the tongue display unit (TDU; Bach-y-Rita et al. 1998). The TDU transmits visual information via the tongue using electrotactile stimulation; it reproduces 'visual patterns' on a 144-pixel square matrix applied on the tongue. These sensory substitution systems provide analogue encoding of visual information (i.e. the spatial arrangement of the elements in a perceived scene is transposed onto the skin by a matrix of 'tactors' that stimulates the somatosensory receptors in a defined skin area). Other devices using wearable vibrotactile belts (Haptic Belt; McDaniel et al. 2008) or gloves (VibroGlove; Krishna et al. 2010) enable people who are blind to perceive social situational information. Both technologies use miniature cameras that are mounted on a pair of glasses worn by the user who is blind. The Haptic Belt provides vibrations that convey the direction and distance at which a person is standing in front of a user, while the VibroGlove uses spatio-temporal mapping of vibration patterns to convey facial expressions of the interaction partner.

Visual-to-auditory substitution devices

Alternatives to the tactile systems include auditory devices such as the vOICe (Meijer 1992), the prosthesis substituting vision with audition (PSVA; Capelle et al. 1998); the Cronly-Dillon algorithm (Cronly-Dillon et al. 1999) and the versatile vision-to-audition sensory substitution device (VIBE) (Hanneton et al. 2010). These allow online translation of visual patterns into sounds that the subject hears through headphones. We describe these below.

THE VOICE

The vOICe (with the three capital letters referring to 'Oh I see') converts live camera views from a video camera into 'soundscapes' (Meijer 1992). A 'soundscape' is an auditory signal that represents the components of the visual scene. The vOICe system uses general video-to-audio mapping by associating height with pitch, and brightness with loudness, in a left-to-right scan of any video frame. In other words, if the visual scene contains an object at height, which is also bright, the corresponding sound will be high in pitch and loud. The left-to-right scanning means that objects in the left-hand visual field are 'sounded' before objects in the right. Views are typically refreshed about once per second with a typical image resolution of up to 60 x 60 pixels, as can be proven by spectrographic analysis. More information about the vOICe device can be found at www.seeingwithsound.com.

THE PSVA

The prosthesis substituting vision with audition (PSVA) translates real-time monochrome images from a miniature head-mounted video camera (frame rate: 12.5 hertz) into sounds using a pixel–frequency relationship (Capelle et al. 1998). The camera image is pixelated according to a simplified dual resolution model of the human retina. This artificial retina consists of a square matrix of 8 x 8 large pixels with the four central ones replaced by 8 x 8 smaller pixels representing the fovea. Therefore, the fovea has four times the resolution of the periphery. A single sinusoidal tone is assigned to each pixel of the artificial retina with frequencies increasing from left to right and from bottom to top; frequencies range between 50 and 12,526 Hz. The grey-scale level of each pixel modulates the amplitude of its corresponding sine wave. The final auditory output of the PSVA is the real-time weighted sum of all 124 sine waves. With head movements, visual frames are grabbed in real time and then transformed into a set of corresponding complex sounds, enabling the wearer to ultimately recognize the scene. A demonstration of the sound produced by a single pixel or a bar when detected by the system is available at www.perceptionweb.com/perc0899/arno.html.

THE VIBE

With the versatile vision-to-audition sensory substitution device (VIBE), the sound produced by this software is also a mixture of sinusoidal sounds produced by the 'translation' of an image into sounds. The visual scene is divided into sections or 'receptive fields' that are each translated into a sine wave of a specific frequency according to its location (Hanneton et al. 2010). Each receptive field is a set of localized pixels. The sound's amplitude is determined by the mean luminosity of the pixels of the corresponding receptive field. In other words, brighter objects are translated into louder sounds. The frequency and the stimulation intensity in each individual ear (inter-aural disparity) are determined by the location of the object in the receptive fields of the system.

In contrast to tactile displays, devices that substitute audio for vision usually use an arbitrary code to translate images into sounds, though some of the key characteristics are quite intuitive and can be understood with little or no prior explanation (e.g. stimulation intensity difference between ears codes for the location of the object in the perceptual field; the left part of the perceptual field renders sounds mainly in the left ear). Despite this difference, both types of vision substitution systems (i.e. auditory and tactile displays) offer similar perceptual possibilities such as shape recognition (Arno et al. 2001a; Ptito et al. 2005; Amedi et al. 2007), object localization and distance estimation (Auvray et al. 2007; Proulx et al. 2008; Renier and De Volder 2010; Chebat et al. 2011) or depth perception (Renier et al. 2005a; Segond et al. 2005). It is worth noting that these modern sensory substitution devices generate elaborated perception that shares close similarities with vision (O'Regan and Noë 2001; Renier and De Volder 2010). For instance, distance estimation using a system with a video camera is based on visual pictorial (or monocular) cues such as the relative size, the height in the perceptual field, occlusion effects, or linear perspective (Renier et al. 2005b; Renier and De Volder 2005), and they recruit specialized visual brain areas (Renier et al. 2005a; Amedi et al. 2007). O'Regan and Noë (2001) also put a lot of emphasis on the fact that head movements, which are usually linked to visual changes in normal conditions, become artificially associated with equivalent changes in the auditory or tactile modality when using a vision sensory substitution system.

2.2.2 Hearing substitution

While there is no tactile-auditory substitution system currently available (i.e. no system that replaces environmental by touch signals), recent experiments show that vibrotactile stimuli can be used to facilitate hearing in normal and hearing-impaired people and may activate the auditory cortex (Schurmann et al. 2006). Schurmann and his collaborators tested subjects while stimulating their fingers and palms with vibration bursts and their finger tips with tactile pressure. They found that tactile stimulation of the fingers led to activation of the auditory cortex, which suggests that there is a relationship between audition and touch. It makes sense to investigate the likelihood of a tactile-auditory sensory substitution system in the future.

2.2.3 Vestibular system substitution

Some people with balance disorders or adverse reactions to antibiotics suffer from bilateral vestibular damage. They experience difficulty with standing and in maintaining posture. Tyler and collaborators (2003) investigated the restitution of postural control through a tactile-for-vestibular sensory substitution. Using a head-mounted accelerometer (i.e. an instrument for measuring acceleration) and a brain–machine interface that employs electrotactile stimulation on the tongue, information about head–body orientation is relayed to the patient so that a new source of data is available to orient himself and maintain good posture (Tyler et al. 2003). The original version of the vestibular substitution system used the tongue display unit (TDU; Bach-y-Rita et al. 1998) and a miniature two-axis accelerometer that was mounted on a hat. Anterior-posterior and medial-lateral angular displacement data (derived by double integration of the acceleration data) were fed to the TDU, which generated a patterned stimulus on a 144-point electrotactile array (12 x 12 matrix) held against the superior, anterior surface of the tongue. Studies demonstrated that providing an open-loop human control system allowed rapid and significant improvements in all tested patients; after three to five days of training with the device, the head–body postural coordination was restored by means of vestibular substitution (Bach-y-Rita et al. 2005). Moreover, postural stability remained for a couple of days after removing the vestibular substitution, after which the open-loop instability reappeared.

2.3 Processes Underlying Sensory Substitution

One of the main questions raised by sensory substitution concerns the exact nature of the related perceptions. What exactly *are* perceptions, and how can they be defined given that sensory substitution devices serve to separate the modality of the stimulus and the modality of the derived sensory experience? And what is that sensory experience *like*? From a general perspective, this problem asks: what are the actual determinants of the nature of a perception? Is it the sensory organ used to receive the information? Or the pathway over which the sensory information is carried (Müller 1835; Norrsell et al. 1999)? Is it the sensory modality of the original stimulus? Is it the nature of the information conveyed? For instance, distance and spatiality are thought to be more specifically related to vision than to any other sense in human beings. Is it the character of the cognitive and/or brain processing that determines its nature? According to Bach-y-Rita, perception is created within the brain and is relatively independent from the sensory modality of the stimulus, or the sense organ that receives it (Bach-y-Rita 1972). Several researchers have proposed that perception based on vision substitution by another sense (e.g. touch/sound signals) is visual since subjects using this type of device generally report visual rather than tactual or auditory sensations, and perceive objects as externally localized rather than on the skin, say (Epstein et al. 1986; Auvray et al. 2005; Ward and Meijer 2010). Supporting this viewpoint, Morgan (1977) underlined the fact that both vision and its sensory substitution provide access to the same kind of information and give rise to similar behavioural responses. It is worth noting that perception by means of sensory substitution of vision fits quite well with most of the definitions of visual perception. For instance, Rock et al. defined visual perception as the '*process of acquiring knowledge about environmental objects and events by extracting information from the light they emit or reflect*' (1999: 5). The above referenced 'modern' vision substitution devices were developed to acquire environmental information in a similar way, namely, the extraction of information conveyed by the light, but providing this information to the user through another sense. O'Regan and Noë (2001) further pointed out the similarities regarding some sensorimotor contingencies of vision and those of sensory substitution devices that used a head-mounted camera. According to these authors, the nature of perception is mainly determined by the relationship between motor actions (e.g. reaching to touch an object) and their sensory consequences (the resultant tactile sensation), the so-called sensorimotor contingencies. They concluded that provided the sensation changes related to head movements occur in the auditory or tactile modality instead of the visual modality, the users of such sensory substitution devices should have visual experiences. Moreover, there are additional arguments that do account for the cognitive aspects of visual perception, in which visual information is interpreted beyond solely the available information in the visual receptive field (e.g. as in optical illusions). For instance, Renier et al. (2005b, 2006) demonstrated the possibility of perceiving pure visual phenomena using the PSVA (the prosthesis substituting vision with audition, a visual-to-auditory substitution device described above). Sighted subjects using the PSVA while blindfolded were sensitive to the Ponzo illusion (Renier et al. 2005b) and the vertical-horizontal illusion (Renier et al. 2006) and were able to interpret visual depth cues when using the PSVA to estimate the distance to an object (Renier and De Volder 2010). This illustrates the top-down influences of visual processes in full accordance with theoretical models of visual perception (Gregory 1997). It clearly indicates the existence of a visual-like processing of sensory information gathered by the PSVA. In addition, previous visual experience was demonstrated to influence perception with the PSVA, since early blind subjects were not sensitive to visual illusions or to visual perspective (Renier et al. 2005b). In addition to subjective reports and observed behavioural performance, results from brain imaging studies highlighted other similarities between vision and perception by sensory substitution of vision. Several brain imaging studies demonstrated a recruitment of visual brain areas in sighted but blindfolded subjects who used a tactile (Ptito et al. 2005) or an auditory (Arno et al. 2001b; Amedi et al. 2007; Reich et al. 2011; Plaza et al. 2012; Striem-Amit et al. 2012) vision sensory substitution device to recognize two-dimensional figures. Furthermore, modulation of some of these brain activation foci according to what was perceived (i.e. two-dimensional versus three-dimensional scene) was also observed with the PSVA, as in vision (Renier et al. 2005a).

2.4 Does Sensory Substitution Provide Artificial (Synthetic) Synaesthesia?

Sensory substitution artificially extends the natural cross-modal perception possibilities of normal subjects by allowing them to process information normally related to one sense by another one (e.g. 'hearing' object shapes). This new type of cross-modal perception fundamentally changed the classical distinction between senses, making their natural boundaries vanish. However, gaining access to environmental information is still different from feeling or experiencing sensations related to another modality. For instance, are blind users able to experience visual sensations (what philosophers call visual qualia) when they use a vision-to-hearing substitution device? Or do they just 'hear' it? Ward and Meijer (2010) recently reported that through extensive use of the vOICe, some blind users described having experienced specifically *visual* sensations. Therefore, using a sensory substitution device to perceive objects would not only be a matter of conveying information in a general sense, but would also generate the corresponding subjective experience inherent to the substituted modality. In addition, after a period of training, some of these proficient blind users reported starting to experience visual sensations in response to environmental sounds while they were *not* using the vOICe. This leads to the suggestion that the blind users had acquired synaesthesia after having used a vision substitution device based on sounds (Ward and Meijer 2010; see also Proulx 2010). This observation is in line with previous observations made by other researchers (Bach-y-Rita 1972; Morgan 1977; Epstein et al. 1986; O'Regan and Noë 2001; Auvray et al. 2005): the perception provided to the user is regarded by the proficient user as 'real', and often outside the body, instead of imagined in the mind's eye. Its reality and vividness are what makes this perception so new, and the related artificial synaesthesia so interesting in its violation of conventional notions of perception. In this way, this type of 'artificial synaesthesia' is a deliberately evoked or induced sensory fusion in which the real information of one sense is accompanied by a perception in another sense through the use of a cross-modal mapping device. This phenomenon is also known as 'virtual synaesthesia' or 'synthetic synaesthesia'. However, it is the use of a *device* to map one type of sensory information stream into an information stream for another sensory modality which clearly distinguishes artificial synaesthesia from spontaneous synaesthesia or developmental synaesthesia as well as from cross-modal associations in non-synaesthetes for normal sensory inputs (see www.seeingwithsound.com/asynesth.htm). In other words, we are dealing with a form of learned synaesthesia (acquired synaesthesia) that might result from machine-generated cross-modal mappings, and this might be particularly relevant in studying the feasibility of developing useful artificial auditory (or tactile)-to-visual synaesthesia for blind people. In contrast to 'natural' synaesthetes who usually report relatively simple or non-generic visual percepts of colour, textures or shapes in association with certain sounds, and where different synaesthetes report different percepts (Ward and Meijer 2010), here we are faced with the fascinating perspective of being able to promote virtually all kinds of learned auditory-induced or tactile-induced visual percepts, and thereby provide a form of synaesthetic experience in each and everybody.

2.5 Sensory Substitution and Cross-Modal Plasticity in Sensorily Impaired Subjects

Studying sensory substitution in blindness (or in deafness) presents a unique opportunity for understanding how the brain adapts itself when it processes visual-like (or auditory-like) information after an extended period of sensory deprivation, or the complete absence of visual (or auditory) information since birth. Therefore, it is not surprising that brain plasticity rapidly became the most studied topic using sensory substitution devices (e.g. Arno et al. 2001a). Early visual deprivation gives rise to a reorganization of the visual cortex (e.g. Rauschecker 1995; Bavelier and Neville 2002; Pascual-Leone et al. 2005; Renier et al. 2013a), and to the emergence of compensatory mechanisms that make early blind people more efficient at achieving certain perceptual tasks, including sensory substitution (Pascual-Leone and Torres 1993; Lessard et al. 1998; Röder et al. 1999; Arno et al. 2001b; Cuevas et al. 2009). Using functional imaging of the brain in congenitally blind subjects, a cross-modal recruitment of the occipital cortex was observed during speech processing and verbal memory (Röder et al. 2002; Amedi et al. 2003; Reich et al. 2011; Bedny et al. 2011), mental imagery tasks (De Volder et al. 2001), Braille reading (Sadato et al. 1996; Büchel et al. 1998; Burton et al. 2012), tactile perception (Pietrini et al. 2004; Renier et al. 2010), sound localization (Kujala et al. 1992; Weeks et al. 2000; Gougoux et al. 2005) and olfactory processing (Renier et al. 2013b). The functional specialization of the ventral, temporo-occipital and dorsal, parieto-occipital stream seems well preserved and developed in early blind subjects, as demonstrated by studies on mental imagery (De Volder et al. 2001; Vanlierde et al. 2003), working memory (Bonino et al. 2008) and auditory and tactile perception (Poirier et al. 2006; Saenz et al. 2008; Renier and De Volder 2010; Renier et al. 2013a). The main contribution of sensory substitution studies was the demonstration of a recruitment of the occipital cortex in early blind subjects, during the processing of auditory or tactile encoded visual information (Arno et al. 2001a; Ptito et al. 2005). This functional role of the occipital cortex of blind subjects in non-visual tasks was also shown using transcranial magnetic stimulation to induce virtual lesions in the brain that interfered with Braille reading (Cohen et al. 1997), speech processing (Amedi et al. 2003), sound lateralization and sensory substitution (Collignon et al. 2007; Merabet et al. 2009). Interestingly, Kupers et al. (2006) showed that transcranial magnetic stimulation applied on the occipital pole induced tactile sensations referred to the tongue in blind subjects who were trained to use the TDU, demonstrating further the cross-modal plasticity mechanisms that develop after a relatively short learning phase. More recently, we demonstrated that early blind subjects could learn visual perspectives while using the PSVA (Renier and De Volder 2010). One may hypothesize that the occipital cortex of blind people is the neural substrate of the compensatory perceptual mechanisms and that it contributes to the subjective visual phenomenology experienced by them.

2.6 Sensory Substitution and Vision Rehabilitation

The very first vision substitution methods, i.e. the long cane and Braille, were developed exclusively in a rehabilitation context. These assistive systems have given birth to electronic versions (e.g. Kay 1961) which are currently used all around the world by blind people. In contrast to Braille or the long cane, which aimed to restore only one function of vision (reading or obstacle detection), sensory substitution systems are intended to simultaneously restore several functions of vision (e.g. spatial localization and shape recognition; Bach-y-Rita 1972). As mentioned above, sensory substitution appeared gradually in basic research, but the idea of creating devices to assist blind people in their everyday life is one of recent interest (e.g. Bach-y-Rita and Kercel 2003; Veraart et al. 2004). Sensory substitution devices are quite adapted to different uses and situations and seem able to respond to most of the needs of blind people for object localization and recognition outside the proximal space. These characteristics can potentially facilitate their mobility and improve the quality of their interactions with the environment in general. Sensory substitution has significant advantages over visual prostheses, such as retinal implants and implanted electrodes that stimulate electrically the optic nerve or the visual cortex (Brindley et al. 1968; Dobelle et al. 1979; Humayun et al. 1996; Brelén et al. 2005). Sensory substitution systems are completely non-invasive (avoiding all the potential problems associated with implanted electrodes). They are suitable even for people with optic nerve damage and hypothetically also appropriate when sensory loss is a consequence of a cortical lesion. Another advantage is that they can be used after a very short training phase (i.e. a few hours). However, despite these qualities, very few sensory substitution devices are currently used by blind people in their daily life, though some of them, such as the vOICe, are available for free on the internet and do not necessitate a lot of equipment to use them. A reason for this limited use of these devices by the blind may still be the relatively poor information conveyed to the users by these devices as compared to vision. Nevertheless, sensory substitution is still a promising alternative to the traditional aids for blind people, implanted visual prostheses and other assistive technologies.

2.7 Conclusions

Although many technological hurdles remain before these devices can be used in daily life, sensory substitution is demonstrably suitable for many tasks such as spatial localization, distance estimation, and shape recognition. Thus these devices could aid mobility and object-grasping. However, despite these very encouraging prospects for rehabilitation, the main interest of sensory substitution still remains in basic research. Throughout the years, by demonstrating valuable practical possibilities to replace some of the key functions of vision, sensory substitution has become a vast and attractive research field in cognitive neuroscience. Although many issues remain yet to be investigated and better understood, studies on sensory substitution have demonstrated valuable contributions to the understanding of human perception, sensory interactions and integration, natural versus artificial synaesthesia and brain plasticity.

References

Amedi, Amir, Noa Raz, Pazit Pianka, Rafael Malach and Ehud Zohary (2003) Early 'visual' cortex activation correlates with superior verbal memory performance in the blind. *Nature Neuroscience* 6: 758–766.

Amedi, Amir, William M. Stern, Joan A. Camprodon, Felix Bermpohl, Lotfi Merabet, Stephen Rotman, Christopher Hemond, Peter Meijer and Alvaro Pascual-Leone (2007)

Shape conveyed by visual-to-auditory sensory substitution activates the lateral occipital complex. *Nature Neuroscience* 10(6): 687–689.

Arno, Patricia, Christian Capelle, Marie-Chantale Wanet-Defalque, Mitzi Catalan-Ahumada and Claude Veraart (1999) Auditory coding of visual patterns for the blind. *Perception* 28: 1013–1029.

Arno, Patricia, Anne G. De Volder, Annick Vanlierde, Marie-Chantal Wanet-Defalque, Emmanuel Streel, Annie Robert, Sandra Sanabria-Bohorquez and Claude Veraart (2001a) Occipital activation by pattern recognition in the Early Blind using auditory substitution of vision. *NeuroImage* 13: 632–645.

Arno, Patricia, Annick Vanlierde, Emmanuel Streel, Marie-Chantal Wanet-Defalque, Sandra Sanabria-Bohorquez and Claude Veraart (2001b) Auditory substitution of vision: pattern recognition by the blind. *Applied Cognitive Psychology* 15: 509–519.

Auvray, Malika, Sylvain Hanneton, Charles Lenay and Kevin O'Regan (2005) There is something out there: distal attribution in sensory substitution, twenty years later. *Journal of Integrative Neuroscience* 4(4): 505–521.

Auvray, Malika, Sylvain Hanneton and Kevin O'Regan (2007) Learning to perceive with a visuo-auditory substitution system: localisation and object recognition with 'the vOICe'. *Perception* 36(3): 416–430.

Bach-y-Rita, Paul (1972) *Brain Mechanisms in Sensory Substitution*. San Diego, CA: Academic Press.

Bach-y-Rita, Paul and Stephen W. Kercel (2003) Sensory substitution and the human-machine interface. *Trends in Cognitive Science* 7: 541–546.

Bach-y-Rita, Paul, Carter C. Collins, Frank Saunders, Benjamin White and Lawrence Scadden (1969) Vision substitution by tactile image projection. *Nature* 221: 963–964.

Bach-y-Rita, Paul, Kurt A. Kaczmarek, Mitchell E. Tyler and Jorge Garcia-Lara (1998) Form perception with a 49-point electrotactile stimulus array on the tongue: a technical note. *Journal of Rehabilitation Research and Development* 35: 427–430.

Bach-y-Rita, Paul, Yuri P. Danilov, Mitchell E. Tyler and Robert J. Grimm (2005) Late human brain plasticity: vestibular substitution with a tongue BrainPort human-machine interface. *Intellectica* 40: 115–122.

Bavelier, Daphne and Helen J. Neville (2002) Cross-modal plasticity: where and how? *Nature Reviews Neuroscience* 3(6): 443–452.

Bedny, Marina, Alvaro Pascual-Leone, David Dodell-Feder, Evelina Fedorenko and Rebecca Saxe (2011) Language processing in the occipital cortex of congenitally blind adults. *Proceedings of the National Academy of Sciences USA* 108(11): 4429–4434.

Bonino, Daniela, Emiliano Ricciardi, Lorenzo Sani, Claudio Gentili, Nicola Vanello, Mario Guazzelli, Tomaso Vecchi and Pietro Pietrini (2008) Tactile spatial working memory activates the dorsal extrastriate cortical pathway in congenitally blind individuals. *Archives Italiennes de Biologie* 146(3–4): 133–146.

Brelén, Marten E., Florence Duret, Benoît Gérard, Jean Delbeke and Claude Veraart (2005) Creating a meaningful visual perception in blind volunteers by optic nerve stimulation. *Journal of Neural Engineering* 2(1): S22–S28.

Brindley, Giles S. and W. S. Lewin (1968) The sensations produced by electrical stimulation of the visual cortex. *Journal of Physiology* 96: 479–493.

Büchel, Christian, Cathy Price, Richard S. J. Frackowiak and Karl Friston (1998) Different activation patterns in the visual cortex of late and congenitally blind subjects. *Brain* 121: 409–419.

Burton, Harold, Robert J. Sinclair and Alvin Agato (2012) Recognition memory for Braille or spoken words: an fMRI study in early blind. *Brain Research* 1438: 22–34.

Capelle, Christian, Charles Trullemans, Patricia Arno and Claude Veraart (1998) Real time experimental prototype for enhancement of vision rehabilitation using auditory substitution. *IEEE Transactions on Biomedical Engineering* 45: 1279–1293.

Chebat, Daniel R., Fabien C. Schneider, Ron Kupers and Maurice Ptito (2011) Navigation without vision: detection and avoidance of obstacles using sensory substitution device. *Neuroreport* 22(7): 342–347.

Cohen, Leonardo G., Pablo Celnik, Alvaro Pascual-Leone, Brian Corwell, Lala Faiz, James Dambrosia, Manabu Honda, Norihiro Sadato, Christaian Gerloff, M. Dolores Catalá and Mark Hallett (1997) Functional relevance of cross-modal plasticity in blind humans. *Nature* 389(6647): 180–183.

Collignon, Olivier, Maryse Lassonde, Franco Lepore, Danielle Bastien and Claude Veraart (2007) Functional cerebral reorganization for auditory spatial processing and auditory substitution of vision in early blind subjects. *Cerebral Cortex* 17(2): 457–465.

Cronly-Dillon, John, Krishna Persaud and Richard P. Gregory (1999) The perception of visual images encoded in musical form: a study in crossmodality information transfer. *Proceedings of the Royal Society of London B: Biological Sciences* 266: 2427–2433.

Cuevas, I., P. Plaza, P. Rombaux, A. G. De Volder and L. Renier (2009) Odour discrimination and identification are improved in early blindness. *Neuropsychologia* 47(14): 3079–3083.

De Volder, Anne G., Hinako Toyama, Yuichi Kimura, Motohiro Kiyosawa, Hideki Nakano, Annick Vanlierde, Marie-Chantal Wanet-Defalque, Masahiro Mishina, Keiichi Oda, Kiichi Ishiwata and Michio Senda (2001) Auditory triggered mental imagery of shape involves visual association areas in early blind humans. *NeuroImage* 14: 129–139.

Dobelle, William H., J. Turkel, D. C. Henderson and J. R. Evans (1979) Mapping the representation of the visual-field by electrical-stimulation of human visual cortex. *American Journal of Ophthalmology* 88: 727–735.

Epstein, William, Barry Hugues, Sandra Schneider and Paul Bach-y-Rita (1986) Is there anything out there? A study of distal attribution in response to vibro-tactile stimulation. *Perception* 15: 275–284.

Farmer, Leicester W. (1978) Mobility devices. *Bulletin of Prosthetics Research* 14: 47–118.

Gougoux, Frédéric, Robert J. Zatorre, Maryse Lassonde, Patrice Voss and Franco Lepore (2005) A functional neuroimaging study of sound localization: visual cortex activity predicts performance in early-blind individuals. *PLoS Biology* 3(2): e27.

Gregory, Richard L. (1997) *Eye and Brain: The Psychology of Seeing*, 5th edn. Princeton, NJ: Princeton University Press.

Hanneton, Sylvain, Malika Auvray and Barthélémy Durette (2010) The Vibe: a versatile vision-to-audition sensory substitution device. *Applied Bionics and Biomechanics* 7(4): 269–276.

Hoover, R. E. (1950) The cane as a travel aid. In P. A. Zahl (ed.) *Blindness*. Princeton, NJ: Princeton University Press, 589.

Humayun, Mark S., Eugene de Juan, Gislin Dagnelie, Robert J. Greenburg, Roy H. Propst and Howard Phillips (1996) Visual perception elicited by electrical stimulation of retina in blind humans. *Archives of Ophthalmology* 114: 40–46.

Kaczmarek, Kurt A., John G. Webster, Paul Bach-y-Rita and Willis J. Tompkins (1991) Electrotactile and vibrotactile displays for sensory substitution systems. *IEEE Transactions on Biomedical Engineering* 38: 1–16.

Kay, Leslie (1961) Orientation of bats and men by ultrasonic echo-location. *British Communications and Electronics* 8: 582–586.

Kay, Leslie (1974) A sonar aid to enhance spatial perception of the blind: engineering design and evaluation. *Radio and Electronic Engineer* 44: 605–627.

Krishna, S., S. Bala, T. McDaniel, S. McGuire and S. Panchanathan (2010) VibroGlove: an assistive technology aid for conveying facial expressions. Proceedings of the 28th Annual CHI Conference on Human Factors in Computing Systems, Atlanta, Georgia, USA, pp. 3637–3642.

Kujala, Teija, Kimmo Alho, Petri Paavilainen, Heikki Summala and Risto Näätänen (1992) Neural plasticity in processing of sound location by the early blind: an event-related potential study. *Electroencephalography and Clinical Neurophysiol*ogy 84(5): 469–472.

Kupers, Ron, Arnaud Fumal, Alain Maertens de Noordhout, Albert Gjedde, Jean Schoenen and Maurice Ptito (2006) Transcranial magnetic stimulation of the visual cortex induces somatotopically organized qualia in blind subjects. *Proceedings of the National Academy of Sciences USA* 103(35): 13256–13260.

Kupers, Ron, Pietro Pietrini, Emiliano Ricciardi and Maurice Ptito (2011) The nature of consciousness in the visually deprived brain. *Frontiers in Psychol*ogy 2: 19.

Lessard, Nadia, M. Pare, Franco Lepore and Maryse Lassonde (1998) Early-blind human subjects localize sound sources better than sighted subjects. *Nature* 395: 278–280.

McDaniel, T., S. Krishna, V. Balasubramanian, D. Colbry and S. Panchanathan (2008) Using a haptic belt to convey non-verbal communication cues during social interactions to individuals who are blind. IEEE International Workshop on Haptic, Audio and Visual Environments and Games, 13–18.

Meijer, Peter B. L. (1992) An experimental system for auditory image representations. *IEEE Transactions on Biomedical Engineering* 39: 112–121.

Mellor, C. M (2008) *Louis Braille: Le génie au bout des doigts*. Paris: Éditions du patrimoine.

Merabet, Lotfi, Lorella Battelli, Souzana Obretenova, Sara Maguire, Peter Meijer and Alvaro Pascual-Leone (2009) Functional recruitment of visual cortex for sound encoded object identification in the blind. *Neuroreport* 20(2): 132–138.

Monnier, R. (1989) Haüy Valentin, *Dictionnaire historique de la Révolution française*. Paris: Presses universitaires de France (reprinted Quadrige, 2005).

Morgan, Michael J. (1977) *Molyneux's Question*. Cambridge: Cambridge University Press.

Müller, Johannes P. (1835) *Handbuch der Physiologie des Menschen für Vorlesungen*, in E. Clarke, and C. D. O'Malley (1968) *The Human Brain and Spinal Cord. A Historical Study Illustrated by Writings from Antiquity to the Twentieth Century*, 2nd edn. Berkeley: University of California Press.

Nielson, L., M. Mahowald and C. Mead (1989) 'SeeHear.' In C. Mead, *Analog VLSI and Neural Systems*. Reading: Addison-Wesley, ch. 13, 207–227.

Norrsell, Ulf, Stanley Finger and Clara Lajonchere (1999) Cutaneous sensory spots and the 'law of specific nerve energies': history and development of ideas. *Brain Research Bulletin* 48(5): 457–465.

O'Regan, J. Kevin and Alva Noë (2001) A sensorimotor account of vision and visual consciousness. *Behavioral and Brain Sciences* 24: 939–1011.

Pascual-Leone, Alvaro and Fernando Torres (1993) Plasticity of the sensorimotor cortex representation of the reading finger in Braille readers. *Brain* 116(Pt 1): 39–52.

Pascual-Leone, Alvaro, Amir Amedi, Felipe Fregni and Lotfi B. Merabet (2005) The plastic human brain cortex. *Annual Review of Neuroscience* 28: 377–401.

Pietrini, Pietro, Maura L. Furey, Emiliano Ricciardi, M. Ida Gobbini, W.-H. Carolyn Wu, Leonardo Cohen, Mario Guazzelli and James V. Haxby (2004) Beyond sensory images: object-based representation in the human ventral pathway. *Proceedings of the National Academy of Sciences USA* 101: 5658–5663.

Plaza, Paula, I. Cuevas, C. Grandin, A. De Volder and L. Renier (2012) Looking into task-specific activation using a Prosthesis Substituting Vision with Audition. *ISRN Rehabilitation*, ID490950.

Poirier, Colline, Olivier Collignon, Christian Scheiber, Laurent Renier, Annick Vanlierde, Dai Tranduy, Claude Veraart and Anne G. De Volder (2006) Auditory motion perception activates visual motion areas in early blind subjects. *NeuroImage* 31(1): 279–285.

Proulx, Michael J. (2010) Synthetic synaesthesia and sensory substitution. *Consciousness and Cognition* 19(1): 501–503.

Proulx, Michael J., Petra Stoerig, Eva Ludowig and Inna Knoll (2008) Seeing 'where' through the ears: effects of learning-by-doing and long-term sensory deprivation on localization based on image-to-sound substitution. *PLoS One* 3(3): e1840.

Ptito, Maurice, Solvej M. Moesgaard, Albert Gjedde and Ron Kupers (2005) Cross-modal plasticity revealed by electrotactile stimulation of the tongue in the congenitally blind. *Brain* 128: 606–614.

Rauschecker, Josef P. (1995) Compensatory plasticity and sensory substitution in the cerebral cortex. *Trends in Neuroscience* 18: 36–43.

Reich, Lior, Marcin Szwed, Laurent Cohen and Amir Amedi (2011) A ventral visual stream reading center independent of visual experience. *Current Biology* 21(5): 363–368.

Renier, Laurent and Anne G. De Volder (2005) Cognitive and brain mechanisms in sensory substitution of vision: a contribution to the study of human perception. *Journal of Integrative Neuroscience* 4(4): 489–503.

Renier, Laurent and Anne G. De Volder (2010) Vision substitution and depth perception: early blind subjects experience visual perspective through their ears. *Disability and Rehabilitation: Assistive Technology* 5(3): 175–183.

Renier, Laurent, Olivier Collignon, Colline Poirier, Dai Tranduy, Annick Vanlierde, Anne Bol, Claude Veraart and Anne G. De Volder (2005a) Cross-modal activation of visual cortex during depth perception using auditory substitution of vision. *NeuroImage* 26: 573–580.

Renier, Laurent, Cédric Laloyaux, Olivier Collignon, Dai Tranduy, Annick Vanlierde, Raymond Bruyer and Anne G. De Volder (2005b) The Ponzo illusion with auditory substitution of vision in sighted and early blind subjects. *Perception* 34: 851–867.

Renier, Laurent, Raymond Bruyer and Anne G. De Volder (2006) Vertical-horizontal illusion present for sighted but not early blind humans using auditory substitution of vision. *Perception and Psychophysics* 68(4): 535–542.

Renier, L., I. Cuevas, C. B. Grandin, L. Dricot, P. Plaza, E. Lerens, P. Rombaux and A. G. De Volder (2013b) Right occipital cortex activation correlates with superior odor processing performance in the early blind. *PLoS One* 8(8): e71907.

Renier, L., A. G. De Volder and J. P. Rauschecker (2013a) Cortical plasticity and preserved function in early blindness. *Neuroscience and Biobehavioral Reviews*. doi: pii: S0149-7634(13)00032-8. 10.1016/j.neubiorev.2013.01.025. [Epub ahead of print].

Rock, Irvin, Jack Gallant and Paul Kube (1999) An introduction to vision science. In Stephen E. Palmer (ed.) *Vision Science*. Cambridge, MA: MIT Press.

Röder, Brigitte, Wolfgang Teder-Salejarvi, Anette Sterr, Frank Rösler, Steven A. Hillyard and Helen G. Neville (1999) Improved auditory spatial tuning in blind humans. *Nature* 400: 162–166.

Röder, Brigitte, Olivier Stock, Siegfried Bien, Helen Neville and Frank Rösler (2002) Speech processing activates visual cortex in congenitally blind humans. *European Journal of Neuroscience* 16: 930–936.

Sadato, Nohiro, Alvaro Pascual-Leone, Jordan Grafman, Vincente Ibanez, Marie-Pierre Deiber, George Dold and Mark Hallett (1996) Activation of the primary visual cortex by Braille reading in blind subjects. *Nature* 380: 526–528.

Saenz, Melissa, Lindsay B. Lewis, Alexander G. Huth, Ione Fine and Christof Koch (2008) Visual motion area MT+/V5 responds to auditory motion in human sight-recovery subjects. *Journal of Neuroscience* 28(20): 5141–5148.

Schurmann, Martin, Gina Caetano, Yevhen Hlushchuk, Veikko Jousmaki and Rita Hari (2006) Touch activates human auditory cortex. *NeuroImage* 30: 1325–1331.

Segond, Hervé, Déborah Weiss and Eliana Sampaio (2005) Human spatial navigation via a visuo-tactile sensory substitution system. *Perception* 34(10): 1231–1249.

Striem-Amit, Ella, Ornella Dakwar, Lior Reich and Amir Amedi (2012) The large-scale organization of 'visual' streams emerges without visual experience. *Cerebral Cortex* 22(7): 1698–1709.

Supa, Michael, Milton Cotzin and Karl M. Dallenbach (1944) 'Facial vision': the perception of obstacles by the blind. *American Journal of Psychology* 57: 133–183.

Thaler, Lore, Stephen R. Arnott and Melvyn A. Goodale (2011) Neural correlates of natural human echolocation in early and late blind echolocation experts. *PLoS One* 6: e20162. doi: 10.1371/journal.pone.0020162.

Tyler, Mitchell, Yuri Danilov and Paul Bach-y-Rita (2003) Closing an open-loop control system: vestibular substitution through the tongue. *Journal of Integrative Neuroscience* 2: 159–164.

Vanlierde, Annick, Anne G. De Volder, Marie-Chantal Wanet-Defalque and Claude Veraart (2003) Occipito-parietal cortex activation during visuo-spatial imagery in early blind humans. *NeuroImage* 19: 698–709.

Veraart, Claude, Florence Duret, Marten Brelen, Medhi Oozeer and Jean Delbeek (2004) Vision rehabilitation in case of blindness. *Expert Review of Medical Devices* 1: 139–153.

Ward, Jamie and Peter Meijer (2010) Visual experiences in the blind induced by an auditory sensory substitution device. *Consciousness and Cognition* 19(1): 492–500.

Weeks, Robert, Barry Horwitz, Ali Aziz-Sultan, Biao Tian, C. Mark Wessinger, Leonardo G. Cohen, Mark Hallett and Josef P. Rauschecker (2000) A positron emission tomographic study of auditory localization in the congenitally blind. *Journal of Neuroscience* 20: 2664–2672.

Zappe, Anne-Catherin, Thorsten Maucher, Karlheinz Meier and Christian Scheiber (2004) Evaluation of a pneumatically driven stimulator device for vision substitution during fMRI studies. *Magnetic Resonance in Medicine* 51: 828–834.

3

Sensory Substitution and the Transparency of Visual Experience

Comments on Laurent Renier

BARRY C. SMITH

Abstract Sensory substitution devices make use of information in one sensory modality to deliver information usually provided by another. But when information usually presented visually is presented to a subject in an auditory or haptic way, is the resulting experience in any sense visual? Or does sensory substitution show that dimensions of experience—about the spatial layout of objects and properties in the environment—that were previously taken to be essentially visual can be experienced in other modalities too? I will consider this question by looking at whether a property such as the transparency of visual experience can be transferred to, and enhance, experience in other modalities.

WHAT IS SENSORY SUBSTITUTION and in what way is it possible? In attempting to answer this question we might hope to cast light on a larger question: namely, what can the possibility of sensory substitution tell us about how we should think of perception and the senses? This is the question that is at the heart of Laurent Renier's illuminating and informative paper on recent work in this area, and it is something to which he believes his own and others' work makes a contribution. I will explore the precise nature of those claims in what follows.

But first, how should we think about sensory substitution? Renier defines it as follows (see p. 43).

> The term 'sensory substitution' was introduced at the end of the 1960s to indicate the use of one sensory modality to supply environmental information normally gathered by another sense (e.g. the use of sound to provide information about visual scenes; Bach-y-Rita et al. 1969).

Very often, people are not as careful in defining sensory substitution as Renier is here. In fact, Renier himself says, when commenting on the work of others, that

Proceedings of the British Academy, **219**, 60–65.

'what would usually be *visual information* is fed to the senses in the form of touch or sound' (p. 45, italics mine). And again, in discussing the tongue display unit, he says the 'TDU transmits *visual information* via the tongue using electrotactile stimulations; it reproduces "visual patterns" on a 144-pixel square matrix applied on the tongue' (p. 45, italics mine). More cautiously, we might want to put things like this:

> It is not visual information but environmental layout or spatial information that is usually harvested effortlessly and encoded in part by the visual system that is put together piecemeal, and at first effortfully, and is encoded in part by the tactile or auditory system.

This way of putting things avoids saying straight off that it is visual information that turns up in the other sensory modalities. That possibility may still exist but we want to leave the question open. We can then ask, are we seeing with hearing or touch, or are we doing something with hearing or touch that we usually do with vision? Even if it is the latter, this would still be an important finding: i.e. to show that through the use of certain sensory substitution devices we are presenting to the subject of experience features of the world in a way that we thought were exclusive to vision. Such a result would show that what we previously thought was definitional of seeing turned out not to be essentially part of vision but could be delivered by a re-working of the other senses.

So, to leave this possibility open, we should say:

> The TDU doesn't transmit visual information, it transmits information usually gathered and encoded visually and re-codes it into vibrotactile information, which it is hoped the subject, or the brain of the subject, can make use of to access that information.

What Renier says is this:

> These sensory substitution systems provide analogue encoding of visual information (i.e. the spatial arrangement of the elements in a perceived scene is transposed onto the skin by a matrix of 'tactors' that stimulates the somatosensory receptors in a defined skin area).
>
> (p. 45)

That's better than the formulation of the previous quotes, but it is still not quite right. It is not the encoding of visual information, but the encoding of what is written in brackets: the spatial arrangements of elements. That's what's encoded.

So we might say that these devices provide an anologue encoding on the skin or the tongue of information normally gathered visually and encoded in (some) visual format for immediate use by other systems: information about a scene, about spatial layout, shape recognition, and depth perception.

Again, we are told in the case of the sensory substitution device, vOICe, there is a transformation of visual landscapes into soundscapes, where 'a "soundscape" is an auditory signal that represents the components of the visual scene'. That's fine so long as we understand this way of talking as meaning the output of the device represents certain components of a scene, most of whose components are normally conveyed visually. Once again, we need to be careful with such formulations.

Going back to the improved definition with which we started, one sense modality is supplying environmental information normally conveyed by another sense modality, while still preserving some of the key functions of the original sense. What are these key functions? Are they in any way visual? This is the issue we need to address, and we need to find a way to address it. In his essay, Renier appeals to the phenomenology of the perceiver. However, subjects are not that good at knowing the modal signatures of their own sensory experiences. The classic case is tasting, where subjects are notoriously bad at recognizing which senses are involved in having the experiences that tasting gives rise to. Most people think that when they are tasting they are just having experiences in a single modality, namely taste, based on information given by the tongue. But in fact the sort of experiences tasting gives rise to, namely flavour experiences, depend on inputs from touch, taste, smell and perhaps trigeminal irritation that are integrated into a unified flavour percept. Thus, what subjects say about the character of their own experiences may not be a good guide to the type of sensory experience they are undergoing.

What is it for subjects to claim to know the modal signature of their perceptual experiences? Is this supposed to be revealed by the experiences themselves, or is it something to figure out? Certainly, subjects report their own experiences using sensory substitution devices by saying things like, 'I can *see* in depth'. 'I can see to the bottom of the box'. So after training with such a device, are they really having visual experiences through an auditory or tactile channel? Renier tells us that

> subjects using this type of device generally report visual rather than tactual or auditory sensations, and perceive objects as externally localized rather than on the skin, say (Epstein et al. 1986; Auvray et al. 2005; Ward and Meijer 2010).
>
> (p. 49)

This talk of subjects having *visual sensations* while perceiving features of the environment is where the appeal to phenomenology comes in. But there is a problem here. What does it mean to have visual sensations, even in normal visual experience? There is a way to understand talk of visual sensations if we talk about phosphenes or blurred vision. But normally, we are not usually aware of the feel of visual experience. We just see things. We just look and take in the scene around us without any awareness of the medium of seeing. So the talk of visual sensations is somewhat questionable, at least philosophically.

Nevertheless, we can still ask whether the new experiences created with the help of a visual-to-auditory sensory substitution device are partly visual. For instance, does the presence of optical illusions in the substituting modality serve Renier's case for the preservation of distinctly visual features of experience any better? Or what about neural imaging data? It's unclear. The occipital cortex can take on the function of odour detection in the congenitally blind (Kupers and Ptito 2013) and tactile reading of Braille in the early blind, so the involvement of what are normally visual areas of the cortex to process signals from a visual-to-tactile or visual-to-auditory device merely shows the neural plasticity of the brain, or shows that the so-called visual cortex is used to encode features of the scene normally gathered visually.

What about the preservation of optical illusions like the Ponzo illusion in auditory substitution demonstrated by Renier and colleagues (Renier et al. 2005)? This may appear to make the case that the phenomenology and new modality of the experience created by the substituting auditory device are in some sense visual. However, this depends on whether the visual information encoded by the visual input device, which is then translated into an auditory code, picks up on the features of distance and depth and thus provides the means to represent the world as it appears to be with seemingly converging parallel lines going into the distance, which then codes this apparent shape as having that perspectival character. Of course, if the optical device does not build in such assumptions but the character of this *visual* illusion is preserved, it is a strong argument for Renier's position. Note, however, that evidence is restricted to visually able subjects and the early blind.

What about evidence from neuroimaging and transcranial magnetic stimulation? Renier cites many cases where there is occipital lobe activity when performing tasks using the substitution device, or where transcranial magnetic stimulation applied to the occipital cortex can disrupt performance. He tells us:

> The main contribution of sensory substitution studies was the demonstration of a recruitment of the occipital cortex in early blind subjects, during the processing of auditory or tactile encoded visual information (Arno et al. 2001a; Ptito et al. 2005).

However, as he acknowledges:

> This functional role of the occipital cortex of blind subjects in non-visual tasks was also shown using transcranial magnetic stimulation to induce virtual lesions in the brain that interfered with Braille reading (Cohen et al. 1997), speech processing (Amedi et al. 2003), sound lateralization and sensory substitution (Collignon et al. 2007; Merabet et al. 2009).
>
> (p. 52)

He also tells us that:

> Interestingly, Kupers et al. (2006) showed that transcranial magnetic stimulation applied on the occipital pole induced tactile sensations referred to the tongue in blind subjects who were trained to use the TDU.
>
> (ibid.)

From this range of evidence he concludes that:

> the occipital cortex of blind people is the neural substrate of the compensatory perceptual mechanisms and that it contributes to the subjective visual phenomenology experienced by them.
>
> (ibid.)

But why think it contributes to 'visual' phenomenology? It would be equally plausible, given the plasticity of the brain, to infer from the evidence that the occipital cortex can be recruited for many tasks, and contribute to experiences of many kinds. It may simply be a mistake to think of it exclusively as the *visual* cortex. Or it could be that the occipital cortex is used to encode information about spatial layout that is normally input visually.

When using visual-to-auditory or visual-to-tactile sensory substitution devices, subjects are getting information about their environment that they normally get visually. So when in receipt of information about the scene or spatial layout in front of them that they normally get visually, it is not surprising that many of them talk, think and take this information to be visual. That is the cloak it is usually wrapped in. But none of this by itself shows that the experience itself is in any way visual. Another conclusion would be that such information about the layout of items in the environment, their distance, shape and so forth, isn't essentially visual; arguably, this is just what sensory substitution shows.

The above considerations may lead us to ask whether the key functions of vision, some of which certain sensory substitution devices aim to preserve, concern purely visual features. It is a feature of visual perception, or experiences of seeing, that they seem transparent (Harman 1990; Tye 1992). You are not aware of the means by which you are seeing, you just take in the world around you, seeing people, tables and chairs. You don't see visual images, but rather, take in, all at once, an environment of physical objects in a spatial array. This openness to the world is characteristic of visual experience and it is something that is developed very early in visual perception; though it is not obviously a feature of the other senses. So, we might wonder whether this transparency of experience is exclusive to visual experience. After all, vision may be quite unlike the other senses; which is why it is a pity that so many philosophers tend to rely on vision alone when talking about perception in general. However, if training with sensory substitution devices for vision creates a way in which this feature of transparency migrates to other sense modalities, so that subjects no longer have the feeling of the proximal stimuli but only of distal objects, then that would help to show that such transparency was not an exclusive, but merely a typical, feature of visual perception. In effect, such devices would not be transferring a visual feature of experience to audition or somatosensation, but rather, enhancing those other modalities to take on functions that are typically performed by vision, but are not exclusively visual in nature.

Sensory substitution can, I think, capture these key functions of vision, not by providing visual phenomenology or visual characteristics for the experiences produced by the substituting modality, but by *enhancing* those experiences so that they take on aspects of transparency that are usually characteristic of visual experiences. By training on tasks with visual input from a camera, we are giving these other, substituting modalities outward-looking and world-involving dimensions that are usually delivered by vision; namely, transparency. The enhanced experiences give us openness to a world we are engaging with but without noticing how we are doing it. But sensory substitution does not give someone the qualitative feel of the original modality in the new sense modality. You still get the qualitative feel of the substituting modality. And that may be why taste and smell are so hard to replicate in another modality. You can get information about what you are tasting or smelling from the new modality. Due to their cross-modal associations, you may learn how sweet or bitter something is by hearing a congruent and corresponding sound, but that would not be the same thing as experiencing the sweetness or the bitterness, and it is very hard to get the substituting modality to become an experience of a taste or a smell. You don't get the migration of the modal feel of a sense experience. For that reason I would want to resist the idea that there is visual phenomenology or visual sensation in the experiences created by using a sensory substitution device. What we are arguing about is whether what does migrate to the new experiences or the substituting modality is in some sense visual.

In conclusion, we can ask, what is achieved by sensory substitution? To answer the question accurately it is important to recognize that we don't actually substitute one sensory modality with another. Rather, we make the 'substituting' modality take on some of the functions of the 'substituted' modality, have the former present information that the latter usually presents, making the two modalities more like each other, or, better, making the larger perceptual experiences they each support more like each other.

References

Harman, Gilbert (1990) The intrinsic quality of experience. In J. Tomberlin (ed.) *Philosophical Perspectives*, vol. 4. Atascadero, CA: Ridgeview, 31–52.

Kupers, R. and M. Ptito (2013) Compensatory plasticity and cross-modal reorganization following early visual deprivation. *Neuroscience and Biobehavioral Reviews* 7634: 191–197.

Renier, Laurent, Cédric Laloyaux, Olivier Collignon, Dai Tranduy, Annick Vanlierde, Raymond Bruyer and Anne G. De Volder (2005) The Ponzo illusion with auditory substitution of vision in sighted and early blind subjects. *Perception* 34: 851–867.

Tye, M. (1992) Visual qualia and visual content. In T. Crane (ed.) *The Contents of Experience*. Cambridge: Cambridge University Press, 158–176.

4

Disambiguating the Perceptual Assumption

JENNIFER CORNS

Abstract Deroy and Auvray (2012, 2014) together with Ptito et al. (this volume) have argued against what they dub 'the perceptual assumption', which they claim underlies all previous research into sensory substitution devices (SSDs). In this chapter, I argue that the perceptual assumption needs to be disambiguated in three distinct ways: (A) SSD use is best modelled as a known, 'natural' modality; (B) SSD use is best modelled as a unique sensory modality *full stop*; and (C) SSD use is best modelled as a perceptual process. Different theorists are variously committed to these distinct claims. More importantly, evaluating A, B, or C for rejection depends on distinct evidence of difference between SSD use and (A) each natural modality, (B) any modality, and (C) perceptual processing. I argue that even if the offered evidence of difference for A–C is granted, Auvray and Deroy's advocated rejections are not entailed; it remains to be shown that the identified differences undermine the appropriate use of the corresponding models.

As THEIR NAME SUGGESTS, sensory substitution devices (SSDs) are devices developed with the aim of enabling humans to use one of their sensory modalities to substitute for the workings of another. The modality being substituted for is often therefore called the *substituted* modality and that being used to substitute for it is often referred to as the *substituting* modality. The development and use of these devices raises interesting philosophical questions. One among many that has engendered significant attention is how to appropriately characterize the sensory modality employed in successful SSD use: as the substituting or the substituted modality. Like others (e.g. Macpherson 2011), Deroy and Auvray (2012, 2014) together with Ptito et al. (this volume) hold that successful SSD use resembles typical uses of both the substituting and substituted modality, such that it is inappropriate to exclusively characterize successful SSD use as either. Uniquely, however, they argue that the differences between perceptual processing and

Proceedings of the British Academy, **219**, 66–72. © The British Academy 2018.

ideally successful SSD use are such that the latter is not appropriately characterized as perceptual.

According to Auvray and Deroy, all previous research into SSDs in both the sciences and humanities rests on an unjustified assumption that successful SSD use is a perceptual process and should, accordingly, be modelled perceptually. This they dub the 'perceptual assumption'. They argue that careful comparison of what is involved in perception using our 'natural' modalities with what is involved in successful SSD use (both real and idealized) supports rejecting the perceptual assumption.

Even as we are encouraged to reject the perceptual assumption, we are invited to instead embrace the idea of successful SSD use as the acquisition of a cognitively mediated skill. Skills built on top of pre-existing perceptual capacities are considered *vertical*, whereas the pre-existing perceptual processes on which they are based are considered *horizontal*. SSD use has been assumed to fall in the latter, perceptual camp, but Auvray and Deroy argue that it belongs in the former. Thus, in a characteristic passage, they write:

> The best way . . . is to think about the integrated use of an SSD being something closer to a new set of automatic recognition abilities arising from a trained rewiring between other sensory modalities, and eventually other pre-existing capacities . . . SSDs are modes of access and delivery that fundamentally arise—technologically and cognitively—and get crafted on the existing senses.
>
> (Deroy and Auvray 2014: 345)

The perceptual assumption should be rejected, they argue, because adequately modelling successful SSD use requires a non-perceptual, i.e. non-horizontal, model that represents the vertical integration of novel cognitive skills onto pre-existing sensory pathways.

Their proposed vertical model of SSD use is explicitly inspired by a proposed analogy with reading. Like reading, they argue, SSD use requires appropriating a conventionally designed symbolic coding system, e.g. vertical sensations on the tongue are designed to code vertical edges of a target object via a conventionally developed symbolic system. Like learning to read, learning to decode these symbols takes training and practice. Also like reading, SSD use relies on pre-existing sensory modalities through which the symbols of the new symbolic coding system can be transduced and ultimately decoded. Auvray and Deroy push the analogy yet further by pointing out that when the new skills have been successfully acquired, the only apparently automatic resultant process is subject to characteristic breakdowns: reading breaks down into seeing mere marks and squiggles, and SSD use breaks down into mere stimulations in the so-called substituting modality.

Though I return briefly to the proposed vertical model below, of present interest is the proffered rejection of the perceptual assumption. What is purportedly being assumed and why it should be rejected both admit of further clarification.

The perceptual assumption is subject to at least three distinct interpretations. From strongest to weakest, these are:

A SSD use is appropriately modelled as a known, 'natural' sensory modality; i.e. as the substituting or substituted modality.
B SSD use is appropriately modelled as a novel sensory modality; i.e. as a distinct, 'emergent' modality, akin to but distinct from the 'natural' modalities.
C SSD use is appropriately modelled as a perceptual process; e.g. as a process of informational acquisition involving the use of multiple modalities.

The first thing to notice about these three disambiguations of the perceptual assumption is that it is unlikely that they are equally widespread. Though the initial aim of these devices may have been, and may even remain, to allow the blind to 'see with the skin' or 'see with the brain', it does not follow that anyone assumed that we should model SSD use as, say, vision. It certainly does not follow that *everyone* now maintains that we should do so. As Auvray and Deroy are undoubtedly aware, controversy continues between distinct advocates (if not assumers) of A and B. I suspect that most researchers from both the humanities and the sciences accept C, but it is not clear that everyone who thinks that we should model successful SSD use as a perceptual process (C) thinks that successful SSD use is best modelled as a single modality—either emergent (B) *or* 'natural' (A). One anyway *may* hold that SSD use is best modelled perceptually (C), but deny that it is a unimodal process. Disambiguating the perceptual assumption allows us to avoid mistaken attributions, e.g. interpreting someone who merely holds C as assuming A or B.

More important is that distinct evidence is relevant for the warranted rejection of each disambiguation. Rejecting A appropriately depends on evidence of differences between (successful) SSD use and each 'natural' sensory modality. Rejecting B appropriately depends on evidence of differences between (successful) SSD use and every 'natural' sensory modality. Rejecting C appropriately depends on evidence of differences between (successful) SSD use and perceptual processes. And, of course, the weaker the claim, the stronger the evidence appropriately required to reject it.

In many passages, it is unclear whether Auvray and Deroy are offering supposed evidence against A, B, or C. For instance, are the appealed-to differences in associated affect between SSD use and visual perception taken to undermine A, B, or C (Deroy and Auvray 2012)? Similarly, which version of the perceptual assumption is supposedly undermined by the fact that SSD use relies on a series of inter-dependent stimuli, whereas perception via a 'natural' modality supposedly does not (the 'stimulation criterion'; Deroy and Auvray 2014)? Similar questions arise for much of the discussed evidence. Once the perceptual assumption is disambiguated, it will be easier to consistently make clear which disambiguation is under attack and whether the attack is successful.

In yet other passages, however, the offered evidence is clearly relevant to particular disambiguations of the assumption.

Some of the offered evidence is clearly relevant only to interpretation A of the assumption. For instance, they write:

> Each dimension in the lacking modality needs to be translated into another dimension in the intact modality, and in this instance it appears a real impossibility to map all visual dimensions simultaneously in modalities that have less dimensions such as touch . . .
>
> (Deroy and Auvray 2014: 342)

An identified mismatch between the dimensions of the substituting and substituted modality is taken to show that the resulting process is not appropriately modelled as either. And Auvray and Deroy indeed hold that SSD use differs from *each* known sensory modality such that it is not appropriately modelled as any one. That is, they reject A. Taken alone, however, this provides no reason to deny that SSD use is best modelled as a modality *full stop* (B) or as perceptual *full stop* (C).

If not explicitly distinguished as such, evidence best targeted at B is also offered. Thus, they write:

> several elements contradict the fact that sensory substitution behaves like a classical sensory channeling of information. In terms of results or outputs, sensory substitution is much more limited . . .
>
> (Deroy and Auvray 2012: 5)

The limitations of even successful SSD use are taken to be evidence that SSD use should not be modelled as a modality. And Auvray and Deroy indeed maintain that SSD use differs from *all* sensory modalities, such that it is not best modelled as a distinct, novel one. That is, they reject B. This entails likewise rejecting the weaker A, but continues to leave C undisturbed.

Evidence for difference between SSD use and perception as such is also offered. In a typical passage they write:

> the very necessity of training, which has been in the background of the studies investigating performance, is also forced into the perceptual framework, and this despite an apparent tension with the common-sense notion of perception.
>
> (Deroy and Auvray 2012: 4)

The idea here is that perception does not require cognitive training, but successful SSD use does. Apparently, Auvray and Deroy think that it is part of both our best theories and our common-sense understanding of perception that it is automatic with no (anyway, no cognitive) training required. The necessity of cognitive training for successful SSD use is therefore taken to undermine modelling SSD use as perceptual; that is, as evidence for rejecting C. And rejecting C, unlike A or B, entails rejecting the perceptual assumption in all three forms.

Indeed, perhaps Auvray and Deroy do not disambiguate A–C not only because they think that all three should be rejected, but that all three stand and fall together. Some passages suggest such an interpretation. Thus, they write:

> The problem with the perceptual assumption is not only that it delivers an unstable verdict regarding the exact sensory modality to which a certain device should be ascribed. A more fundamental problem than to decide whether using a device is closer to seeing or hearing, is to examine whether the theorizing concerning these devices should remain bound to the perceptual framework where, canonically, perceiving means channeling information through a single, dedicated route.
>
> (Deroy and Auvray 2012: 3)

The idea here seems to be that differences between SSD use and perception through each 'natural' modality appropriately raise the question of whether SSD use is perceptual at all—since perception just is ('perceiving *means*') receiving information through a single dedicated route. For rejecting B, also needed would be the assumption that the five canonical modalities are the only such single, dedicated routes. Perception, then, would be exhausted by the canonical exercise of the five canonical modalities. On this interpretation, the perceptual assumption, in all three forms, should be rejected on the basis of difference between SSD use and each 'natural' modality.

Instead of rejecting any interpretation of the perceptual assumption, however, we might instead revise the relevant antecedent conceptions. In the light of successful SSD use we might revise our conception of a particular sense modality or sensory modalities as such. For instance, we might revise our conception of taction, now allowing that it can provide colour information—and resist rejecting A. Or we might revise our conception of modalities as such, granting that modularity is not necessary—and resist rejecting B. Similarly and more likely than these examples, instead of rejecting C, we might be advised to revise our antecedent understanding of perception and its relationship(s) to cognition.

Questions concerning the relationship between perception and cognition are particularly timely. As noted above, the difference Auvray and Deroy most emphasize between successful SSD use and perception is the reliance of the former on cognitive training. But perhaps all the offered evidence should be interpreted to show that perception is more cognitive—more 'vertical'—than some theorists have thought. Contemporary discussions about cognitive penetration and evaluative perception are thriving. It is not simply obvious that perception (or perceptual experience) is exhausted by a modular, bottom-up, process through one of five canonically identified channels. It has, I suspect, not been obvious for some time.

Moreover, the perceptual assumptions concern how SSD use is appropriately modelled. Even as we might revise the relevant concepts, we might revise our categorizing of the corresponding models: even as one might hold that perception is (at least sometimes) vertical, one might hold that vertical models are (at least sometimes) perceptual models. Consider again the analogy with reading and models thereof. If it is allowed that perception (at least sometimes) includes the cognitively mediated acquisition of a conventional symbolic system, then the offered model is, after all, a perceptual model. If perceptual processes are sometimes cognitively mediated, then perceptual processes might be appropriately modelled both 'vertically' and 'horizontally'.

In short, Auvray and Deroy's identified differences may warrant revision without warranting rejection of any, much less every, version of the perceptual assumption. Whether revision or rejection is warranted turns on issues that cannot be settled in this space. I mean only to establish that there *are* issues of such relevance—live ones of current debate.

Yet further, even resisting all revision one may likewise evade any rejection by denying that the identified differences undermine the appropriateness of the corresponding models. As a general matter: identifying differences between two types of things is not enough to show that they are not both appropriately modelled as the same type of thing for many purposes. Identified similarities often outweigh identified differences relative to purpose. Cars and bikes are different types of things, but they might both be appropriately modelled as transportation for some purposes. Auvray and Deroy's offered evidence of difference may be granted, while identified similarities nonetheless vindicate the appropriateness of the corresponding model.

All three versions of the perceptual assumption may be plausibly defended in this way. For version A, for instance: one might accept that there are more visual than tactile dimensions, but maintain that successful use of TVSS should nonetheless be modelled as vision because of the types of tasks it facilitates and the subset of visual dimensions that are captured. Similarly, in defending version B for instance: one might accept that SSD use yields unavoidably relatively limited results and outputs, but maintain that it should nonetheless be modelled as an emergent modality because of the results and outputs that it *does* facilitate. As a final for instance, defenders of C might admit the necessity of cognitive training for successful SSD use, but maintain that it should nonetheless be modelled as a perceptual process since information is being sensorily transduced and decoded to facilitate objective identification and action. Again, the general strategy is to identify similarities that vindicate the corresponding models despite granting the identified differences.

In summary, I have been arguing that the following six questions warrant independent consideration:

1 How does successful SSD use differ from successful employment of each of the five canonical sensory modalities?
2 Do the differences between successful SSD use and each of the five canonical sensory modalities undermine modelling the former as any of the latter?
3 How does successful SSD use differ from successful employment of any sensory modality?

4 Do the differences between successful SSD use and the successful employment of a sensory modality undermine modelling the former as the latter?
5 How does successful SSD use differ from perception?
6 Do the differences between successful SSD use and perception undermine modelling the former as the latter?

If not distinguished as such, Auvray and Deroy have made important contributions to 1, 3, and 5. Affirmative answers to 2, 4, and 6, however, require further argument.

Despite these gaps, Auvray and Deroy's discussions, joined by Ptito et al. (this volume), have provided a wealth of insights that are useful for improved modelling of SSD use. Their work invites us to transform our assumptions about perception and the sensory modalities into reasoned positions—or to reject them. The invitation is worth accepting.

References

Deroy, O. and Auvray, M. (2012) Reading the world through the skin and ears: a new perspective on sensory substitution. *Frontiers in Psychology* 3: 457. doi: 10.3389/fpsyg.2012.00457.

Deroy, O. and Auvray, M. (2014) A crossmodal perspective on sensory substitution. In D. Stokes, M. Matthen and S. Briggs (eds) *Perception and Its Modalities*. Oxford: Oxford University Press.

Macpherson, F. (2011) Individuating the senses. In F. Macpherson (ed.) *The Senses: Classical and Contemporary Readings*. Oxford: Oxford University Press.

5

Sensory Substitution and the Challenge of Acclimatization

PAUL NOORDHOF

Abstract I defend a refined characterization of sensory substitution that allows for its existence while denying that the substituting sense plus sensory substitution device is always appropriately classified as the substituted sense. Accepting that there are genuine cases of sensory substitution of this kind implies that acclimatization to a sensory substitution device may provide presentations of properties. Externalist accounts of experience together with objectivist characterizations of such properties have the upshot that properties putatively proprietary to a sense modality can be presented in another modality in cases of substitution. I consider three objections to this argument. I close by explaining how reflection on the phenomena of sensory substitution and, in particular, acclimatization is important for the development of any kind of representationalist or relationist theory of phenomenal properties or, at the very least, suggests we need to refine the idea of certain properties—rather than particular ways in which their presentation is bundled together—being proprietary to the particular senses.

In the present essay, I am going to explain how the possibility, indeed actuality, of sensory substitution devices presents a distinctive challenge to a certain combination of views, namely various externalist accounts of how we experience objects and properties in the world together with an objectivist characterization of properties which are, intuitively, proprietary to a particular sense modality. In addition, I will explain how reflection on the phenomena of sensory substitution and, in particular, acclimatization is important for the development of any kind of representationalist or relationist theory of phenomenal properties. The overall argument cannot be demonstrative because the correct thing to conclude from the experience of subjects with sensory substitution devices is, as yet, by no means clear. Equally, it is conceivable that the detail of some externalist account of how we experience objects and properties may provide some room for manoeuvre (although I doubt it). Rather, by constructing this network of considerations, I hope to

Proceedings of the British Academy, **219**, 73–93.

indicate the further philosophical interest that work on sensory substitution devices possesses.

The essay takes the following structure. I begin by giving a characterization of sensory substitution which, I hope, is a refinement of that which is usually offered in the literature. I compare it with other ways in which it may have been developed and seek to motivate my preferred version. In considering alternative ways in which sensory substitution might be characterized, I consider the various accounts of how senses should be individuated which, it might be thought, place constraints upon when a sense may be thought to be genuinely substituted. I argue against such constraints. For the purposes of the argument I develop in the later parts of the essay, the key results of this section are first that my characterization of sensory substitution is plausible and, second, crucially, the resultant sense is not appropriately characterized as the substituted sense. Thus, it is not the case that, when a sensory substitution device for vision is used, the result is that we have visual experiences. It is this gap between the conditions for sensory *substitution* and a complete alternative realization of a particular sense that is the basis for the subsequent argument.

In the second section, I give some famous examples of what it is like to acclimatize oneself to a sensory substitution device and draw on observations by subjects (and experimenters) about the proper way to characterize it. Although there is some robustness to these observations, obviously they may be mistaken and represent an important point of weakness in the discussion. I then construct the argument which these cases suggest against the twin theses identified at the beginning. I consider three responses to this argument—in effect, three responses to interpreting the consequences of acclimatization in the way that I have suggested in the third section of the essay. I close by outlining how further reflection on acclimatization, and the resultant sensory experience, has implications for the successful development of relational and representationalist theories of phenomenal properties.

5.1 Sensory Substitution

It is plausible to characterize sensory substitution devices in the following way.

> Sensory substitution devices provide inputs to a particular sense modality M (e.g. touch) conveying information which is standardly, and perhaps more readily, available through a distinct sense modality M* (e.g. vision) in a way that may be integrated with a subject's responses to sense modality M while reflecting the functional role of a subject's responses to such information in M*.

Two famous examples of sensory substitution devices are Paul Bach-y-Rita et al.'s Tactual Visual Sensory Substitution device (TVSS) and Meijer's vOICe, substituting sounds for vision (Bach-y-Rita et al. 1969; Meijer 1992). Many descriptions are available of the workings of these two devices, some available in this volume. In brief, the TVSS takes visual input to a camera and changes it into vibrotactor stimulation on a subject's back reflecting the spatial distribution of light signals. The vOICe converts camera input into sounds heard through headphones with changes in pitch corresponding to objects' vertical position higher (high pitch) or lower (low pitch); and the ear to which the sound is presented corresponding to the object being to left or right, and loudness corresponding to brightness.

Let me offer a few comments to explain features of the characterization of sensory substitution just given. First, it does not require that the information conveyed to the substituting sense by the sensory substitution device must only be available to the substituted sense and, thereby, unavailable to the substituting sense without the device in question. Sensory substitution devices have often been used to provide spatial information. Spatial properties are arguably common sensibles; that is, properties available to more than one sense. In which case, a characterization of sensory substitution which insisted that the information must be unavailable to the substituting sense without the sensory substitution device would be ruling out this class of cases.

Perhaps some refinement can deal with this issue. For example, it might be insisted that, in particular, only visual experience can provide us with depth information, or information about the shape of objects at some distance from the perceiver. These points, though, seem to draw on special features of visual substitution when touch is the substituting sense. Auditory perception picks up information about objects some distance from the perceiver. Depth information is not just presented visually but aurally and tactually.

My talk of the information conveyed through M being 'integrated with a subject's responses to sense modality M while reflecting the functional role of a subject's responses to such information in M*' is meant to address the following observation. One way in which a subject can receive information through M which, for example, is more readily available through M*, is by reading material or testimony. Suppose I instant message you information about the sounds I hear in my room with you some distance away in yours. This is information you take in visually by reading my text. We don't have a case of sensory substitution. Likewise, if you are blind and I tell you what I see in front of you, and you pick up this information by my testimony, once more this isn't a case of sensory substitution. There are devices available to the blind which similarly fail to count as intuitive cases of sensory substitution, for example, a colour detector which outputs spoken words that blind subjects can understand relating to the colour of objects.[1]

My thought is that, while in all of these cases a subject is able to respond to the information, it is not in a way which reflects the functional role of a subject's responses when he or she is the recipient of information as part of a sensory space,

[1] I'm grateful to Helen Bradley for drawing my attention to such devices.

within which certain sensory properties are instantiated, or in the ways in which the information is typically bundled together, for example, shape and size (Bach-y-Rita and Kercel (2003: 542) emphasize the continuities in response between substituting and substituted sense). Instead, gaining information by reading or testimony conveys the information in relatively isolated chunks mediated by a particular perceptual-cognitive activity, the understanding of speech and writing, activated by the way in which the information is conveyed (e.g. text).

Of course, it would be possible to loosen our notion of sensory substitution to allow these latter cases to count as examples of it. Indeed, Bach-y-Rita and Kercel talk of reading being an early sensory substitution device (Bach-y-Rita and Kercel 2003: 541). Nevertheless, this would not alter the fact that there is an important discontinuity between these cases and the central cases mentioned above and upon which I shall say more below, specifically under the heading of acclimatization. Indeed, the 'reading' objection to my argument below depends upon emphasizing this discontinuity.

The final comment about this characterization is to note that I have drawn it in terms of providing additional information to a sense modality, which information then plays a certain functional role, rather than in terms of phenomenology, sensory structure, or any other way one might characterize sensory substitution drawn from various ways in which philosophers have sought to demarcate the senses from each other (see, for example, Grice 1962).

To describe some of the alternatives, it is helpful to introduce some terms of art which will be of use to our later discussion as well. Let us characterize the phenomenal content of our mental lives—others talk in terms of phenomenal character—as what it is like to have the mental states or events which characterize our mental lives. Focusing on the senses, that means: what it is like to visually experience an elephant waving its trunk, what it is like to hear a baby's cry (a sound which can go right through you), what it is like to feel someone stroking your hand, and so on. The phenomenal properties of an experience, we may stipulate, are those properties which determine what the phenomenal content of that experience is.

Here it pays to have a distinction. Let the manifest objects and properties be those that constitute the phenomenal content of a subject's mental state or event. For example, if the subject were visually experiencing the elephant waving its trunk, then amongst the manifest objects would be the elephant and amongst the manifest properties would be that of being grey. Phenomenal properties determine the phenomenal content of a mental state in the following sense. They do not constitute the phenomenal content but it is in virtue of them that the state in question has the manifest objects and properties that it does, amongst other things. A certain kind of representationalist holds that phenomenal properties are representational properties of a particular kind. Such representationalists think of representational properties as those properties which yield truth conditions in the case of beliefs, satisfaction conditions in the case of desire, and veridicality conditions in the case of perceptions. For them, the phenomenal properties of a mental state will determine its phenomenal content by settling what is represented by the state in question. It should not be assumed, though, that the phenomenal contents of mental states and events are exhausted by their manifest objects and properties. It may be true but it would be the outcome of establishing certain views about the nature of phenomenal properties.

With these terms in place, attempts to individuate the senses by phenomenology will suggest that two sense modalities M and M* are different if they have substantially and systematically different kinds of phenomenal contents. It is certainly not enough simply to require that they have different phenomenal contents because the result would be a veritable plethora of different senses. My visual experiences of elephants have different phenomenal contents from those of aquatic creatures but I don't have, as a result, two senses: elephant and aquatic vision. Nor is it satisfactory to talk about senses being different in so far as they have different phenomenal contents because that would suggest that differences between sense modalities are on a continuum with differences between what is sensed in a particular modality.

It would be a mistake to insist that a sensory substitution device should be responsible for the provision of the same kinds of phenomenal contents as the sense for which it is trying to substitute (rather than the differences of information to which I appealed). Successful provision of the phenomenal content of the substituted sense is very unlikely to occur. If a subject becomes acclimatized to such devices, they will typically have to integrate the information that they receive by them with the information they typically receive from a very different, substituting, modality into some overall perceptual experience. Even if efforts are made to isolate all other input—as in the case of the vOICe where a subject wears headphones and just receives the auditory signal from the sensory stimulation device—information in the substituted sense is being made available to a substituting sense with a very different way of structuring sensory information. As a result of this, one would expect there to be substantial phenomenal differences in what is provided by the sensory substitution device. Nevertheless, it may be entirely appropriate to conclude that sensory substitution has taken place if additional information has been provided properly integrated with the subject's responses.

If that is right, then a corollary of this point is that such a means of individuation of the senses would more than likely force the conclusion that the appropriate classification of the sense which results from say M plus sensory substitution device would be a new kind of sense. We are not simply extending the powers of a sense modality, M; for example, extending the powers of vision by putting better lenses in glasses.

Relatedly, sensory substitution devices may fail to reproduce all the structural features of the sense for which they are seeking to substitute and yet still count as legitimate substitutions for a particular sense. There will be, at least, two dimensions of this. First, once more, because they are providing information which is going to be integrated into the information already provided by the substituting sense, there will be a new set of relations set up. Second, the means by which the sensory substitution device conveys the information—e.g. patterns of tactual stimulation, certain kinds of tone—will have their own distinctive structural features only some of which will be relevant to the information they convey.

A third way in which the differences between the senses have been characterized is in terms of differences in what can be represented by them. So it is argued that vision has, as a proprietary property, colour; audition, sound; and so on. This is closely related to the way I have chosen to characterize sensory substitution in terms of information, but my preferred characterization is, importantly, weaker. It is open to a theoretician to claim that, in the case of sensory substitution, our tactual sense doesn't *now* represent (say) the distance of objects, where it failed to do so before. Instead it receives input from a device which, while the device, itself, conveys (natural) information about these properties (and so, in an extended sense, represents them), is not enough for the *substituting* sense to count as representing them. It is to keep this theoretical option open that I have characterized sensory substitution in the way that I have.

Setting aside this point, if we sought to understand sensory substitution in terms of providing information about the proprietary properties of another sense, then none of the famous cases of sensory substitution devices appear to pass muster. The TVSS and vOICe are both taken to be sensory substitution devices for vision but neither provides colour information.

There is an important distinction between the proprietary properties of the senses and the way in which information is conveyed by the senses. The latter need not, though could, be understood in a way unsympathetic to representationalism. The way information may be conveyed by a particular sense modality could be, as the representationalist would prefer, characterized in terms of how the information is bundled—e.g. surfaces presented simultaneously as opposed to sequentially—or it might be characterized in terms of distinctive non-representational modes of sensing. Sensory substitution devices may reproduce the way in which the information is bundled to a limited extent while failing to convey the proprietary properties of the substituted sense. Indeed, rather than requiring even reproduction of the way in which the information is bundled, it may be enough that there should be substantial overlap in the way in which the information is conveyed in M* for it to be substituted for by a sensory substitution device feeding into M. Given the point made earlier, about how the structural features of M plus the device will differ from those of either M or M* in isolation, and, for that matter, the failure to convey information about proprietary properties of a sense, it is clear that, once more, such cases will be ones in which the sensory substitution device feeding into M will give rise to a new sense.

A fourth way of understanding differences between the senses is in terms of the kind of stimuli they receive, for example, patterns of light or sound waves, as a result of the sense organ involved (e.g. Heil 1983: 7–10). I have chosen to characterize sensory substitution in terms of inputs conveying information rather than in terms of the kind of stimuli received because it is an open question whether—say—in TVSS the input to the camera should count as one of the stimuli of the tactual sense. It might be argued that taking something to be the stimulus for a certain sense is for it—the stimulus—to be in the appropriate form to be perceptually processed along the proprietary processing path of a particular sense. Light waves are not in the appropriate form; they need to be converted into something which is. By contrast, there is no denying that the sensory substitution device provides inputs which convey certain information.

As far as the classification of the resultant sense is concerned—M plus sensory substitution device—it is certainly true that it shares a proper subset of the stimuli of the substituted sense. Equally, it would be wrong to insist that, say, the full stimuli to the human visual system should be reproduced, to count as being substituted for, since other animals are counted as seeing things even though they lack sensitivity to stimuli that we have, for example, colours in the case of dogs. Nevertheless, the substituting sense also has a range of its own stimuli which, in sensory substitution experiments, experimenters often go to some efforts to dampen (e.g. by headphones). This makes it implausible to suppose that the resulting sense is simply the substituted sense. Similar remarks would apply to a development of this position which emphasizes not merely the kind of input but how this depends upon motor activity (the sensorimotor approach to the senses championed by O'Regan and Noë (2001), and others).

A final way of understanding the differences between the senses is in terms of proprietary processing in the brain. According to such an approach, a sensory substitution device would be one which converts inputs in the to-be-substituted sense into inputs for the substituting sense in such a way as to enlist the proprietary processing of the latter to extract information more readily available in the former. This makes the presence or absence of sensory substitution devices hostage to evidence which is equivocal at best.

There are indications that some acclimatized/trained users of visual-to-auditory sensory substitution devices use what are normally thought to be visual areas of the brain to pick up information from the auditory stimulation. Anne De Volder et al. discovered that there was recruitment of the visual pathways in the case of early blind subjects, but not in normal blindfolded subjects, trained to use the same sensory substitution device (De Volder et al. 1979; see also Ptito et al. 2005). For the particular case of depth perception using a visual-auditory sensory substitution device, Laurent Renier et al. discovered recruitment of the visual pathways for blindfolded *sighted* subjects (Renier et al. 2005). If it is insisted that we only have a genuine case of visual sensory substitution if inputs to the auditory sense enlist the auditory areas alone (thereby, as it were, running visual information extraction through an auditory processing pathway), then these results might suggest that sensory substitution according to this last view is not so much substitution, or certainly not *just* substitution, but rather a non-standard way of enlisting the visual sense.

There is, however, an intriguing alternative. After training congenitally blind subjects with the tongue display unit (TDU, a visual-tactile sensory substitution device), Ron Kupers et al. found that if they stimulated, by transcranial magnetic stimulation, the areas responsible for visual processing in us, but triggered when processing TDU stimulation in the trained subjects, some of these subjects reported *tactual* sensations (Kupers et al. 2006). These reports were not made by these subjects prior to training. This suggests that there is no straightforward answer to the question of whether a certain part of the brain is for visual processing or for the processing of some other kind of sense like touch. Rather than have a non-standard enlistment of visual processing, we have an extension of tactual processing. For such subjects, we would have—according to this account of the individuation of the senses—extended tactual perception that enabled them to obtain information more readily available visually. Nevertheless, as I have already noted, there is considerable variation between subjects and so many cases will not be extensions to tactual perception but the creation of a distinct sense.

I have argued that successful sensory substitution should not require more than that it conveys information standardly available in the substituted sense in a way that reflects the functional role of the substituted sense. Nevertheless, discussion of other accounts of the individuation of the senses favour recognition of sensory substitution as supplying a new sense rather than simply touch extended or supplanted by vision. If instead of taking them individually, we take them as a group indicative of whether or not a new sense is present, then this conclusion is reinforced (for further sophisticated discussion, see Deroy and Auvray (2015)). So we may conclude that experiences that result from typical sensory substitution devices we have considered are neither experiences of touch or vision.

5.2 Cases of Sensory Substitution and the Argument from Acclimatization

In order to appreciate the challenge of the argument I am about to present, we need a bit more information about subjects acclimatized to sensory substitution devices. Take the case of TVSS. As Ophelia Deroy and Malika Auvray observe, after an hour or so, most users are able to walk around and navigate their environment. Soon acclimatized subjects start to locate objects in space. After nine hours of training, users of the tongue display unit could describe the shapes of objects (Sampaio et al. 2001; Kaczmarek and Haase 2003) and users of a TVSS on the back or forehead could locate them in space (Jansson 1983).

More striking still, over time, is the experience of *distal attribution* (as it has been called) (Bach-y-Rita et al. 1969; White et al. 1970; Bach-y-Rita and Kercel

2003). This is a change in the phenomenal content of the users' experiences. Users no longer take stimulation on their skin as part of this content, but rather just suppose that they have been stimulated by the properties of distant objects. For example, in Bach-y-Rita et al. (1969), it is noted:

> Our subjects spontaneously report the external localisation of stimuli, in that sensory information seems to come from in front of the camera, rather than from the vibrotactors on their back. Thus, after sufficient experience, the use of the vision substitution system seems to become an extension of the sensory apparatus.

And again, another subject who experienced TVSS reported:

> Very soon after I had learned how to scan, the sensations no longer felt as if they were on my back, and I became less and less aware that vibrating pins were making contact with my skin. By this time objects had come to have a top and a bottom; a right side and a left; but no depth—they existed in an ordered two dimensional space.
> (Guarniero 1974)

The remarks of one subject using the vOICe (a visual-auditory sensory substitution device) are even more striking. After having used the vOICe immersively for many months, PF, an experimental subject, says:

> I've developed it where one day I was washing dishes and without thinking I grabbed the towel, washed my hands, and looked down into the sink to make sure that the water had got out and I realised 'Oh! I can see down. I can see depth.' And I stepped back from that sink and looked down again to make sure that I wasn't fooling myself, and I walked slowly through my house looking into the rooms and it was like incredible. I could see into the room. That flat drawing now has depth to it. I can sense it. I can't tell you what is across the other end of the room but I can tell you that it is across from me.
> (Ward and Meijer 2010: 496)

These experiences seemed to depend upon giving the subjects the ability to move around the sensory substitution device to scan over objects rather than just receiving its input in a passive fashion.

The phenomenon of distal attribution seems very close to what some philosophers call the transparency or diaphanousness of visual, and perhaps other kinds of, experiences. Indeed, some psychologists pick up this description (Siegle and Warren 2010). Others distinguish distal attribution from transparency but it is not clear what difference they have in mind (e.g. Deroy and Auvray 2015). Distal attribution involves no longer being aware of the stimulation of the sensory substitution device but rather the source of its inputs. The properties perceived by the aid of the device are taken to be properties of a distal object. A natural way of understanding this is to suggest that their experiences present no properties of experience but go right through to the manifest objects and properties of the experience. In any event, I shall not distinguish between the phenomena here.

It should be noted that not all subjects report the same experiences. It is unclear whether this is a consequence of subjects having different capacities for acclimatization or different ways in which they prefer to characterize their experience. As a result, the argument I am going to construct, extrapolating a little from these empirical observations, can, at best, only be understood as a challenge. It is, of course, open to me to claim that thought experiments will back up the premises where actual observations do not. The reason why I prefer not to go down this path is that I doubt whether we can engage in thought experiments of the relevant type with sufficient confidence in the security of the assumptions needed to frame the possibilities in question. Indeed, the consequences of the argument from acclimatization for certain theories about the character of phenomenal properties suggest that these assumptions will be seen as questionable. The reports of actual subjects, with no theoretical axe to grind, therefore add plausibility to the argument.

The argument from acclimatization begins with what many might view as a datum and, at the least, as a strikingly plausible claim.

(1) *Colour as proprietary property for vision*: Auditory/tactual sensory substitution devices for vision can't give the subjects who use them substitute sensory experiences of colour: that is, redness/greenness etc. showing up in the phenomenal content of auditory or tactual experiences, or of extensions thereof, or of new sensory modes based upon them (see Peacocke 1983: 35; and Smith 1990: 239, for commitment to this).

We saw from the previous section that visual sensory substitution devices don't produce visual experiences. So if colours were to be experienced, then they wouldn't be experienced visually. If (1) is correct, then this is not possible.

The *colour as proprietary property* claim can only be explained in one of two ways. It either reflects something about the nature of colour or it reflects something about the nature of visual experience. The rest of the argument develops in terms of premises which rule out certain kinds of explanation of the *colour as proprietary property* claim. The first of these is a claim about colour itself:

(2) *Objectivism about colour*: Colours exist in nature with a character independent of, and not characterized in terms of, their effects upon our perceptual experiences.

Dispositional theories of colour might be claimed to be one form of objectivism since dispositions certainly exist in nature and are mind-independent. Even if an object is red if and only if it is disposed to cause red experiences in us, the existence of this disposition does not require the existence of any of us. That is not the kind of objectivism I have in mind and hence my formulation has deliberately attempted to rule it out. Instead, objectivism about colour in the sense which is relevant for the argument from acclimatization is that colour is either some intrinsic physical property of an object, some property which is realized by a disjunction of intrinsic physical properties, or a simple property of the world, as the colour primitivists attest.

Understanding colours in this way rules out one kind of explanation for the claim that colour is a proprietary property of vision. According to this ruled-out explanation, we can only experience colours by vision because they are dispositions, or relations, characterized in terms of properties only instantiated in visual experiences. This might appear to replace one thing which needs explaining with another. It might be pressed: why can't certain properties of a subject show up in other experiences than visual ones? The answer that the proponent of this kind of explanation will give is that one of the constraints on what it is to be a visual experience, as opposed to another kind of experience, is that these properties are characteristic of it. I return to this matter at the end.

The third premise in the argument is likely to be the most contentious because, although it identifies a condition which, in fact, is hard to resist, many theories of phenomenal properties are inexplicit on the matter and might, thereby, seem to avoid commitment to it.

(3) Subjects will experience colours if they stand in a certain kind of causal relation to the colours.

Obviously not any kind of causal relation will make subjects experience colours. For a start, the causal relations should hold between colours and the properties of a subject which must be present in order for the subject to be in a conscious mental state. Many philosophers hold that, for a state to be conscious, it must be either the object of a higher-order thought or display a certain kind of availability to other mental states (see, for example, Rosenthal 1990; Armstrong 1981). Michael Tye, for example, talks in terms of the state being poised for the belief-desire system (Tye 1995: 138). When I talk in terms of a certain kind of causal relation, part of its characterization will appeal to conditions inside the subject that support these kind of views, or others, about what makes a state conscious.

Nevertheless, another important element in the characterization of the kind of causal relationship will be the relations which must hold between the subject and the colours. Externalist representationalist theories take these relations to be required for the representation to take place. To fix preliminary ideas, consider once more the position of Tye. He holds that a certain kind of experience will represent a certain kind of property if it causally covaries with that property in optimal circumstances and is present because of that property. As he puts it, S represents that P = df If optimal conditions obtain, S is tokened in x if and only if P and because P (Tye 1995: 101). For Tye, there must be a certain kind of general dependency and, presumably, to experience a particular instance of a colour, an actual case of a causal relation. Other theories of representational properties appeal to various different external relations. Such appeals might get quite complex and involve a host of background conditions and contextual factors. Nevertheless, all of this complexity simply speaks to the complex, and possibility non-reductive, kind of causal relations to which premise (3) is addressed. When causal relations hold in these conditions, then such theories will say that subjects experience colours.

Let us now consider relationist accounts of phenomenal properties (e.g. Campbell 2002). According to relationists, the manifest objects and properties of an experience are settled by relations of brute awareness constitutive of the experience. This relation of brute awareness is usually taken to be a primitive. Certainly there can be no causal relation between the colours and experiences, taken *in toto*, so understood. Nevertheless, it is very hard to resist the thought that these relations of brute awareness will be realized by the colours, relations between the colours and the subject, and certain kinds of internal properties of the subject. Even if these relations cannot be reduced—probably in much the same way talk of optimal conditions is hard to reduce—the realizing relations are very plausibly thought to provide a context in which causal relations between the colours and internal states of the subject will make the subject brutely aware of the colours. In this context, what makes a subject brutely aware of a particular instance of a colour is that the particular instance is a cause of some internal state of the subject. There may be no way of specifying the contextually specified kind of causal relations upon which brute awareness depends (or, as Kalderon (2011: 256–257) calls it, partial perspective). There may be more than one type of such relation which can underpin any particular type of brute awareness. But, when all is said and done, there are types of causal relations where, if they hold, a subject is brutely aware of the colours. Note, the claim is not that subjects are aware of the colours in virtue of being aware of the internal states in question. That would be anathema to relationists. It is simply that, to put it roughly, metaphysically necessarily, if S is in a certain internal state, that state stands in certain relations to the environment, and a token colour c_1 causes the internal state, then S is brutely aware of c_1.

This brings me to the last premise.

(4) If subjects acclimatize to a sensory substitution device which can detect colours, amongst other things, then they will experience colours by some sense other than visual experience.

Obviously (1) to (4) are consistent as they stand. The conflict arises only if we can see no reason to deny that subjects may acclimatize to a sensory substitution device which can detect colours. The problem is that premises (2) and (3) together with the reports about acclimatization in the experimental work on sensory substitution make it very difficult to see how one could resist the claim that subjects may acclimatize to a sensory substitution device that can detect colours.

Once more, to fix preliminary ideas, it helps to think about Tye's theory. Let there be a visual-tactile sensory substitution device that takes as inputs information about light and, as outputs, generates tactile stimulation. As a subject gets acclimatized to the device, it is plausible that two things hold. First, that, rather than have the outputs available to the subject, the information the outputs convey becomes poised for the subject. Second, along with the acclimatization, there comes a characterization of optimal conditions in which the sensory substitution device's working counts as part of the optimal conditions. The challenge is simply this. If the outputs are tactual stimulation then there seems to be nothing to differentiate tactual stimulation which conveys information about colours and tactual stimulation which conveys information about, say, spatial properties, that makes it plausible one cannot acclimatize to the former but can to the latter. If colours are objective in the sense I have specified, then why shouldn't there be a sensory substitution device which takes the relevant colour stimulation and turns it into tactual stimulation? Indeed, there have been some attempts to do just this which don't seem to raise problems of principle (Aiello 1998).

It is harder to argue the same point for relationists, but once more there seem to be no structural features of their position which give them a line of resistance to the argument. After all, they are not going to deny, one might argue, that acclimatization is possible in order to perceive some properties by a sensory substitution device. When it happens, we get the kind of direct awareness of properties that they have taken to characterize the nature of experience. They cannot claim, either, that the fact that the tactual stimulations were originally intermediaries means that the relations of brute awareness cannot hold between the subject and the inputs of the sensory substitution device. There are many intermediaries in the causal chain between the manifest objects and properties of the experience and those internal properties of a subject in virtue of which, taken *in toto*, the relation of brute awareness holds. These do not vitiate the picture.

Thus, I conclude that either (1) must be abandoned or one or both of (2) and (3) must be. In the next section, I consider three lines of response to the argument and I close with indicating my preferred verdict.

5.3 Three Objections to the Argument from Acclimatization

The first objection to the argument is to say that sensory substitution devices show nothing about perceptual experience in general because, while our favourite theory (whatever that happens to be) is true of perceptual experience, as sensory substitution devices provide outputs which are inputs to a particular sense, sense datum theory is true of this particular combination of substituting sense and substitution device. By sense datum theory, I mean, loosely, any theory that holds that there is an intermediary, between the experiencing subject and the objects and properties of the world the experience concerns, such that the subject is aware of these objects and properties in virtue of being aware of the intermediary (see, for example, Jackson 1977: 16–20). These intermediaries, obviously, can occur without the objects and properties being present and it is because of this that we have an explanation of the possibility of hallucination, and so on.

Proponents of the first objection might develop their line of resistance to the argument as follows. They would say that whatever acclimatization involves, it cannot involve experience of colours because the existence of (say) *tactile* intermediaries in the case of a visual-tactual sensory substitution device shows that the right kind of causal relations can't hold to the colours. So (4) is false.

The problem with this response is that it seems to conflict with the reports of subjects regarding distal attribution. The subjects are not aware of the tactile stimulation, for example, but rather attribute what they experience as properties of objects. This phenomenon of distal attribution has, in other terminology, been directly responsible for the apparent attractiveness of representationalist and relationist theories of phenomenal properties. Each have emphasized that it is part of our everyday experience that we come across no properties of experience but rather are taken through to objects and properties in the world. This is the so-called transparency or diaphanousness of experience. My point is not that this notion is sufficiently well worked out to motivate representationalist or relationist theories. I don't need that for the present argument. Rather, my claim is that relationists and representationalists will have problems motivating their own theories if, in the face of apparent transparency in the case of sensory substitution, they insist that, in fact, the tactual stimulations are intermediaries. But if the right kind of causal relations can hold in cases of acclimatization to visual-tactual substitution devices relating to depth, then there is no reason for denying it in the case of colour on these grounds.

Let me, at this point, forestall a misunderstanding. The transparency thesis is compatible with being neutral about what the manifest objects and properties of experience are. They can be objects and properties in the world or they can be mental objects and properties as the sense datum theorist envisages them. Since G. E. Moore, often taken as one of the people who first identified the transparency/diaphanousness of experience, endorsed a sense datum theory, it is no surprise that this putative feature of experience does not decide between the theories (Moore 1903: 30). The fact it does not, it may be urged, undermines the objection I have just offered to what we may dub the 'sense datum theory' reply to the argument. Transparency is compatible with the tactual stimulation being the object of immediate awareness.

The problem with this objection to the reply is that it misses one dimension of the first response to the acclimatization argument. The point was supposed to be this. Sensory substitution devices cannot give us experiences of colour because the intermediaries—the sense data—have other properties, viz. tactile or auditory ones. It was the claim that sensory substitution devices give a different kind of input, when coupled with the observation about sense datum theory, which constituted the response to the acclimatization argument. My response was that the way in which acclimatized subjects were putatively transparently presented with *depth* properties showed why it could not be argued that, since tactual stimulation was the object of immediate awareness, we could not experience colour by such sensory substitution devices.

Interesting experimental work to support the transparency of experience due to sensory substitution devices has been done by Siegle and Warren (2010). They compare two models. First, there is the idea that, in the case of sensory substitution devices, the immediate objects of perception are the outputs of these devices. From these outputs, subjects infer properties relating to distal objects. Second, there is the idea that we are directly presented with distal objects and properties. They compare the performance of subjects asked to focus on their proximal stimulation with that of subjects asked to focus on their distal stimulation for making distance judgements on the basis of a visual-tactual sensory substitution device. They found that subjects who focused on their distal stimulation were more successful than those who focused on their proximal stimulation. If subjects were inferring what was the case distally from their proximal stimulation, you would not expect this difference in performance. Therefore, we have evidence that they have experiences of the distal objects and properties (Siegle and Warren 2010: 220–221).

The second objection to the argument is drawn from the position defended by Ophelia Deroy and Malika Auvray (2012). They argue that, in sensory substitution, the correct model is not to think of the device as something which creates a new kind of perceptual experience in us but rather something which we become adept at reading.

The analogy with reading is meant seriously. Reading is learning to access words through vision rather than audition. It is not an independent visual route to having auditory perception. We don't perceive auditory objects—such as sounds—by reading. According to a dual-route model of reading—which Deroy and Auvray endorse—the capacity to read is not an autonomous perceptual system but rather a second route grafted onto an auditory route, specifically that involving speech perception (see, for example, Coltheart and Rastle 1994: 1198). The second route maps known written signs onto phonemes and, thereby, onto meanings. When we learn to read, there is a change in subjective experience. We perceive the colours and shapes of words as meaningful.

If the analogy with reading is successful, then we have another way in which premise (4) of the argument can be false. When subjects acclimatize to sensory substitution devices, they don't have experiences characterized in terms of the manifest objects and properties that they might obtain from another sense modality. Instead, they can interpret what the output of the sensory substitution device means, for example, what a certain pattern of auditory stimulation means in terms of visual shape.

There are, no doubt, important similarities with reading, and thinking these through is likely to help us understand the nature of sensory substitution more. Nevertheless, there is one important disanalogy which vitiates this alternative model as an objection to the argument and, indeed, throws into question whether sensory substitution can really involve something akin to reading. In reading, there is no presentation of properties but only of meanings—as Deroy and Auvray acknowledge. However, this does not seem to be the case in sensory substitution. Acclimatized subjects do not experience the output as meaningful and, unlike the written word, struggle to attend to the proximal stimulation at all. Instead, they take themselves to be presented with properties.

Reading is held to be a perceptual-cognitive skill. Presumably the cognitive part is that which is responsible for seeing patterns on the page as having certain meanings. If so, then the fact that, when subjects acclimatize to sensory substitution devices, they don't see something as meaningful, but rather take themselves to be presented with certain kinds of properties, suggests that acclimatization is not properly understood as cognitive. Rather the outputs of a particular sensory substitution device become integrated with our perceptual processing in a particular way in order to yield either the presentation of distinctive kinds of properties or a distinctive way of being presented with information about objects and properties which is, perhaps, also available through other senses.

The last objection I am going to consider is drawn from a particular way of understanding colour objectivism. According to this perspectival view of colour, espoused in different ways by John Campbell and Mark Kalderon, although colours are objective, they require particular kinds of sensory apparatus in order to be experienced (e.g. Kalderon 2007: 594; Campbell 1993, where this is shown by his denial that colours figure in the absolute conception). We can only understand the nature of colours by being capable of having the kind of experience in which they show up. Colours are objective because the conditions under which they are seen—the enabling conditions—are metaphysically independent of the colour an object has. Thus, unlike dispositional accounts of colour, there is no way in which, if an object is experienced to have a certain colour under normal conditions—the enabling conditions—then it follows the object must have the colour in question simply from the nature of colour. However, it does follow from the nature of experience. If the enabling conditions are met, then the subject stands in a certain brute relation of awareness to a particular colour—let it be red. Experiences of red, and the other colours, derive their nature from their manifest properties. So if a subject is experiencing red when the enabling conditions are met, the object must be red. If it were a different colour, there would a different experience in its stead with that colour constituting its phenomenal content. The metaphysical independence of colours from the enabling conditions is not explained in terms of it being metaphysically possible for subjects to experience colours, when the enabling conditions are met, and yet objects not have the colours in question. Ruling out this possibility is common ground between the dispositionalist and the perspectival view. Rather the independence is captured by the difference in explanation of how this possibility is ruled out. For the perspectivalist, it derives from a thesis concerning what makes an experience of a colour rather than the nature of colour (as the dispositionalist proposes) (Campbell 1993: 261–267).

Such a view of colour would question premise (4) for a different reason. It would deny that there could be a sensory substitution device for colour to which a subject could acclimatize. Colours just wouldn't be detectable by anything else but visual systems. In putting it this way, I am setting aside the question of whether there are different kinds of equally good visual systems—belonging to different creatures—which pick up different colour ranges in the world, so that all objects are multiply, compatibly coloured (Kalderon 2007). Rather I am focusing on the kernel idea that would seem to threaten the argument above. If there were different colour ranges, then the issue would be reformulated in terms of whether sensory substitution devices would enable us to acclimatize to each (or, indeed, whether it would be possible for one of the range which would be interesting in itself). The key features of the response wouldn't change.

There are significant difficulties with this line of objection to possibility of acclimatization however. The first point to make is that sensory substitution devices are devices which assist a sense modality, which might not normally obtain information about a certain property, to obtain information about that property. So, it might be said, we can agree that normally only visual systems can detect colours, and so colours only show up in visual experience. However, sensory substitution devices appeal to the fact that the causal path which enables a subject to experience the colour in question is one which can be exploited by a device which takes as input the same as the visual system but then converts it into another format. If our tactual system can acclimatize to these outputs in the format suitable for it, then we should experience the colours via tactile stimulation.

The way in which I put the last point does not presume that explanations appealing to wavelengths and physiology—as Campbell puts it—are in some way explanatorily primary leaving the colours with little (i.e. no) causal work to do. As Campbell acknowledges, the explanation at the wavelength/physiological level and that in terms of colours and experiences may be intimately related but not in explanatory competition (Campbell 2002: 262). This intimate connection may be just as much present relating colours to our tactual experiences mediated by the sensory substitution device. Sensory substitution devices just introduce new enabling conditions which were not available before. So the argument from acclimatization is a way of challenging the attempt to characterize a perceiver-relative notion of objectivity in a way which captures the truth of (1) rather than a failure to take into account the particular features of this position on the nature of colours. In brief, the position seems committed to denying that a subject's tactual system together with a sensory substitution device can enable a subject to experience colour even though the subject is sensitive to the presence of colour and the tactual system processes this sensitivity in a way which allows for acclimatization. This creates an explanatory burden which is hard to discharge.

5.4 Concluding Remarks

One conclusion one could draw from the argument of the previous section is that (1) is false. There are no proprietary properties for visual, or any other, experiences, although there may be properties which are, in fact, only detected by certain kinds of senses as things are. Perhaps what is proprietary to particular senses is not particular properties but particular ways in which information about properties may be bundled. This, in itself, would be an interesting result.

However, if we persist in finding it plausible that colour is a proprietary property for visual experience, then it seems to me that we have two options. The first is to recognize that we need to refine our notion of acclimatization and distinguish between the kind of direct awareness that acclimatization to sensory substitution devices may give us of properties and that direct awareness which is typical of visual and other experiences. Any theory of awareness, or the integration of representations into a perceptual process, or characterization of how a relation of brute awareness may be realized, which failed to differentiate itself from the acclimatization subjects undergo in sensory substitution will be, according to this option, incomplete. Reading is one thing, acclimatization another, and the kind of integration that is required for a perceptual process to make us aware of objects and properties in the way that the human senses do, a third. According to this view, the argument does not defeat externalist accounts of phenomenal properties—externalist representationalisms or appeal to brute relations of awareness—it simply identifies an explanatory debt, I hope a little more sharply than before.

The second option is to recognize a new way in which representationalism can be developed. Once more, to fix ideas, since there are complexities I do not have space to go into, suppose that a determinate shade of red, red_3 is the disposition to give rise to certain internal properties in a subject's head, intuitively, properties of the visual system. Call those properties $m(red_3)$. Then these properties can, in principle, be used by the subject's brain to identify the presence of a certain disposition in the environment, a disposition to bring about them. Whether or not $m(red_3)$ is used to *represent* the presence of the disposition will turn on whether they play the right functional role. There is a functional story of some kind or another about what makes a certain bundle of properties into something which is a representation. However, with this functional role in place, what makes $m(red_3)$ represent the disposition it does is its own character. Just as there might be a functional story to explain why the colour squares on a colour chart, or swatches of material in a tailor's book, represent the colours in which you can get paint, or material in which you can get suits made, the representation of which colour, or which material, still remains done by the character of the colour or material in question.

If representationalism is developed in this way, then we have a natural explanation of why colours are proprietary for a particular sense modality: they are dispositions to give rise to properties which are characteristic of the processing of that modality. In saying this, we leave open the question of the nature of these properties. They may, themselves, be relational, functional, or intrinsic non-functional properties (as the analogy with colour squares or swatches of material suggests). It is quite compatible with this position that there might be considerable neural plasticity. The point is simply that the argument of the first section showed that, because the substituting sense plus sensory substitution extension were not properly classified as, for example, vision, the subject could not experience by these means properties characterized in terms of their disposition to put the visual system into certain states.

Of course, the representationalist component to this story is not mandatory. It would be a sufficient explanation of the fact that colours are proprietary to visual experience, if they were dispositions to give rise to internal properties of a subject's visual system (see, for example, Peacocke 1983: 37–43). These properties need not be representational. Nevertheless, such a truncated theory would face two kinds of problem. The first concerns how visual experiences would come to be of colours so understood. Suppose one took visual experiences to be representational even if one denied representationalism is true of phenomenal properties. Then the question would be: how do visual experiences represent properties which are dispositions to produce the instantiation of properties which are instantiated in the very experiences in question. What theory of representation would have that as a consequence?

Consider, further, the position of Christopher Peacocke back in 1983. He defines sensational properties to be any non-representational properties which serve to characterize what an experience is like (Peacocke 1983: 5). The internal properties which characterize the dispositions mentioned above are one such property. Even if these properties characterize what an experience is like, that is not sufficient to make the experiences represent anything about the presence of the disposition. Yet, they do. How is this achieved?

The need to provide such an account is obscured by talking of these properties as characterizing what an experience is like. That might suggest that in some way colours are presented in experience. It cannot be ruled out that this is so since talk of *presentation* is hard to pin down. The important point is simply that we have no story as yet about how they are *represented* in experience if that is the picture with which we are working. Note also that Peacocke characterizes these sensational properties—'red', blue' and so on—in terms of how red things (say) are presented in normal circumstances in the visual field. This seems to make them fall on the manifest side of the distinction between manifest objects and properties on the one hand, and phenomenal properties on the other. In which case, they are not to be understood as properties of a subject's visual system. Rather, sensational properties so understood figure in the phenomenal content of a subject's visual system in virtue of properties of the subject's visual system. There only seems to be no worry about how colours show up in experience—understood Peacocke's way—because their location (as manifest properties) disguises the fact that an answer has already been assumed without being provided.

The second problem for the truncated theory follows on from the problem of representation just identified. Why wouldn't using the experience's properties to represent the disposition to produce them be a compelling, indeed the only plausible, answer to the explanatory challenge the first question posed? What's wrong with it? Those who insist on a truncated version of the second option need an answer. In the absence of an answer, I conclude that the other option is to recognize a kind of intrinsic representationality.

Sensory substitution devices, therefore, are not just of significant interest to psychological researchers of vision and those who seek to provide new sources of sensory information for those suffering from sensory deficits. Reflection on their performance brings to light inadequacies in our current understanding of direct awareness in experience, or the nature of representational properties, or, perhaps, both.

References

Aiello, Gaetao L. (1998) Multidimensional electrocutaneous stimulation. *IEEE Transactions on Rehabilitation Engineering* 6(1): 95–101.

Armstrong, D. M. (1981) What is consciousness? In D. M. Armstrong, *The Nature of Mind*. Brighton: Harvester Press, 55–67; reprinted in Ned Block, Owen Flanagan and Güven Güzeldere (eds) *The Nature of Consciousness*. Cambridge, MA: MIT Press, 1997, 721–728.

Bach-y-Rita, Paul and Stephen W. Kercel (2003) Sensory substitution and the human-machine interface. *Trends in Cognitive Sciences* 7(12): 541–546.

Bach-y-Rita, Paul, Carter C. Collins, Frank A. Saunders, Benjamin White and Lawrence Scadden (1969) Vision substitution by tactile image projection. *Nature* 221: 963–964.

Campbell, John (1993) A simple view of colour. In John Haldane and Crispin Wright (eds) *Realism, Representation and Projection*. Oxford: Oxford University Press, 257–268.

Campbell, John (2002) *Reference and Consciousness*. Oxford: Oxford University Press.

Coltheart, Max and Kathleen Rastle (1994) Serial processing in reading aloud: evidence for dual-route models of reading. *Journal of Experimental Psychology, Human Perception and Performance* 20(6): 1197–1211.

Deroy, Ophelia and Malika Auvray (2012) Reading the world through the skin and ears: a new perspective on sensory substitution. *Frontiers in Psychology* 3, Article 457.

Deroy, Ophelia and Malika Auvray (2015) A crossmodal perspective on sensory substitution. In D. Stokes, M. Matthen and S. Biggs (eds) *Perception and its Modalities*. Oxford: Oxford University Press, 327–347.

De Volder, Anne G., Mitzi Catalan-Ahumada, Annie Robert, Anne Bol, Daniel Labar, Anne Coppens, Christian Michel and Claude Veraart (1979) Changes in occipital cortex activity in early blind humans using a sensory substitution device. *Brain Research* 826: 128–134.

Grice, H. P. (1962) Some remarks about the senses. In R. J. Butler (ed.) *Analytical Philosophy*. Oxford: Blackwell; and in H. P. Grice (1989) *Studies in the Way of Words*. Cambridge, MA: Harvard University Press, 248–268; and in Fiona Macpherson (ed.) (2011) *The Senses*. Oxford: Oxford University Press, 83–100.

Guarniero, G. (1974) Experience of tactile vision. *Perception* 3: 101–104.

Heil, John (1983) *Perception and Cognition*. Berkeley: University of California Press.

Jackson, Frank (1977) *Perception*. Cambridge: Cambridge University Press.

Jansson, G. (1983) Tactile guidance of movement. *International Journal of Neuroscience* 19: 37–46.

Kaczmarek, K. A. and S. J. Haase (2003) Pattern identification and perceived stimulus quality as a function of stimulation current on a fingertip scanned electrotactile display. *IEEE Transactions on Neural Systems and Rehabilitation Engineering* 11: 6–16.

Kalderon, Mark (2007) Colour pluralism. *The Philosophical Review* 116(4): 563–601.

Kalderon, Mark Eli (2011) The multiply qualitative. *Mind* 120(478): 239–262.

Kupers, Ron, Arnaud Furnal, Alain Maertens de Noordhout, Albert Gjedde, Jean Schoenen and Maurice Ptito (2006) Transcranial magnetic stimulation of the visual cortex induces somatotopically organised qualia in blind subjects. *Proceedings of the National Academy of Sciences USA* 103(41): 13256–13260.

Meijer, Peter B. L. (1992) An experimental system for auditory image representations. *IEEE Transactions on Biomedical Engineering* 29(2): 112–121.

Moore, G. E. (1903) The refutation of idealism. *Mind*, NS, xii; reprinted in G. E. Moore (1922) *Philosophical Studies*. London: Routledge & Kegan Paul, 1–30.

O'Regan, J. Kevin and Alva Noë (2001) A sensorimotor account of vision and visual consciousness. *Behavioural and Brain Sciences* 24: 939–1031 (including comments and response).

Peacocke, Christopher (1983) *Sense and Content*. Oxford: Oxford University Press.

Ptito, Maurice, Solvej M. Moesgaard, Albert Gjedde and Ron Kupers (2005) Cross-modal plasticity revealed by electrotactile stimulation of the tongue in the congenitally blind. *Brain* 128: 606–614.

Renier, Laurent, Oliver Collignon, Colline Poirier, Dai Tranduy, Annick Vanlierde, Anne Bol, Claude Veraart and Anne G. De Volder (2005) Cross-modal activation of visual cortex during depth perception using auditory substitution of vision. *NeuroImage* 26: 573–580.

Rosenthal, David M. (1990) A theory of consciousness. *ZiF Technical Report*, Bielefeld, Germany; reprinted in Ned Block, Owen Flanagan and Güven Güzeldere (eds) *The Nature of Consciousness*. Cambridge, MA: MIT Press, 1997, 729–753.

Sampaio, Eliana, Stephane Maris and Paul Bach-y-Rita (2001) Brain plasticity: 'visual' acuity of blind persons via the tongue. *Brain Research* 908: 204–207.

Siegle, Joshua H. and William H. Warren (2010) Distal attribution and distance perception in sensory substitution. *Perception* 39: 208–223.

Smith, A. D. (1990) Of primary and secondary qualities. *The Philosophical Review* 99(2): 221–254.

Tye, Michael (1995) *Ten Problems of Consciousness*. Cambridge, MA: MIT Press.

Ward, Jamie and Peter Meijer (2010) Visual experiences in the blind induced by an auditory sensory substitution device. *Consciousness and Cognition* 19: 492–500.

White, Benjamin, Frank A. Saunders, Lawrence Scadden, Paul Bach-y-Rita and Carter C. Collins (1970) Seeing with the skin. *Perception and Psychophysics* 7(1): 23–27.

6

What Can Sensory Substitution Tell Us about the Organization of the Brain?

SARAH HILLENBRAND, DINA RAVEH AND AMIR AMEDI

Abstract We discuss how sensory substitution devices (SSDs) can be used to study the organization of the brain. To do so we look at the use of SSDs in the blind and how SSDs can be used to identify sensory-dependent and sensory-independent brain function. Cross-modal interactions may represent new patterns of connectivity or the unmasking of pre-existing associations. We show how the blind brain can be a window into cross-modal plasticity and can dissociate intrinsic and experience-dependent brain functions. We argue that the brain is a sensory-independent task machine and explain the implications for the rehabilitation of blind people.

6.1 Introduction

JOHN LILLY, AUTHOR OF *The Deep Self: Consciousness Exploration in the Isolation Tank*, was an early pioneer of sensory deprivation experiments in the 1950s. He enclosed himself in flotation tanks in total darkness and silence, simply floating and introspecting, for hours at a time. Lilly wanted to know what the mind did when it wasn't being stimulated. With no outside input to fuel thought, would the workings of the mind grind to a halt, or would it develop a deeper sensitivity to even the slightest stimulation? He was convinced that by shutting out all sensory stimulation he would ultimately come to know the structure of the mind itself.

Lilly's obsession points to an important problem in the study of the mind: the need to dissociate the brain's computations from its inputs. Since phrenology was first proposed as a way to explain why lesions to different brain areas produced different pathologies (Gall and Spurzheim 1835), the brain has been thought of as a collection of modular regions, each with a specific function (Pascual-Leone and Hamilton 2001). Association cortices are thought to handle abstract computations performed on information relayed from different sensory systems, with each

Proceedings of the British Academy, **219**, 94–121.

sensory cortex processing inputs from a single sensory modality. Somehow, through the interaction of parallel unimodal sensory systems and multimodal association cortical regions, we get our thoughts.

But the line between sensory and abstract is blurry. For instance, it is difficult for a sighted person to identify an abstract thought that isn't in some way shaped by their sense of vision. Even our most abstract thoughts are shaped by the limits of our biological senses (Lakoff 1980). Trying to disentangle which properties of our minds are intrinsically determined and which are moulded by experience is a difficult endeavour. What would our minds be like in the absence of stimulation? How much of the structure of thought would remain were it not for our experiences?

These questions have blindness as an intriguing test case. The blind brain, after all, seems like the perfect example of a brain that has had to acquire its function and structure in the absence of sensory input. Anatomically, the visual cortex of the blind appears similar to that of sighted controls (Wanet-Defalque et al. 1988). If you were presented with two images, one depicting a brain with a high level of activity in visual cortex and one with little or no activity in visual cortex, it would seem safe to guess that the former belongs to a sighted individual and the latter to a blind individual. Counterintuitively, however, you would be wrong. Functionally, the visual cortex of the blind is anything but dormant. Positron emission tomography (PET) imaging shows that the blind brain exhibits higher levels of glucose metabolism in the visual cortex (Phelps et al. 1981). This presents a puzzle: What, exactly, does visual cortex do when it's not doing vision?

Blindness results in massive cross-modal plasticity. Plasticity refers to the re-wiring of connections between neurons in the brain in response to some change, like sensory deprivation. The brain is constantly forming new connections as we learn, and in general, the experiences we have shape the way our brain gets wired. Pascual-Leone and colleagues point out that 'Plasticity is an intrinsic property of the human brain and represents human evolution's invention to enable the nervous system to escape the restrictions of its own genome and thus adapt to environmental pressures, physiologic changes, and experience' (2005: 377).

Cross-modal plasticity, specifically, refers to plasticity between the neural underpinnings of multiple senses. For example, when one source of sensory input is lost, the brain areas normally responsible for processing these inputs may take on the task of processing information coming in from other sources. In the blind, it has been found that the visual cortex is involved in such activities as reading Braille (Phelps et al. 1981; Reich et al. 2011), which relies on touch. This leads to another set of questions: Just how flexible is the 'unemployed' cortex in the sorts of tasks it takes on? It seems to be able to take on not just new sensory processing computations, but computations well outside the realm of sensory processing, like memory (Amedi et al. 2003). Where does this flexibility come from? How does it help or hinder the blind as they negotiate their environments?

Recent advances in the creation and use of sensory substitution devices (SSDs) have given researchers a powerful new tool with which to approach these questions. SSDs rely on the intact senses of the blind (most usefully, touch and hearing) to communicate information about the spatial layout of the world. Typically, sighted individuals rely heavily on vision for this information. By presenting this information via an atypical pathway, we can begin to delineate which computations require certain inputs (sensory-dependent) and which do not (sensory-independent). We can use measures of sensory dependence to find the border between the hard-wired and the experiencc-dependent plastic properties of the human brain. Here we explore the insights into cross-modal plasticity and the structure of thought that can be gained from the study of blind participants using SSDs, and the potential applications of these insights for clinical rehabilitation.

6.2 How Can SSDs Be Used to Study the Organization of the Brain?

6.2.1 The use of sensory substitution devices in the blind

The blind use a variety of adaptations to allow their intact senses to take in information about the world. In the tactile domain, for instance, canes are used for navigation and Braille for reading. Sensory substitution devices rely on an input sensor, a processing unit, and an output human–machine interface (Bach-y-Rita et al. 1969; Bach-y-Rita and Kercel 2003; and for review, see Maidenbaum et al. 2014) to take in visual or spatial information and translate it into something interpretable by a subject's remaining senses.

One such device, called the vOICe, translates information in the visual field from luminance to loudness, pitch to vertical location, and time to horizontal location (Meijer 1992; seeingwithsound.com). A good way to conceptualize what this might sound like is to know that a white vertical line on a black background in the left half of the screen would sound like a single blast of many tones, early in a one-second sweep of the visual scene. A white horizontal line, on the other hand, would sound like an extended pure tone whose pitch rises with the vertical location of the line, and if it's in the right half of the screen, that pure tone will come late in the sweep. The recently developed 'EyeMusic' SSD provides pleasant musical image representations that seamlessly integrate colour information while preserving shape information (Abboud et al. 2014; brain.huji.ac.il/EM.html).

6.2.2 How can SSDs be used to identify sensory-dependent and sensory-independent brain function?

SSDs provide a unique opportunity to experimentally dissociate two of the most stubbornly confounded variables of brain function: sensory input modality and computation. Because we are such visual creatures, a large proportion of our brain is given over to visual processing. Previously, it had been very difficult to say whether this visual dominance represented some intrinsic property of brain structure, hard-wired into our genetic code, or whether the brain has the capacity to process information more flexibly, and it is simply the overwhelmingly superior spatial resolution of visual input that drives the brain to take on so much visual function.

SSDs provide experimental conditions to investigate cross-modal activation in primary sensory areas as they allow the same visual stimuli to be presented in image form or via auditory substitution to both sighted and blind subjects. Furthermore, by comparing meaningful and meaningless stimuli it is possible to identify association cortices that encode conceptual information but show no preference for how stimuli are communicated. In this way, the sensory-dependent and sensory-independent factors contributing to brain function can be distinguished.

Where blind brains differ from sighted brains, despite a common sensory input (both groups using SSDs), we can infer that compensatory plasticity has occurred in the blind that allows them to process the stimulus differently. Where their brains differ despite common semantic input (the sighted using vision and the blind using audition), we can infer that it is possible that multiple sensory modalities may be processed in tandem or flexibly by the same brain regions. Furthermore, certain brain functions require that connections be established before, or during, a critical period. If, for example, visual input is withheld from a developing organism, the visual cortex does not have the proper instruction to wire up its normal organizational features (Hubel and Wiesel 1963). The brains of early, late, and congenitally blind participants may be compared to learn about the roles of experience and critical periods.

SSDs can be used to corroborate and expand upon what is known about the blind brain. In the next section, we will discuss the mechanisms of plasticity. In the following section, we will discuss whether sensory and higher-level cognitive functions are assigned differently in the brain.

6.3 Cross-Modal Interactions May Represent New Patterns of Connectivity or the Unmasking of Pre-Existing Associations

Before discussing how cross-modal plasticity interacts with extant brain connectivity, it is important to form a clear picture of how each of the two mechanisms works. We will first review some seminal examples of cross-modal plasticity, and then move on to some examples of the sorts of cross-modal interactions that occur normally in the sighted brain.

6.3.1 Extreme cross-modal plasticity: re-wiring experiments in animals

Cross-modal plasticity was demonstrated in animal studies when researchers surgically detached the optic nerve from the primary visual cortex (V1) in young animals and rerouted it to the primary somatosensory cortex (S1), which normally processes touch (Métin and Frost 1989). This allowed them to ask whether brain areas specialized for processing information from a certain sensory modality were hard-wired to do so, or whether they were moulded that way by experience. They found that in the adult animals, S1 had taken on V1-like properties in response to the rerouted visual input. In a similar experiment, using ferrets, the optic nerve was rerouted to the primary auditory cortex (A1) (Roe et al. 1992). Again, neuronal properties typically seen in the visual system appeared. These included ocular dominance, a proportionally V1-like mix of simple and complex receptive neuron fields, orientation tuning, direction selectivity, and velocity tuning. In both experiments the cells were driven by their new sensory inputs and took on the functions typically carried out by visual cortex.

These experiments demonstrate that the patterns of local organization seen in visual cortex emerge as the result of the statistics of the stimulus, rather than as an intrinsic property of the cortex. It is important to remember that this reorganization was induced surgically as part of an experiment, and as such, making the case for such a process to occur in nature would require an explanation of the underlying mechanism. Nevertheless, they are striking examples of experience-driven cross-modal plasticity.

6.3.2 Normal multisensory connectivity: experiments in the sighted

Blindfolded sighted participants were used to test for the presence of extant connectivity. After five days of continuous blindfolding, V1 was recruited to process tactile and auditory stimuli (Pascuale-Leone and Hamilton 2001). Five days is too short a period to re-wire the cortex, so the connections between the tactile (S1) and auditory (A1) input pathways and the visual (V1) cortex must already have been in place. Alternatively, blindfolding could lead to release from inhibition normally placed on visual cortex on the processing of other sensory modalities.

Cross-modal inhibition can arise when sensory inputs conflict or compete: for instance, if you are trying to understand spoken words in a noisy environment, your brain helpfully attenuates responses in the visual cortex. Similarly, if you are engaged in visual imagery the auditory cortex is inhibited (Kuchinsky et al. 2012). This indicates that our primary sensory cortices are linked functionally and perhaps also anatomically, and that these links can be modulated in a context-dependent way. Thus both extant connectivity and cross-modal plasticity are viable mechanisms by which non-traditional sensory responses may arise.

6.4 The Blind Brain as a Window into Cross-Modal Plasticity

The unemployed visual cortex and higher visual areas of the blind are capable of taking on a variety of functions. Primary sensory cortices specialize in processing a single input modality, and association cortices support integration among the sensory modalities and higher cognitive functions (Calvert and Thesen 2004). However, it is unclear how cortex becomes one kind or the other, whether this division is itself plastic or not, and how blindness can alter this process.

6.4.1 The visual cortex is involved in reading Braille in the blind

In a 1996 PET study, Sadato and colleagues scanned the brains of blind and sighted participants as they read Braille. The primary visual cortex of the blind participants was activated, whereas it was deactivated in sighted participants. This is good correlational evidence for the role of blind visual cortex in processing Braille. Patient and transcranial magnetic stimulation (TMS) studies can provide causal evidence. One blind patient, proficient in Braille reading, was rendered unable to read Braille by a stroke which damaged her occipital cortex bilaterally (Hamilton et al. 2000). This is corroborated by studies where TMS was used to induce a temporary, virtual lesion (Pascuale-Leone et al. 2000). TMS allows researchers to isolate the effect of the virtual lesion from other confounding factors such as long-term compensatory plasticity in patients with brain lesions.

TMS administered to occipital cortex impairs identification of Braille or embossed Roman letters in the blind but not in the sighted (Cohen et al. 1997; Hamilton and Pascual-Leone 1998). Blind participants knew they were touching Braille words but were unable to identify them, saying they felt ‘different’ or ‘less sharp, less well-defined’. They occasionally reported ‘phantom’ Braille dots or distorted perceptions. This indicates that the occipital cortex plays a role in processing the Braille stimuli in the blind.

6.4.2 The visual cortex is recruited for higher cognitive functions in the blind

It is thought the blind compensate for their lack of vision with an increased reliance on verbal memory. Anecdotally, in ancient times, blind individuals were often considered 'living databases'. A blind person quoting the bible was considered much more reliable than a sighted person (Amedi et al. 2003). Amir Amedi and colleagues investigated whether they might be using the 'unemployed' visual cortex to produce this adaptation. They found that the degree to which the blind recruited primary visual cortex correlated positively with their performance on a verbal memory task (Amedi et al. 2003). The sighted did not activate their V1 during this task, and had inferior memory. This suggests that primary visual cortex had been moulded to perform a new function: memory.

In a verbal memory task, participants recalled words memorized from a list six months prior. Importantly, simply recalling the words covertly required no tactile or auditory sensory input. The participants were all congenitally blind and all of the words were intentionally abstract, to eliminate the possibility that they were relying on visual imagery. The acquisition of a higher-level cognitive function by visual cortex raises challenges for explaining the flexibility of cortex. It begins to seem that the brain does not merely swap out visual input for somatosensory input, but can also reorganize itself to process both sensory and abstract information.

6.4.3 The lateral occipital complex (LOC): a multimodal shape processor in the sighted brain

It is important to acknowledge the multimodal nature of the brain's responses in the sighted as well as in the blind. While some of the new functions of 'visual' regions in the blind arise as the result of *de novo* compensatory cross-modal plasticity, not all do. Some simply reflect the strengthening of extant connectivity that becomes unmasked by visual deprivation.

One location that is instructive in differentiating these processes is a visual region known as the lateral occipital complex (LOC). The LOC responds preferentially to objects compared to scrambled objects or textures. Amedi and colleagues found that a portion of this area also prefers objects over textures when objects are presented to be palpated with the hand rather than presented visually (Amedi et al. 2001). Calling this area LOtv (tactile/visual), they reasoned that it must be involved in representing graspable objects in a multimodally integrated way. Subsequently, the region's sensory-independent responsiveness to objects was tested using auditory input. Participants listened to the sound an object typically makes (for example, the sound of a bottle opening to identify a bottle), but this auditory stimulation did not evoke responses in the LOC (Amedi et al. 2002).

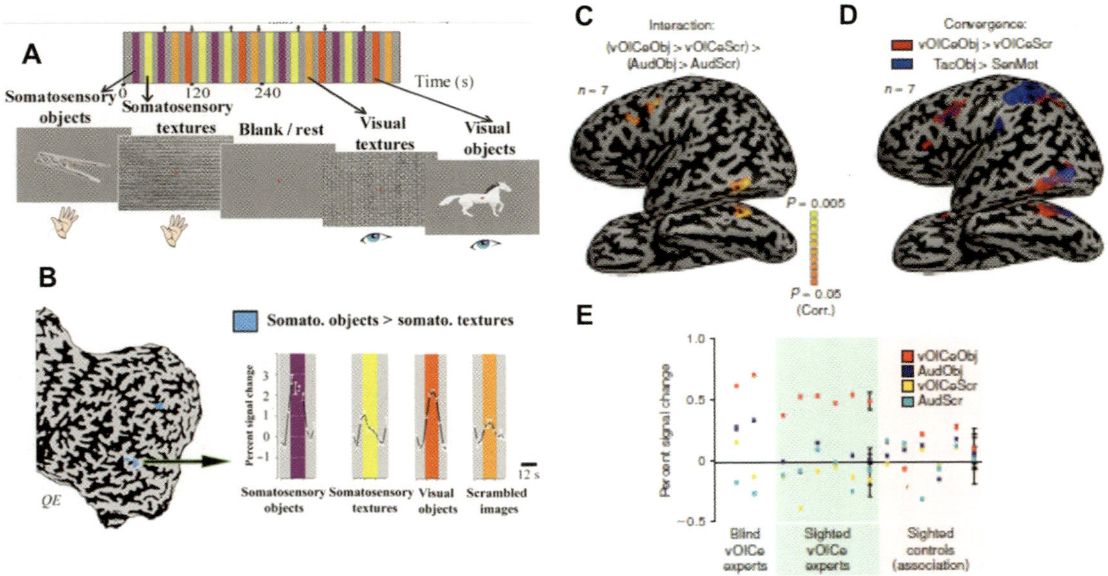

Figure 6.1 Area LOtv is the earliest studied and most well-characterized sensory-independent, task-specific metamodal area. The lateral occipital tactile-visual area (LOtv), situated in the LO object recognition complex, activates selectively during tasks that involve the processing of geometric information.

A The experimental protocol included four conditions presented in an interleaved fashion in a block design. Stimuli were visual and somatosensory objects as well as scrambled images and somatosensory textures. Small upward arrows represent eye openings; small downward arrows represent eye closings. Adapted from Amedi et al. 2001.

B Left: Flattened cortical map with somatosensory object-selective voxels highlighted in blue. Right: Timecourse of activation, averaged across repetitions of each condition, in somatosensory object-selective voxels. Note that the comparison of interest revealed a preference for somatosensory objects over somatosensory textures, although these voxels also demonstrated a preference for visual objects over scrambled visual objects. Adapted from Amedi et al. 2001.

C The lateral occipital area (LO) shows a greater preference for objects (over scrambled objects) presented using the vOICe than for objects (over scrambled objects) presented in the auditory modality. Adapted from Amedi et al. 2007.

D Red areas prefer vOICe objects over vOICe scrambled objects, and blue clusters prefer tactile objects over the sensorimotor control condition. Purple areas indicate where these areas overlap. Adapted from Amedi et al. 2007.

E Dots indicate the amount of activity in left LOtv for all non-tactile conditions. Both blind and sighted vOICe experts showed greater activity for vOICe objects (in red) than sighted controls. Adapted from Amedi et al. 2007.

6.5 The Use of SSDs to Dissociate Intrinsic and Experience-Dependent Brain Functions

The LOC is one example of an area whose multimodal response properties have been revisited using SSDs (Amedi et al. 2007). Soundscapes presented using the vOICe (Meijer 1992; seeingwithsound.com) were used to convey information about the shape of the objects. The LOC was activated by this input in both sighted and blind participants. The subtle distinction between listening to an object's typical sound and hearing information about its geometric shape conveyed through sound made all the difference. Hearing a bird tweet, after all, tells you nothing about its shape. The region seems to truly be specialized for extracting geometric shape information from the statistics of the stimulus itself rather than by merely forming associations. This lends support to the idea that this region, in the sighted as well as in the blind, is intrinsically suited to perform a certain computation regardless of sensory input. Increasingly, SSDs are revealing similar predilections across many other visually responsive regions.

6.5.1 SSDs have been used to reveal the intrinsic computations of what only appear to be visual areas

The visual system is organized into two streams, the ventral and dorsal streams (Ungerleider and Mishkin 1982). The ventral stream was dubbed the 'what' stream and the dorsal stream the 'where' stream, later referred to as the 'where/how' stream (Goodale and Milner 1992). The ventral 'what' stream is involved in object recognition and detailed visual processing of, for example, colour and shape. The lateral occipital complex, described here earlier, is part of the ventral stream. The dorsal 'where/how' stream is involved in visuospatial perception, visually guided movements, and generally determining the location of objects.

The vOICe SSD (Meijer 1992; seeingwithsound.com) was used to determine whether this organization is experience-dependent, arising only in the brains of people who have experienced visual input, or intrinsic, arising even in the absence of visual input. Congenitally blind and blindfolded sighted participants performed tasks in which they were required to discern either the shape (angular or round) or location (left or right) of a stimulus presented via the vOICe's soundscapes (Striem-Amit et al. 2012b). Critically, this was done with only a brief period of training to rule out the effect of long-term practice-induced changes in brain organization.

Across all conditions, the blind participants had higher levels of brain activation compared to controls when listening to the soundscapes. Specifically, the whole of the occipital lobe (along with parts of the emanating dorsal and ventral streams) was activated in the blind, but not in the sighted controls. Two main regions demonstrated preferences for one task over the other: the inferior temporal sulcus, part of the ventral 'what' stream, preferred shape, whereas the precuneus, part of the dorsal 'where/how' stream, preferred location. Importantly, this preference was evident in the brains of both the blind and the sighted. This suggests that the 'what' and 'where/how' streams of processing need not be vision-specific—they are perfectly happy to perform their preferred computations on auditory inputs if need be.

This flexibility suggests that the emergence of the 'what' and 'where' streams in the blind is not the result of long-term compensatory cross-modal plasticity in the blind, but a reflection of extant connectivity whose sensory independence is unmasked in the absence of visual input. In the case of the two streams, it is probable that in the sighted, vision flooded these streams with its superior informational content, causing the streams to appear to be visual in nature.

6.5.2 SSDs can be used to study the flexible weighting and combination of multiple sensory inputs

Lacey and colleagues (Lacey et al. 2009) posited that the LOC's representation of geometric shape was modality-independent and could be accessed flexibly by bottom-up sensory inputs or from top-down influences in frontoparietal regions. The brain could modulate the balance between top-down and bottom-up influences based on the familiarity of the object to be recognized. When objects are more familiar, the brain may superimpose templates from visual imagery to aid in the haptic identification of the object. When objects are unfamiliar, identifying them may require a stronger bottom-up input from S1. Such a mechanism is supported by the finding that, behaviourally, humans optimally weight conflicting sensory information according to the reliability of the modality (Ernst and Banks 2002).

Cross-modal attenuations also occur when input from two sensory modalities conflicts. This can manifest as a deactivation in one sensory cortex when an additional sensory cortex is brought online (Laurienti et al. 2002). This may represent top-down influences in attempting to resolve two conflicting sources of sensory information.

Hertz and Amedi (2015) capitalized on this cross-modal attenuation to make inferences about which inputs the brain weights preferentially before and after learning to use the vOICe SSD (Meijer 1992; seeingwithsound.com). Prior to learning, auditory soundscapes were uninformative, but after learning, they became informative and began to attenuate the responses in visual cortex. Non-informative inputs tend to be inhibited by informative stimuli, and when a new input became informative after learning, it then attenuated the 'veteran' sensory input. It is the informativeness of the stimulus, then, that drives the relative weighting of the sensory modality in which it is presented.

In contrast with the sensory cortices, the association cortices changed their actual sensory responses (and not just the relative attenuation) according to the change in context elicited by learning. This suggests that the brain has a stable, bottom-up system that resembles the compartmentalization of functionality seen in dividing the brain up according to sensory modality. It also, however, relies on a dynamic, context-dependent system that modulates the responses of the stable system.

6.5.3 The axis of abstraction is flipped in the ventral temporal lobe of the blind brain

In the sighted, vision is hierarchical. The LOC receives feedforward, bottom-up sensory input from V1 in order to represent complex stimuli. In the blind, however, it does not receive these inputs. Meanwhile, V1 becomes engaged in high-level cognitive functions (Amedi et al. 2003). The gradient of abstraction appears flipped, now running from anterior (where object recognition continues to reside, in the LOC) to posterior (where low-level features are normally analysed, but here memory reigns). What must have happened for the organization of the brain to change so dramatically?

In the sighted, we have seen that the LOC processes visual as well as tactile information. This indicates that it must receive projections from S1, just as it does from V1. The tracks have been laid, so to speak. In the blind, as the LOC increasingly processes tactile information and, in SSD users, auditory information, the connections between S1 or A1 and the LOC may become strengthened. This could explain why the anterior portions of the temporal lobe, where the LOC is located, take on a strong preference for sensory processing.

Amedi proposes that in localizing a strong sensory response there, it may act as an 'anchor' for development of the Braille responses in visual cortex, with tactile functionality creeping backwards into primary visual regions. This 'reverse hierarchical organization' calls into question the innateness of the visual hierarchy in the sighted. The location and organization of sensory and abstract areas in the brain may itself be determined by the nature of the inputs we receive.

In the next section, we explore how blindness results in atypical, but concrete, sensory responses being taken on by typically hierarchically higher visual regions. As with the LOC, in the absence of visual input, corticocortical connections from places like A1 and S1 may 'feed' these specialized areas. This may result in their preserved object selectivity even as V1 is co-opted for more abstract computations like verbal memory.

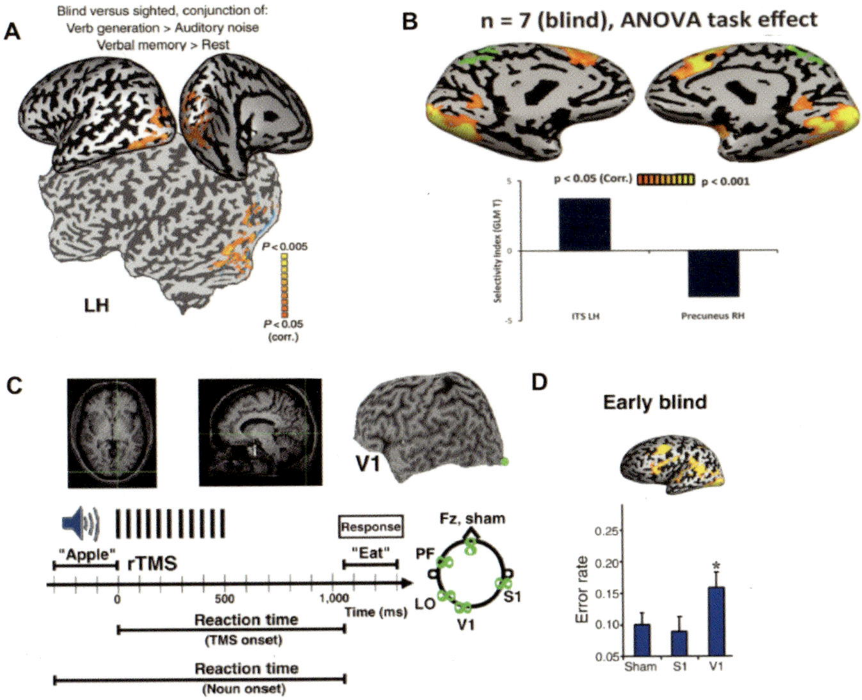

Figure 6.2 Brain scans (fMRI: functional magnetic resonance imaging) and disruptive pulses (rTMS: repetitive transcranial magnetic stimulation) were used to demonstrate brain plasticity. In the visual cortex of the blind, plasticity creates a cross-modal switch in task affinity, from processing vision to processing verbal memory and language. Two streams of visual processing also emerge in the blind brain, suggesting that this organization is not truly tied to vision. Furthermore, disrupting V1 in the blind disrupts non-visual processing.

A Areas highlighted in orange indicate differences between blind and sighted groups when searching for areas that were more active during verb generation than during auditory noise presentation AND more active during verbal memory than rest. Blind subjects relied more on early visual areas in the occipital lobe. Cerebral hemispheres are shown both as an inflated (left hemisphere only) and flattened surface. Adapted from Amedi et al. 2003.

B Top: Congenitally blind participants showed specific task selectivities consistent with the 'where' stream (green) and 'what' stream (orange). Bottom: The left inferior temporal sulcus, a 'what' stream area, prefers shapes, while the right precuneus, a 'where' stream area, prefers location. Adapted from Striem-Amit et al. 2012b.

C Top: An axial (left), saggital (middle), and surface (right) view of the site of TMS stimulation over V1 (primary visual cortex). Bottom (left): The timeline of rTMS trials. Immediately after each noun was presented, rTMS was delivered, and subjects responded with a verb. This allowed reaction times to be computed both from the onset of the noun and of the rTMS pulse. Bottom (right): Schematic of all sites where rTMS was delivered. Adapted from Amedi et al. 2004.

D Top: The pattern of fMRI activation, averaged across blind subjects, during verb generation (Amedi et al. 2003; included here to illustrate the network of rTMS sites: note that the prominent activation in V1 was not present in sighted controls). Bottom: Error rate for all rTMS sites. The star above V1 indicates a difference in the error rate between early blind subjects and sighted controls. Adapted from Amedi et al. 2004.

6.5.4 The visual word form area (VWFA) and extrastriate body area (EBA): complex ventral stream computations performed on SSD input

The visual word form area is a region located in ventral temporal cortex that is selective for words and letters (Cohen et al. 2000). It responds preferentially to words regardless of the script, language, or font used. In this part of the ventral stream, visual information has ascended the hierarchy and is now represented in complex forms.

It has been shown that in the blind the VWFA responds more strongly to Braille letters than to homogeneous Braille dots (Reich et al. 2011). In 2012, the vOICe SSD (Meijer 1992; seeingwithsound.com) was used to further test the sensory modality independence of its responses (Striem-Amit et al. 2012a). In the congenitally blind, the VWFA demonstrated a selectivity for letters presented via soundscapes over spoken words or letters. This effect is reminiscent of the LOC's responsivity to soundscapes of objects but not to the sounds these objects make. This provides evidence of the VWFA being specialized for extracting geometric information from letters in a sensory modality-independent way.

As a stricter test of this area's selectivity for the geometry of letters, the team scanned a patient who had been blind since birth and was proficient in Braille, but had never learned the shape of Hebrew letters. The patient was scanned before and after a training session in which she learned the shapes of letters. Prior to scanning, her VWFA responded robustly to Braille letters over non-letters but did not show such a response to soundscape letters over other types of soundscape. After training, however, the VWFA responded selectively to the letter soundscapes as well. It is striking that this area responded robustly after very brief training. It is even more striking that this response was observed in an adult brain, given the propensity of the brain to take on novel functionality in the absence of stimulation. This area seemed to have been ready for the novel auditory input, despite many years where it responded to tactile stimuli alone. This argues against a critical period for interpretation of the acquisition of letter geometry processing in the VWFA.

The case of the VWFA is instructive because of the high-level status of reading as a cognitive ability. Early critics surmised that it actually performed a variety of functions, as reading was unlikely to have a dedicated module within the brain. However, it seems that its selectivity for the computations underlying reading runs deeper than its selectivity for visual input. It has even been suggested that, through the recycling of object recognition machinery, the forms of the letters that humankind uses to communicate were themselves determined by our perceptual abilities (Dehaene and Cohen 2007, 2011). As highly selective areas like the VWFA may anchor the flipping of the axis of abstraction, they may even anchor the ways in which we produce ways of communicating abstract concepts in the world.

The extrastriate body area (EBA) is another ventral stream area with remarkable selectivity in the sighted: it responds robustly to the presentation of human

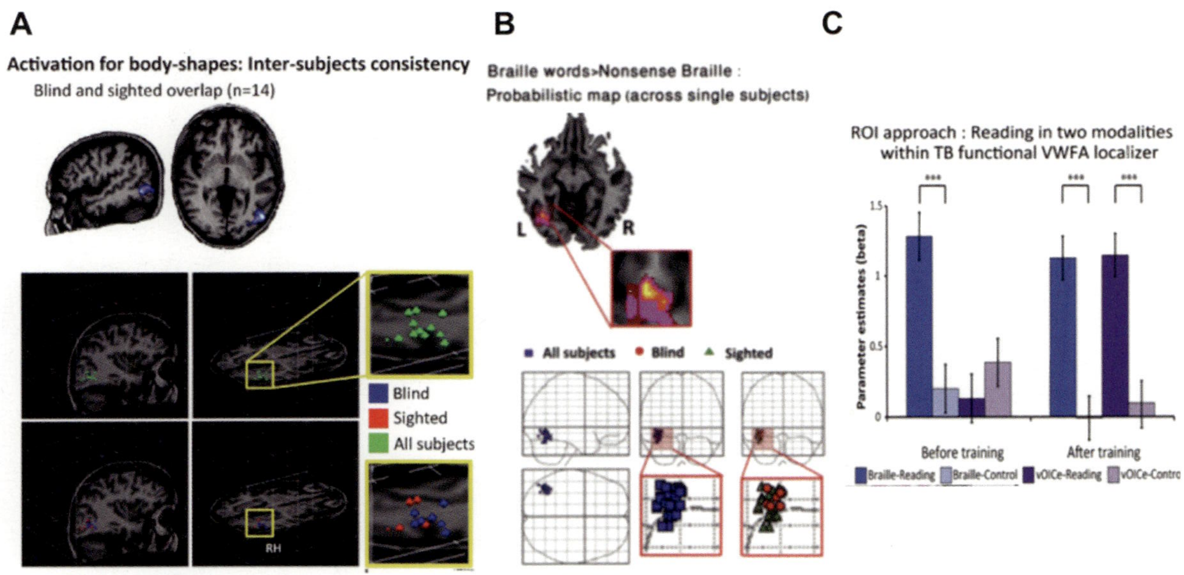

Figure 6.3 Cross-modal, sensory-independent, task-selective plasticity occurs in the extrastriate body area (EBA) for processing body shapes and in the visual word form area (VWFA) for reading visually and in Braille. This suggests that even highly specialized processing and acquired skills like reading capitalize on the brain's information processing capabilities rather than being limited to a given sensory modality.

A Top: Blue area indicates that at the location of the EBA, sighted controls and congenitally blind subjects share common activity when viewing full-body silhouettes and when listening to vOICe silhouettes, respectively. Bottom: Activity peaks for both blind and sighted subjects cluster in the EBA. The tight clustering of these peaks demonstrates the spatial reproducibility of the preference for body processing across both groups. Adapted from Striem-Amit and Amedi 2014.

B Top: A probabilistic map showing that, across all subjects, the area that most consistently showed a preference for Braille words over nonsense Braille words was the VWFA. Adapted from Reich et al. 2011. Bottom: Activity peaks for both blind and sighted subjects cluster in the VWFA, demonstrating anatomical consistency both within and between groups.

C Bars indicate the activation in the VWFA, which is greater for Braille reading before training, and equal for Braille and vOICe reading after training. This indicates that the training induced a selectivity for words in a new sensory modality, a selectivity that was previously absent. Adapted from Striem-Amit et al. 2012a.

body parts (Downing et al. 2001). Unlike reading, the perception of body postures is thought to be present even in infants (Gliga and Dehaene-Lambertz 2005). A recent study used the vOICe SSD to test the selectivity of the EBA in congenitally blind participants and sighted controls (Striem-Amit and Amedi 2014). Participants discriminated between body silhouettes in various postures. Sighted controls perceived the silhouettes visually, while the blind perceived them via soundscape. Despite the differing modality of the sensory input across the two groups, both groups activated the EBA.

In the absence of vision, how might information about the body posture of others benefit the blind? It may be involved in our ability to know the contents of other minds. This ability is referred to as Theory of Mind (ToM), and activities which rely on ToM robustly activate the temporo-parietal junction (TPJ) (Saxe and Kanwisher 2003). As it turns out, the EBA in resting participants showed activity that was highly correlated with that of the TPJ over time (Striem-Amit and Amedi 2014). Because activity in these two regions tends to sync up, it is thought that they may be anatomically connected. Regardless of input modality, the EBA may communicate important data for extracting information about people from their body postures.

The EBA, and the VWFA, serve as examples of what kinds of functions may rely on computations in the ventral stream, but not on the sensory modality of the input. Having seen a range of functions taken on by seemingly visual areas, we can begin to think of the brain as organized not according to sensory input, but according to computation. Importantly, this organization appears in the brains of sighted people, not just as the result of deprivation. In the next section we discuss the ways in which SSDs have shaped our understanding of the brain as a metamodal task machine.

6.6 The Brain as a Sensory-Independent Task Machine

6.6.1 Addressing the role of visual imagery in cross-modal activations

To confirm that the regions we have examined are truly multimodal, it is important to rule out the role of visual imagery in driving this region's responses. People blinded before the age of 6, the age at which Braille is typically learned in the congenitally blind, are considered 'early blind', while those blinded after the age of 6 are considered 'late blind'. The late blind are more likely to have a residual capacity for visual imagery. To address the role of visual imagery in activating visual cortex during auditory or tactile tasks, the late blind are often compared with the congenitally blind (for review, see Amedi et al. 2005).

An example is a verb-generation task where participants were required to generate a verb to accompany a noun presented either as a spoken-word, auditory stimulus, or as a Braille somatosensory stimulus. Sighted participants showed no visual cortex activity, whereas both early and late blind subjects recruited visual cortex (Burton et al. 2002; Burton 2003). In a later study, congenitally blind participants showed tactile responses in V1 as well as in the LOC (Amedi et al. 2010). This confirmed that visual imagery was not necessary for tactile object recognition to activate V1 or LOC. Together, these results make an imagery-based explanation for the cross-modal visual cortex activations unlikely.

One result in particular also suggests that the activations in the early blind were engaged in some work besides imagery. Counterintuitively, visual cortex recruitment was more prominent in the early blind during the cross-modal verb-generation task (Burton et al. 2002; Burton 2003). Despite the early blind participants' more limited experience with mental imagery, they nevertheless increased rather than diminished their reliance on visual cortex. It may be the case that the early blind, unlike the late blind, were blinded before entering some critical period during which cortex becomes defined as visual. This plasticity, which fades with time, may be crucial for allowing undifferentiated cortex to take on functions like memory, leading to additional compensatory recruitment of these regions (Amedi et al. 2003).

6.6.2 Common computations or common semantic content?

Another possible interpretation of the multimodal responses found in the brain is that they simply reflect the processing of shared semantic content. That is, an apple presented visually and via soundscape could simply activate a shared semantic network—the one that encodes the concept of the word *apple*. To test a region's involvement in processing semantic information, responses to meaningful and meaningless stimuli are often compared. Areas selective for meaningful content could arguably be dubbed linguistic areas. A similar test is used to compare sensory-dependent and sensory-independent response properties: If the preference for meaningful stimuli is greater than the preference for a given stimulus modality, it seems safe to say that the area is specialized for a computation rather than processing a certain sensory input. For this reason, many multimodal activations may reflect semantic processing.

There is evidence to suggest that these areas are truly processing sensory input and not semantic information. They tend not to become activated during semantic processing in the absence of sensory input. LOtv, one area thought to be multimodal in its response properties in both the blind and sighted, was not activated during verbal memory tasks in which no sensory stimulus was administered (Amedi et al. 2001, 2010). The LOC was not activated in response to the sound of objects (such as the crow of a rooster), but was activated by the visual or tactile presentation of such stimuli (Amedi et al. 2002). These tasks surely have their participants engaged in a web of semantic processing that would be difficult to voluntarily suppress, and yet they do not activate the areas where multimodal sensory processing is thought to be localized. This argues against a linguistic interpretation of its processing.

Moreover, the VWFA selectively responded to word soundscapes over spoken words. It is also selective for meaningful over meaningless Braille dots, but not meaningful over meaningless pairings in a verb-generation task. This preference seems localized to sensory processing, not semantic processing. Rather, the selective regions seem to be selective for the extraction of the spatial statistics typically conveyed visually.

Regions involved in more abstract processing may recruit these regions to perform the computations needed, using whichever sensory input modality is best. Language requires the integration of information across multiple sensory modalities. It is likely that semantic information is processed in a distributed manner across the entire cortical sheet rather than in certain specialized centres (Huth et al. 2012). Because language may be less localized than previously thought, the function of divisions between cortical areas becomes less clear. The possibility arises that the cortex itself wires up according to the sorts of computations it wants to do rather than being predisposed to any given sensory modality.

6.6.3 The brain: a mosaic of metamodal operators. Intrinsic vs. experience-imposed function

We began with a question: How much of the brain's organization is intrinsic, and how much is imposed by the statistics of the stimulus? In many instances, SSDs have been used to tease apart computations from the sensory inputs on which they are typically performed. Time after time, we have seen that the brain seems to know exactly what to do, no matter what sort of input we feed it. It has taken some doing, but these powerful demonstrations all point to a single hypothesis: The brain is a metamodal task machine, where computations are intrinsic while it is the sensory inputs that are shaped by our experiences.

Hertz and Amedi posit that 'multisensory processing can be both a highly dynamic system and a deterministic and hierarchical one' (2015: 2058). By manipulating the information, novelty, and task relevance of sensory inputs they showed that multisensory processing is comprised of 'a stable, bottom-up system, which is not context-dependent, in line with the classical view, and dynamic context-dependent elements, which modulate the stable system' (Hertz and Amedi 2015: 2058). The bottom-up system seems localized to the sensory cortices, while association cortices modulate the relative weights of their inputs. That they do this according to the informativeness of the stimulus is remarkable. This lends support to the notion that the brain will operate on whichever of its sensory inputs is richest. This flexibility is crucial even in the sighted brain, as it allows us to filter uninformative stimuli and to learn from informative stimuli. In this way, we develop expertise in processing the stimuli that best instruct the brain in how to extract the information it needs.

For as consistent as the architecture of our sensory cortices appears, then, it is surprising that the sculpting of these areas is so contingent on experience. While in some situations, blindness may represent a pathological state that can result in cross-modal plasticity, this plasticity seems to follow paths already laid out in the brain. To explain how these tracks are laid down, we turn to the idea of the brain as a set of metamodal operators (borrowing heavily from Pascual-Leone and Hamilton 2001, and see also Ricciardi et al. 2014).

Pascual-Leone and Hamilton argue that 'the brain might actually represent a metamodal structure organized as operators that execute a given function or computation regardless of sensory input modality' (2001: 427–428). Operators may be predisposed to take a certain sensory input based on how suitable that input is for the computation. This predisposition may be reinforced until each of the operators, performing its own function, becomes named for the function it performs, like 'visual' cortex.

The metamodal brain may acquire distinct functionalities by following a model they base on Robert Jacobs' Mixture of Experts (ME) architecture (Jacobs 1999). In the model, different brain networks act as 'experts' in some computation. Each time a network gets you one step closer to something useful, it learns something. Just like a person would learn something by selecting the right door in a game show, or learn from throwing a ball to hit a target spot-on. Once you've done it, you gain information about what it's like to do it. And so you get better. A network, similarly, becomes an expert in processing the stimulus that works best. The senses are differentiated competitively, with a second set of brain networks acting as 'gating' networks. The gating networks mediate the competition between the expert networks. Pascual-Leone and Hamilton write:

> If ME architecture bears any resemblance to the development of functional brain modules, it may not be the visual cortex that determines what the act of seeing will be like. Rather, it is the task of seeing that instructs the functional modules of the developing brain regarding what vision will be like, and how it must be processed. (2001: 443)

This model helps explain how our different faculties come to be, emphasizing the extent to which they rely on the inputs we receive. Because vision provides a rich substrate for computations, it comes to dominate major portions of the brain. We see the consequences of this process most clearly when vision is removed from competition, but it is likely that what we are seeing reflects a subtle, but present, pattern of wiring that exists even in visually dominated brains.

In situations where primary sensory cortices take on responsivity to a new sensory modality, it is likely that this represents true *de novo* cross-modal plasticity.

However, for instance, when a region like the LOC responds during haptic object recognition while the primary visual cortex does the work of verbal memory, we see changes in extant wiring lead to plasticity. The two processes form a continuum. In this case, the ventral temporal object-selective cortex, cut off from visual input, is allowed to strengthen its connections to somatosensory and (using SSDs) auditory cortex. This may happen by cortical mechanisms as when one modality's 'territory' encroaches onto that of another modality (for example, Klinge et al. 2010). This process parallels intramodal plasticity, such as when the representation of the reading index finger in the brains of Braille readers becomes enlarged despite the fingerpad being no more sensitive to the stimulation as measured by a sensory threshold test (Pascual-Leone and Torres 1993). In corticocortical cross-modal plasticity, the functionality of cortex devoted to one modality creeps into areas usually devoted to a different modality.

In the example of the LOC, its intensified tactile responsivity is thought to 'anchor' sensory processing in this region. The hierarchy of increasingly abstract processing that usually emanates from V1 now emanates from the LOC, spreading its abstractions back into the unemployed primary visual cortex. While it is true that this constitutes a novel formation of wiring, it did not come from nowhere. Pascual-Leone and Hamilton suggest:

> [T]he many studies that demonstrate processing of sensory information outside of the classically reorganized cortical boundaries for that modality may not be examples of the brain being redundant or 'getting its wires crossed,' but instead may represent the workings of an efficient metamodal brain, which uses inputs to those cortical regions (operators) that seem best suited to execute their computations successfully.
>
> (2001: 443)

It is this continuum, from the extant, sensory-independent predispositions of the uninstructed cortex to the information carried by sensory modalities, along which we see the push and pull of intrinsic and experience-dependent factors. SSDs used in the blind have served to chart this territory, mapping the spectrum of what is possible rather than what is considered normal.

It is here that we can find the answer to a very old problem of neuroscience and philosophy known as Molyneux's question (as described in Pascual-Leone and Hamilton 2001). Posed in a 1688 letter to John Locke, Molyneux's famous question asks whether a blind person whose sight were to suddenly be restored would be able to recognize objects based on the similarities between the new visual representation and their other representations. Would they, for instance, be able to point to which of the two objects they had just palpated was the globe, and which the cube? Even if their visual apparati could be made perfect, would their perception and their recollection know how to line up in the brain? In the next section, we will explore the ways in which SSDs may be used in future rehabilitation work, particularly in restoring functionality following sight restoration surgery.

The insights about the brain which we have gained so far may serve as the basis for the development of new techniques.

6.7 Implications for Rehabilitation

6.7.1 SSDs are improving the quality of life of blind users

SSDs can provide their users with a greatly improved quality of life. Using SSDs, blind people can point to targets, recognize patterns, perform motion discrimination and tracking tasks, extract depth cues, estimate object distance, recognize objects, and detect and avoid obstacles in a course (Reich et al. 2012). Users are able to exceed the World Health Organization (WHO) threshold for blindness (Striem-Amit et al. 2012c). Some proficient SSD users even report the feeling of visual qualia when using SSDs (Bubic et al. 2010; Ward and Meijer 2010).

Work is being done to improve auditory-to-visual SSDs in three main ways: the aesthetics of the stimuli presented; the accuracy with which their (sighted) users can match sounds and images as a test of the translation's fidelity; and the accuracy with which their users can discriminate between similar images, as a test of acuity (Wright and Ward 2013). EyeMusic, for instance, adds colour information to facilitate object recognition and the accurate segmentation of parts of the visual scene (Abboud et al. 2014). It also conveys this information using pleasant tones that do not fatigue the user as easily as the complex, alien soundscapes of older devices.

6.7.2 SSDs may be used to train circuits in preparation for sight restoration surgery

However, the utility of SSDs is not limited to their stand-alone use. They may also be used in tandem with sight restoration surgery to facilitate rehabilitation of visual function. Advances in surgical and prosthetic means of restoring visual input include the transplantation of photoreceptors (Yang et al. 2010), gene therapy (Busskamp et al. 2010), and retinal prostheses ('bionic eyes') (Ahuja et al. 2011; and for review, see Rizzo 2011). However, just because the visual apparatus provides a new input does not necessarily mean that the brain will be able to interpret it. The brains of the blind may be ill-prepared to process the new input. Molyneux's question seems more relevant than ever in light of these advances: Can a person whose sight has been restored make use of their vision right away, or must they learn to interpret the signals? For objects that have become familiar to them in the tactile or auditory domain, how can they integrate their novel perceptions with their recollections?

As it turns out, not all visual function is acquired equally easily. Pascual-Leone and Hamilton (2001) describe the patient who underwent one of the early surgeries to restore vision in 1728. The boy 'had no idea of space or size, and found it remarkably difficult to recognise and remember the visual form of objects, and had to constantly relate them to his previously acquired tactile impressions'. He was unable to recognize the house cat until he was able to pick it up. At this point, he stared at the cat while palpating it, seeming to try to commit to memory the novel visual information and tie it to his tactile representation. Object recognition abilities, in particular, must be learned through experience.

Dorsal stream functions like orienting to moving stimuli tend to be accessed relatively readily in the newly sighted, but ventral stream processes such as object recognition are more elusive (see Lewis and Maurer 2005 for review). Even after months of training, ventral stream functions can still be deficient (Fine et al. 2003; Gregory 2003; Ostrovsky et al. 2006, 2009). Striem-Amit and colleagues (2012b) demonstrated robust ventral stream activation to shape recognition tasks performed using SSDs. This activation extended into primary visual regions. However, the dorsal stream activations were weaker and did not extend to V1. This may be the result of the dorsal stream completing its development earlier in life (see Lewis and Maurer 2005 for review). The ventral stream is plastic far later in life and has longer periods where it is susceptible to being moulded by its inputs. This makes it more likely that it can quickly reorganize to respond to its new auditory input when listening to soundscapes, for instance (Amedi et al. 2007; Striem-Amit et al. 2012b). However, it also means that the ventral stream of the blind has a long way to go in acquiring visual function that, in the sighted, takes years of experience.

Furthermore, there may be cross-modal plasticity to contend with. The blind brain compensates with new connections and functions which may be impossible to effectively identify and work around. If the goal is to make a region process visual input, it may first have to 'unlearn' whatever sensory modality it has come to specialize in in the absence of vision. It may even have to make the switch from performing abstract, memory-related functions to sensory processing (Amedi et al. 2003). It may be too late, or too difficult, to overcome these changes. In this way, for the blind, plasticity is a double-edged sword: it allows them to compensate for their loss of function, but it is possible that it closes doors for future rehabilitation (Merabet and Pascual-Leone 2010).

The brain fights against both critical periods and cross-modal plasticity in its ability to acquire visual function late in life. However, the readiness with which SSDs can instruct cortex to process new input gives reason for hope. Recall that the auditory cortex of re-wired ferrets was able to take on complex visual response properties, suggesting that the sensory input did not merely influence but actually instructed the cortical circuits in establishing their new organization (Roe et al. 1992).

It is possible, then, that the cortex can be awakened to visual input if it has the proper instruction beforehand. SSDs may be used to shake loose the grip of whatever functions may have encroached on the cortex and trained it to perform new functions. By feeding the cortex information through, for instance, a soundscape, the cortex can 'practise' extracting spatial information. This training may prepare the brain for the kinds of computations it will have to perform on visual inputs. Because of the brain's metamodal organization, it may be possible to exercise an area by having it practise a certain computation. Specific regions may be prepared to extract certain types of information based on the task at hand: for example, the task of reading letters, in the case of the VWFA. In a patient scheduled to undergo sight restoration surgery, extracting the information may teach the cortex to serve as a general 'sensory interpreter' (Striem-Amit et al. 2012b; Maidenbaum et al. 2014). In this role, its job would be to explain the new inputs to other brain networks involved in abstraction, so that the region becomes skilled at matching up its outputs with higher-level conceptual machinery.

6.7.3 SSDs may provide multimodal augmentation following sight restoration surgery

SSDs may also be used after sight restoration surgery to augment the new visual inputs. Whereas a patient's training before surgery could help them match their visual perceptions with their auditory recollections after surgery, they may find it helpful to receive continued auditory input after surgery and may benefit from the continued use of the SSD as a guide to the objects and environments they encounter. Even a patient who begins using the SSD only after surgery may find such augmentation useful, as the coincidences across sensory inputs may themselves be helpful.

Cross-modal enhancement can occur when inputs from two sensory modalities are in accordance. An enhancement refers to a situation where the presence of one sensory input increases the response of another sensory cortex (Fu et al. 2003; Kayser and Logothetis 2007). For example, cross-modal binding can occur to create a unified percept as you watch someone's lips move and simultaneously hear what they are saying, amplifying the auditory cortex's response (Calvert et al. 1999). This can even occur during silent lip-reading (Calvert et al. 1997). Such enhancement could occur via bottom-up coincidence detection. It is possible, then, that such coincidences could speed the acquisition of visual processing skills.

We have seen that SSDs may be useful on their own. They may also be used in preparation for sight restoration. Finally, SSD use following sight restoration may serve to provide computational practice as well as enhance the processing of a new sensory modality by cross-modal enhancement. The more these devices are used, the more information researchers acquire to help target and improve their use. In this way, experimentation and therapy form a mutually beneficial positive feedback loop for progress. Experiments that employ SSDs have shed invaluable new light on how the brain organizes and reorganizes itself. As our understanding of these processes grows more sophisticated, we can in turn apply this knowledge to make improvements that have real benefits for patients the world over.

6.8 Conclusion

We have seen many striking ways in which SSDs have contributed new evidence to either corroborate or disprove previous claims about the organization of function in the brain. Currently, these devices are primarily used in laboratory settings to answer experimental questions. This may change over time. As we amass evidence for the boundaries of *de novo* cross-modal plasticity and plasticity within extant cross-modal pathways, we advance our understanding of how these devices can be used therapeutically.

Because blindness does result in cross-modal plasticity, and because this plasticity can be so remarkably thorough in transforming a given cortical region's functions, it initially seems as though the blind are unique in developing compensatory adaptations. Much of the response taken on by primary visual cortex may in fact reflect *de novo* cross-modal plasticity. However, as we have seen, this plasticity often follows the pathways laid down by the brain's extant cross-modal connections. In this sense, multimodal association areas come to serve as specialists in their remaining sensory inputs, strengthening these connections and ultimately serving as sensory 'anchors' for abstract functions which can become localized in the unemployed primary visual cortex. These processes are far from distinct—they are intimately linked.

The reorganization seen in the blind brain provides a valuable window into the brain's intrinsic computations. In the absence of visual influence, we can find out which processes are contingent on sensory experience, and we can find out which are computations to which the brain is intrinsically predisposed. To this end, SSDs provide a powerful means of manipulating sensory input. It is difficult to imagine a technique better suited for testing these questions than SSDs, as they allow us to tease out the influence of sensory modality. Presenting stimuli in atypical modalities can reveal a region's response invariance across sensory modalities, as can be seen in multimodal sensory cortices. Alternatively, a region may demonstrate pure selectivity for a given stimulus modality, as is seen in the primary sensory cortices of the sighted. A region may respond with something in between abstract and sensory responses if it displays multimodal sensory responses. These regions are well positioned to mediate the transfer of information from sensory to abstract networks, and can often provide flexible bridges between top-down and bottom-up processes. From the continuum from sensory to multimodal sensory to abstract processing regions, we can infer a continuum of stimulus-imposed, sensory- or experience-dependent function at one end, to intrinsic, sensory- and experience-independent function at the other.

Perhaps the greatest surprise that these experiments have revealed is that the brain may not be comprised of specialized sensory modules after all. On the contrary, it seems more committed to performing defined computations than it does to processing specific sensory inputs. The developing brain may wire up according to the results of competition between sensory inputs. By comparing across sighted, congenitally blind, early blind, and late blind participants, we can learn about the role of critical periods in brain development. Which series of events must occur in which critical periods in order for an organism's sensory processing to be on par with that of its conspecifics? What happens when these requirements are not met? How does the brain adapt to its increased reliance on alternative inputs and strategies? What is the role of cross-modal plasticity?

One open question is whether common or distinct mechanisms drive thalamocortical and corticocortical cross-modal plasticity. Cross-modal plasticity induced via thalamocortical means, as in the ferret re-wiring studies, may differ in key ways from corticocortical plasticity, as when neighbouring regions' activity encroaches upon idle territory. By comparing across cleverly designed tasks, we can dissociate situations in which these mechanisms play different roles. This approach comes to us as part of a larger project of dissociating input from computation in the brain. In doing so, we are coming to an ever-clearer understanding of the role of experience in shaping the mind. Thus far, the use of SSDs in service of this dissociation has yielded many insights as to how the brain self-organizes. It does so, in exquisite detail, through a mix of intrinsically suited operators and competing sensory inputs.

References

Abboud, S., Hanassy, S., Levy-Tzedek, S., Maidenbaum, S. and Amedi, A. (2014) EyeMusic: introducing a 'visual' colorful experience for the blind using auditory sensory substitution. *Restorative Neurology and Neuroscience* 32: 247–257.

Ahuja, A. K., Dorn, J. D., Caspi, A., McMahon, M. J., Dagnelie, G., Dacruz, L., Stanga, P., Humayun, M. S., Greenberg, R. J. and Argus II Study Group (2011) Blind subjects implanted with the Argus II retinal prosthesis are able to improve performance in a spatial-motor task. *British Journal of Ophthalmology* 95: 539–543.

Amedi, A., Malach, R., Hendler, T., Peled, S. and Zohary, E. (2001) Visuo-haptic object-related activation in the ventral visual pathway. *Nature Neuroscience* 4: 324–330.

Amedi, A., Jacobson, G., Hendler, T., Malach, R. and Zohary, E. (2002) Convergence of visual and tactile shape processing in the human lateral occipital complex. *Cerebral Cortex* 12: 1202–1212.

Amedi, A., Raz, N., Pianka, P., Malach, R. and Zohary, E. (2003) Early 'visual' cortex activation correlates with superior verbal memory performance in the blind. *Nature Neuroscience* 6: 758–766.

Amedi, A., Floel, A., Knecht, S., Zohary, E. and Cohen, L. G. (2004) Transcranial magnetic stimulation of the occipital pole interferes with verbal processing in blind subjects. *Nature Neuroscience* 7(11): 1266–1270.

Amedi, A., Von Kriegstein, K., Van Atteveldt, N., Beauchamp, M. S. and Naumer, M. J. (2005) Functional imaging of human crossmodal identification and object recognition. *Experimental Brain Research* 166: 559–571.

Amedi, A., Stern, W. M., Camprodon, J. A., Bermpohl, F., Merabet, L., Rotman, S., Hemond, C., Meijer, P. and Pascual-Leone, A. (2007) Shape conveyed by visual-to-auditory sensory substitution activates the lateral occipital complex. *Nature Neuroscience* 10: 687–689.

Amedi, A., Raz, N., Azulay, H., Malach, R. and Zohary, E. (2010) Cortical activity during tactile exploration of objects in blind and sighted humans. *Restorative Neurology and Neuroscience* 28: 143–156.

Bach-y-Rita, P. and Kercel, S. W. (2003) Sensory substitution and the human-machine interface. *Trends in Cognitive Science* 7: 541–546.

Bach-y-Rita, P., Collins, C. C., Saunders, F. A., White, B. and Scadden, L. (1969) Vision substitution by tactile image projection. *Nature* 221: 963–964.

Bubic, A., Striem-Amit, E. and Amedi, A. (2010) Large-scale brain plasticity following blindness and the use of sensory substitution devices. In M. J. Naumer and J. Kaiser (eds) *Multisensory Object Perception in the Primate Brain*. New York: Springer, 351–380.

Burton, H. (2003) Visual cortex activity in early and late blind people. *Journal of Neuroscience* 23: 4005–4011.

Burton, H., Snyder, A. Z., Diamond, J. B. and Raichle, M. E. (2002) Adaptive changes in early and late blind: a fMRI study of verb generation to heard nouns. *Journal of Neurophysiology* 88: 3359–3371.

Busskamp, V., Duebel, J., Balya, D., Fradot, M., Viney, T. J., Siegert, S., Groner, A. C., Cabuy, E., Forster, V., Seeliger, M., Biel, M., Humphries, P., Paques, M., Mohand-Said, S., Trono, D., Deisseroth, K., Sahel, J. A., Picaud, S. and Roska, B. (2010) Genetic reactivation of cone photoreceptors restores visual responses in retinitis pigmentosa. *Science* 329: 413–417.

Calvert, G. A. and Thesen, T. (2004) Multisensory integration: methodological approaches and emerging principles in the human brain. *Journal of Physiology—Paris* 98: 191–205.

Calvert, G. A., Bullmore, E. T., Brammer, M. J., Campbell, R., Williams, S. C., McGuire, P. K., Woodruff, P. W., Iversen, S. D. and David, A. S. (1997) Activation of auditory cortex during silent lipreading. *Science* 276: 593–596.

Calvert, G. A., Brammer, M. J., Bullmore, E. T., Campbell, R., Iversen, S. D. and David, A. S. (1999) Response amplification in sensory-specific cortices during crossmodal binding. *Neuroreport* 10: 2619–2623.

Cohen, L. G., Celnik, P., Pascual-Leone, A., Corwell, B., Falz, L., Dambrosia, J., Honda, M., Sadato, N., Gerloff, C., Catalá, M. D. and Hallett, M. (1997) Functional relevance of cross-modal plasticity in blind humans. *Nature* 389: 180–183.

Cohen, L., Dehaene, S., Naccache, L., Lehéricy, S., Dehaene-Lambertz, G., Hénaff, M. A. and Michel, F. (2000) The visual word form area: spatial and temporal characterisation of an initial stage of reading in normal subjects and posterior split-brain patients. *Brain* 123(Pt 2): 291–307.

Dehaene, S. and Cohen, L. (2007) Cultural recycling of cortical maps. *Neuron* 56: 384–398.

Dehaene, S. and Cohen, L. (2011) The unique role of the visual word form area in reading. *Trends in Cognitive Science* 15: 254–262.

Downing, P. E., Jiang, Y., Shuman, M. and Kanwisher, N. (2001) A cortical area selective for visual processing of the human body. *Science* 293: 2470–2473.

Ernst, M. O. and Banks, M. S. (2002) Humans integrate visual and haptic information in a statistically optimal fashion. *Nature* 415: 429–433.

Fine, I., Wade, A. R., Brewer, A. A., May, M. G., Goodman, D. F., Boynton, G. M., Wandell, B. A. and MacLeod, D.I.A. (2003) Long-term deprivation affects visual perception and cortex. *Nature Neuroscience* 6: 915–916.

Fu, K.-M. G., Johnston, T. A., Shah, A. S., Arnold, L., Smiley, J., Hackett, T. A., Garraghty, P. E. and Schroeder, C. E. (2003) Auditory cortical neurons respond to somatosensory stimulation. *Journal of Neuroscience* 23: 7510–7515.

Gall, F. J. and Spurzheim, J. C. (1835) *On the Function of the Brain and Each of its Parts: with Observations on the Possibility of Determining the Instincts, Propensities and Talents, or the Moral and Intellectual Dispositions of Men and Animals, by the Configuration of the Brain and Head*. Boston: March, Capen, and Lyon.

Gliga, T. and Dehaene-Lambertz, G. (2005) Structural encoding of body and face in human infants and adults. *Journal of Cognitive Neuroscience* 17: 1328–1340.

Goodale, M. A. and Milner, A. D. (1992) Separate visual pathways for perception and action. *Trends in Neuroscience* 15: 20–25.

Gregory, R. L. (2003) Seeing after blindness. *Nature Neuroscience* 6: 909–910.

Hamilton, R. H. and Pascual-Leone, A. (1998) Cortical plasticity associated with Braille learning. *Trends in Cognitive Science* 2: 168–174.

Hamilton, R., Keenan, J. P., Catala, M. and Pascual-Leone, A. (2000) Alexia for Braille following bilateral occipital stroke in an early blind woman. *Neuroreport* 11: 237–240.

Hertz, U. and Amedi, A. (2015) Flexibility and stability in sensory processing revealed using visual-to-auditory sensory substitution. *Cerebral Cortex* 25(8): 2049–2064.

Hubel, D. H. and Wiesel, T. N. (1963) Receptive fields of cells in striate cortex of very young, visually inexperienced kittens. *Journal of Neurophysiology* 26: 994–1002.

Huth, A. G., Nishimoto, S., Vu, A. T. and Gallant, J. L. (2012) A continuous semantic space describes the representation of thousands of object and action categories across the human brain. *Neuron* 76: 1210–1224.

Jacobs, R. (1999) Computational studies of the development of functionally specialised neural modules. *Trends in Cognitive Science* 3: 31–38.

Kayser, C. and Logothetis, N. K. (2007) Do early sensory cortices integrate cross-modal information? *Brain Structure and Function* 212: 121–132.

Klinge, C., Eippert, F., Röder, B. and Büchel, C. (2010) Corticocortical connections mediate primary visual cortex responses to auditory stimulation in the blind. *Journal of Neuroscience* 30: 12798–12805.

Kuchinsky, S. E., Vaden, K. I., Jr, Keren, N. I., Harris, K. C., Ahlstrom, J. B., Dubno, J. R. and Eckert, M. A. (2012) Word intelligibility and age predict visual cortex activity during word listening. *Cerebral Cortex* 22: 1360–1371.

Lacey, S., Tal, N., Amedi, A. and Sathian, K. (2009) A putative model of multisensory object representation. *Brain Topography* 21: 269–274.

Lakoff, G. (1980) *Metaphors We Live By*. Chicago: University of Chicago Press.

Laurienti, P. J., Burdette, J. H., Wallace, M. T., Yen, Y.-F., Field, A. S. and Stein, B. E. (2002) Deactivation of sensory-specific cortex by cross-modal stimuli. *Journal of Cognitive Neuroscience* 14: 420–429.

Lewis, T. L. and Maurer, D. (2005) Multiple sensitive periods in human visual development: evidence from visually deprived children. *Developmental Psychobiology* 46: 163–183.

Lilly, J. (1977) *The Deep Self: Consciousness Exploration in the Isolation Tank*. New York: Simon and Schuster.

Maidenbaum, S., Abboud, S. and Amedi, A. (2014) Sensory substitution: closing the gap between basic research and widespread practical visual rehabilitation. *Neuroscience and Biobehavioral Reviews* 41: 3–15.

Meijer, P. B. (1992) An experimental system for auditory image representations. *IEEE Transactions on Biomedical Engineering* 39: 112–121.

Merabet, L. B. and Pascual-Leone, A. (2010) Neural reorganisation following sensory loss: the opportunity of change. *Nature Reviews Neuroscience* 11: 44–52.

Métin, C. and Frost, D. O. (1989) Visual responses of neurons in somatosensory cortex of hamsters with experimentally induced retinal projections to somatosensory thalamus. *Proceedings of the National Academy of Sciences USA* 86: 357–361.

Ostrovsky, Y., Andalman, A. and Sinha, P. (2006) Vision following extended congenital blindness. *Psychological Science* 17: 1009–1014.

Ostrovsky, Y., Meyers, E., Ganesh, S., Mathur, U. and Sinha, P. (2009) Visual parsing after recovery from blindness. *Psychological Science* 20: 1484–1491.

Pascual-Leone, A. and Hamilton, R. (2001) The metamodal organisation of the brain. *Progress in Brain Research* 134: 427–445.

Pascual-Leone, A. and Torres, F. (1993) Plasticity of the sensorimotor cortex representation of the reading finger in Braille readers. *Brain* 116(Pt 1): 39–52.

Pascual-Leone, A., Walsh, V. and Rothwell, J. (2000) Transcranial magnetic stimulation in cognitive neuroscience—virtual lesion, chronometry, and functional connectivity. *Current Opinion in Neurobiology* 10: 232–237.

Pascual-Leone, A., Amedi, A., Fregni, F. and Merabet, L. B. (2005) The plastic human brain cortex. *Annual Review of Neuroscience* 28: 377–401.

Phelps, M. E., Mazziotta, J. C., Kuhl, D. E., Nuwer, M., Packwood, J., Metter, J. and Engel, J., Jr (1981) Tomographic mapping of human cerebral metabolism visual stimulation and deprivation. *Neurology* 31: 517–529.

Reich, L., Szwed, M., Cohen, L. and Amedi, A. (2011) A ventral visual stream reading center independent of visual experience. *Current Biology* 21: 363–368.

Reich, L., Maidenbaum, S. and Amedi, A. (2012) The brain as a flexible task machine: implications for visual rehabilitation using noninvasive vs. invasive approaches. *Current Opinion in Neurology* 25: 86–95.

Ricciardi, E., Bonino, D., Pellegrini, S. and Pietrini, P. (2014) Mind the blind brain to understand the sighted one! Is there a supramodal cortical functional architecture? *Neuroscience and Biobehavioral Reviews* 41: 64–77.

Rizzo, J. F., 3rd (2011) Update on retinal prosthetic research: the Boston Retinal Implant Project. *Journal of Neuroophthalmology* 31: 160–168.

Roe, A. W., Pallas, S. L., Kwon, Y. H. and Sur, M. (1992) Visual projections routed to the auditory pathway in ferrets: receptive fields of visual neurons in primary auditory cortex. *Journal of Neuroscience* 2: 3651–3664.

Sadato, N., Pascual-Leone, A., Grafman, J., Ibañez, V., Deiber, M. P., Dold, G. and Hallett, M. (1996) Activation of the primary visual cortex by Braille reading in blind subjects. *Nature* 380: 526–528.

Saxe, R. and Kanwisher, N. (2003) People thinking about thinking people. The role of the temporo-parietal junction in 'theory of mind'. *NeuroImage* 19: 1835–1842.

Striem-Amit, E. and Amedi, A. (2014) Visual cortex extrastriate body-selective area activation in congenitally blind people 'seeing' by using sounds. *Current Biology* 24: 687–692.

Striem-Amit, E., Cohen, L., Dehaene, S. and Amedi, A. (2012a) Reading with sounds: sensory substitution selectively activates the visual word form area in the blind. *Neuron* 76: 640–652.

Striem-Amit, E., Dakwar, O., Reich, L. and Amedi, A. (2012b) The large-scale organisation of 'visual' streams emerges without visual experience. *Cerebral Cortex* 22: 1698–1709.

Striem-Amit, E., Guendelman, M. and Amedi, A. (2012c) 'Visual' acuity of the congenitally blind using visual-to-auditory sensory substitution. *PLoS One* 7: e33136.

Ungerleider, L. G. and Mishkin, M. (1982) Two cortical visual systems. In D. J. Ingle, M. A. Goodale and R. J. W. Mansfield (eds) *Analysis of Visual Behavior*. Boston: MIT Press, 549–586.

Wanet-Defalque, M. C., Veraart, C., De Volder, A., Metz, R., Michel, C., Dooms, G. and Goffinet, A. (1988) High metabolic activity in the visual cortex of early blind human subjects. *Brain Research* 446: 369–373.

Ward, J. and Meijer, P. (2010) Visual experiences in the blind induced by an auditory sensory substitution device. *Consciousness and Cognition* 19: 492–500.

Wright, T. and Ward, J. (2013) The evolution of a visual-to-auditory sensory substitution device using interactive genetic algorithms. *Quarterly Journal of Experimental Psychology* (Hove) 66: 1620–1638.

Yang, Y., Mohand-Said, S., Léveillard, T., Fontaine, V., Simonutti, M. and Sahel, J.-A. (2010) Transplantation of photoreceptor and total neural retina preserves cone function in P23H rhodopsin transgenic rat. *PLoS One* 5: e13469.

7

Sensory Substitution Devices and Behavioural Transference: A Commentary on Recent Work from the Lab of Amir Amedi

DEREK BROWN

Abstract Sensory substitution devices (SSDs) are most familiar from their use with subjects who are deficient in a target modality (e.g. congenitally blind subjects), but there is no doubt that the use and potential value of SSDs extend to persons without such deficits. Recent work by Amedi and his team (in particular Levy-Tzedek et al. 2012) has begun to explore this. Their idea is that SSDs may facilitate behavioural transference (BT) across sense modalities. In this case, a motor skill learned through visual perception might be subsequently employed in response to auditory perception, using an SSD as a mediator. They infer from the existence of such BT that the learned skill is amodally represented. After a brief overview I identify ways to more fully test for BT within this experimental paradigm and argue that their conclusion about amodal representation is premature. Additionally, I argue that their preferred SSD (Eyemusic) is of limited value for the project. While my remarks are critical, my intention is to be constructive, particularly in light of the fact that Levy-Tzedek et al. (2012) is, I believe, the first output from Amedi's lab concerning this line of research.

7.1 Introduction

In everyday life many motor skills are learned and implemented in reaction to multimodal stimuli: hunting, driving and most sports typically utilize at least visual, auditory and tactile information; foraging, cooking and gardening utilize at least visual, tactile and olfactory information if not also gustatory information; and so on. This is possible because these behaviours are in reaction to parts of the

Proceedings of the British Academy, **219**, 122–129.

world that are accessible to many modalities. While these are complex behaviours, they are common, and they reinforce a conception of motor skills as skills that are standardly developed and informed by many modalities. By contrast, thinking of specific motor skills as generally developed in alliance with a single modality, while perhaps beneficial for controlled experimentation, seems artificial. In this regard, since the relevant idea of behavioural transference (BT) presumes an initial skill–modality pairing, it presumes a phenomenon that may not be naturally widespread.

Nonetheless, should we antecedently expect BT in the right conditions? If each motor skill were allied with a specific modality, then perhaps we would generally not expect BT. However, given that motor skills are often learned and implemented in reaction to the excitation of multiple modalities, one might expect BT when opportunity arises, however rarely that may be. This is one reason to doubt the hypothesis of Levy-Tzedek et al.,[1] that 'A priori, there is *no reason* to assume that [BT would occur]' in their experiment (p. 1, italics added). The point is not that this area of research is uninteresting or of little value. It is that its value likely doesn't lie in the potential to demonstrate the presence of BT. The interest isn't in the existential question 'Is there transference of learned behaviour across modalities?', for the answer is, antecedently, plausibly yes. The interest is instead in questions that arise from this positive response, questions such as:

(1) How much does this transference occur, across which modalities, and in which directions (section 7.3)?
(2) How important are sensory substitution devices (SSDs) to this area of research (section 7.4)?
(3) What models of storage, retrieval and utilization of learned behaviours are consonant with the data that emerges from studying (1) and (2) (section 7.5)?

7.2 Interlude: Experimental Paradigm

Levy-Tzedek et al. utilized the Eyemusic visual-auditory SSD device. The device plays *soundscapes*, auditory stimuli lasting a few seconds that represent a scan of the subject's immediate frontal environment. It is governed by three mapping rules: the spatial dimension of low–high height (relative to subject) is represented by low–high pitch; the spatial dimension of left–right is represented by earlier–later auditory tones; colours are represented by timbre. For example, a high tone at the beginning of a soundscape represents a feature that is at the top left of the

[1] All references are to: Levy-Tzedek, S., I. Novick, R. Arbel, S. Abboud, S. Maidenbaum, E. Vaadia and A. Amedi (2012) Cross-sensory transfer of sensory-motor information: visuomotor learning affects performance on an audiomotor task, using sensory-substitution. *Scientific Reports* 2: 49. doi: 10.1038/srep00949.

subject's environment, a low tone at the end of a soundscape represents a feature at the bottom right of the subject's environment, and a saxophone might represent blue. Colour–timbre mappings will not be important to our discussion.

Here is a rough summary of the experiment reported in Levy-Tzedek et al. (2012). Subjects were asked to move a *cursor* to a *target* using a quick joystick movement. The task had both a visual (using a computer screen) and an auditory (using Eyemusic) condition, with a crucial difference: in the visual condition subjects received *feedback* in that they could perceive the endpoint reached by the cursor in response to joystick movement; in the auditory condition this feedback was absent. After a baseline was established, a *rotation* was introduced which skewed the effect of joystick movement on the movement of the cursor. In the visual condition, because of the feedback subjects could perceive the rotational skew and learn to compensate; in the auditory they could not. Thus, as subjects learned to compensate for the rotation in the visual condition, the extent to which that learning transferred across modalities to the auditory condition could be measured. If the learned behaviour was modality-specific, it should not impact performance during the auditory condition. By contrast if the learned behaviour was not modality-specific, it should be available for and somewhat impact the auditory condition.

Robust levels of BT were observed.

Using this experimental paradigm as a model for this area of research, two constraints are utilized:

(a) *Multimodal accessibility of stimuli.* The relevant stimuli (cursor and target) must be accessible by more than one modality.
(b) *Feedback variation.* The novel factor that demands behavioural learning (rotational effect) must be perceivable in one modality and not in the other.

The first constraint ensures that the task can be performed via either modality, and the second that the extent to which subjects learn in response to the novel factor is confined to a single modality. Combined, these constraints allow us to measure BT across modalities in an interesting way.

7.3 Transference Magnitude, Breadth and Direction

Let me proceed with a cautionary remark about the experiment. Hand movements are not generally tied to a specific modality. Instead such movements are routinely made using at least visual and auditory (not to mention tactile) perceptions. Videogames (a familiar domain for joysticks) are a fine example of this: trying to play a game with the sound muted after having learned to play it with both visual and auditory cues often yields (anecdotally) at least a temporary performance change. In the experiment, subjects engage in several repetitive small hand movements in response to visual and subsequently to auditory stimuli, knowing (at least implicitly) that feedback is present in the former and not in the latter condition. If in the feedback condition a subject (even if unconsciously) adjusts her behaviour to counteract the novel factor and is then switched to the non-feedback condition, it should *not* be surprising if behavioural adjustments transfer to the latter. Feedback is lacking in the auditory condition, and so to some extent the subject is guessing as to which motion will achieve the desired result, and her best sample for success is the motions she performed in the visual condition where she received feedback. Indeed there should be no expectation that she *disregard* her feedback data and instead try to recall her behaviours from previous non-feedback trials. Instead, 'Do what I did when I had feedback' should be expected in non-feedback conditions. Therefore, as generally argued above, in this paradigm BT across modalities is antecedently expected, and its absence would be surprising. Let me suggest how the paradigm might generate more sophisticated results, in an effort to address (1).

Obvious questions about behavioural transference emerge. Is the magnitude of visual-auditory BT dependent on the specifics of the task? Does BT happen symmetrically (from auditory to visual in addition to visual to auditory)? Does BT happen across other modality pairs, beyond the auditory-visual pair? There is in principle no difficulty in testing these questions, once it is recognized that multimodal accessibility and feedback variation are sufficient constraints for the program. However, doing so requires recognizing the limitations of the Eyemusic device.

Symmetry. To test for the extent to which visual-auditory transference is symmetrical one must design a feedback auditory condition and a non-feedback visual one. The latter is straightforward: simply do not display on the screen where the cursor moves in response to joystick movement. In theory the former is equally straightforward. We require two auditory dimensions to which left–right and forward–back joystick movement can correspond. Many are available, some more suitable for the task than others, including: pitch; perceived left–right location; perceived height location; loudness; timbre; and so on. Consider an example using pitch and perceived left–right location. One could simultaneously play two, sustained spatially-located tones for the subject, one higher-pitched and to the left of the subject, and one lower-pitched and at the subject's location. The latter can serve as cursor and the former as target. The cursor pitch can then move in response to forward–back joystick movement, and the left–right cursor location in response to left–right joystick movement. For ease of reference call this set of abstract constraints auditory feedback system (AFS). The subject's task can be to move the cursor to the target's pitch and location. Subjects can be taught an analogous but non-feedback visual task. After brief training, trials can begin that induce a rotational effect in the auditory task, and behavioural learning and transference from auditory to visual conditions can be measured. We can then compare the results with visual-auditory transference results to begin to assess for symmetry.

Unfortunately, introducing real-time feedback into Eyemusic is difficult. Soundscapes last a few seconds and the earlier-to-later sounds correspond to left-to-right locations in the subject's environment. Thus, a given soundscape is a static picture of what is before the subject. This makes *movement* of environmental objects representable only by comparing soundscapes (S_1, S_2 etc.): left–right object movement corresponds to earlier sound in S_1 followed by later sound in S_2; low–high object movement corresponds to lower pitch in S_1 followed by higher pitch in S_2. Tracking moving objects across soundscapes will generally be difficult for subjects (though might be assisted somewhat by utilizing another dimension such as timbre). In other words, introducing real-time feedback into the auditory condition is not in principle or practice difficult, but is particularly challenging when restricted to Eyemusic because of its reliance on soundscapes.

Further, it should now be plain why Eyemusic is even more limited. The idea that we should test for symmetry is not terribly novel. But if we are to perform such a test then at least some of the visual-auditory and auditory-visual experiments should be as similar as possible, so that we have a control for the type of task being performed. Eyemusic makes this control difficult to achieve, and is thus doubly disadvantageous.

Other modality pairs. An auditory feedback condition is not only important to test for the symmetry of BT between audition and vision. It is important if one wishes to generalize the project to additional modalities, for such gneralizations will demand a feedback and non-feedback condition for each involved modality.

Potential outcomes. Suppose a fairly thorough study of BT and the extent of symmetry is performed for several modality pairs (for simplicity assume subjects with a full set of normally functioning modalities). The picture that emerges can be of various forms. Perhaps BT is robust and robustly symmetrical across all modality pairs. This outcome would be surprising (to me), but it might suggest that amodal representation of learned behaviours is the norm. By contrast perhaps vision is the most useful modality for behavioural learning, and for BT the vision-to-other modality direction is more powerful than any other modality-to-vision direction (i.e. symmetry fails for vision). This outcome might be taken to suggest that visual as opposed to amodal representation of learned behaviours is the norm. In other words, the conclusion of Levy-Tzedek et al., that their results 'give strong support to the hypothesis that neural representations of motor control are sensory-modality-independent', is premature (p. 2). Inferences to the existence or non-existence of amodal representations from BT must be made with greater care. Importantly, this is appreciable without even considering what competing models of neural representation are available, a matter we turn to shortly (section 7.5).

7.4 SSDs, Behaviourism and Eyemusic

If the value of Eyemusic to such a project is rather limited, and systems capable of real-time auditory feedback (e.g. those satisfying AFS) are of greater value, have we shown that in this case SSDs are more of a hindrance than an asset? That depends on how we conceive of SSDs.

Rather than engage in a thorough discussion of the nature of SSDs, consider characterizing SSDs in terms of their use in our topic of behaviour modification. Here a central purpose of SSDs is to elicit behaviours, by stimulating one sense modality, that are normally elicited by stimulating a different sense modality.[2] Note that if this is *the* central feature of SSDs, then AFS is certainly usable as an SSD, as is the computer screen with depicted cursors and targets from the above experiments. More interestingly, Pavlov's bell is too. If a dog is trained to salivate or walk toward a food dish in response to the ring of a bell, then that ring is eliciting a behaviour via audition that is normally elicited via olfaction. And, regardless of how one characterizes SSDs, this serves as a primitive example of BT.

One might worry that this purely behaviouristic way of characterizing SSDs is too broad. Perhaps, in addition to merely eliciting a behaviour via a substituting modality that is normally elicited via the substituted modality, an SSD must contain: (a) the ability to be stimulated via an informational source peculiar to the substituted modality (e.g. photons in the case of vision, soundwaves for audition, etc.); (b) the ability to generate outputs in a form peculiar to the substituting modality; and (c) an internal representational scheme that translates at least some elements of the former into elements of the latter. On this characterization, an SSD utilizing the AFS mappings is possible, but so too is one using Pavlov's bell. In the latter case one requires a means of intaking olfactory information (i.e. the chemical constitutents of odours) and transforming it into an auditory output (i.e. ringing of the bell)—surely a doable task. In the classic experiments, while the bell on its own would not be an SSD, the union of Pavlov and the bell suffice: Pavlov's olfactory system could have provided the needed intake system (a), the bell the needed output system (b), and Pavlov's ability to translate odour recognitions into a wrist flick could have constituted the needed translation scheme (c).

I would, however, like to caution readers against heavy reliance on characterizations of SSDs in terms of (a)–(c). From the behavioural perspective, our goal is behavioural modification. If we develop SSDs to aid blind persons (as Amedi and his team are doing), then successfully modifying subject behaviour in beneficial ways is far more important than doing so via a device that satisfies (a)–(c). If a

[2] E.g. instead of characterizing SSDs in terms of elicited behaviours one might focus on elicited experiences or neural states.

subject learns to, say, stop in response to a bell, then whether that bell encodes information drawn from photons is of little consequence. The important achievement is that she learns to perform a behaviour via audition that by hypothesis is typically performed via vision. In this regard the limits of Eyemusic mentioned above are of considerable importance.

Compare a situation in which a subject receives real-time feedback regarding object movements (AFS) versus one in which she has to infer object movements by waiting for subsequent soundscapes and cognitively comparing them (Eyemusic). All else being equal the former is far more useful, and whether the former provides that feedback via encoding photons or soundwaves is tangential to the project. What is critical is whether the subject can navigate her evironment using audition in ways that approach how well the sighted navigate using vision.

Thus, we should not be too hasty in jettisoning the purely behaviourist conception of SSDs. Focus on creating a device that registers photon patches as retinas do and maps those in some simple way into the auditory analogue of a 'snapshot' of the visual scene—i.e. focus on generating soundscapes or generally on SSDs as devices satisfying (a)–(c)—might prevent us from developing more straightforward ways of benefiting subjects that, at least behaviourally, employ SSDs.

7.5 Models for Behavioural Storage

I have argued that inferences from BT to the existence or non-existence of amodal representations for motor control must be made with greater care than Levy-Tzedek et al. have taken. One reason (section 7.3) is that a richer data set may paint a very different picture than the one Levy-Tzedek et al. suggest. I conclude with another reason, namely that the existence of BT of motor skills across modalities places a constraint on models of motor control representation that can be met in various ways. To illustrate, here are two highly simplified propositions:

[A] *Amodal storage.* Learned motor skills are represented in a modality-free or amodal form. E.g. 'In response to stimulus S perform P', where neither S nor P makes reference to a modality.

[B] *Modal storage.* Learned motor skills are represented in a form that makes reference to the modality used to learn the skill. E.g. 'In response to *visual* stimulus V perform P.'

Our question is whether the existence of BTs 'gives strong support' for [A] (p. 2)? I suggest that it does not.

Suppose the following. A subject learns some behaviour through vision, and [B] obtains. Hence, there is a representation in our subject of the form 'In response to visual stimulus V perform P.' Our subject is now auditorily stimulated in ways to induce and measure BT of that behaviour. In order for her to use this representation she requires a means of translating the relevant parts of the content of 'visual stimulus V' into an auditory form. In theory this is easy to achieve, for example by hypothesizing 'visual stimulus V is equivalent to auditory stimulus A in relevant respects'. She can then discern whether her occurent auditory stimulation is akin to A and decide whether to perform P. In short, provided there is some means of mapping relevant visual content to relevant auditory content, modal representations of learned skills are generally adequate to explain the existence of BT. No amodal representations are required.

For concreteness, consider such a model to explain the Levy-Tzedek et al. experiment. During baseline trials the subject forms the representations 'In response to visual stimulus V_x move joystick in direction D_x' and 'In response to auditory stimulus A_x move joystick in direction D_x.' When rotation is introduced in joystick movement in the visual feedback condition, the subject forms a new representation 'In response to visual stimulus V_x move joystick in direction $D_{x\text{-}30degrees}$.' When rotation is introduced in joystick movement in the auditory *non*-feedback condition, the subject activates the representation 'In response to visual stimulus V_x move joystick in direction $D_{x\text{-}30degrees}$' and maps that into 'In response to auditory stimulus A_x move joystick in direction $D_{x\text{-}30degrees}$' by postulating 'V_x is equivalent to A_x in relevant respects.' Behavioural transference occurs without any purely amodal representations.

Taking the existence of BT in the context of Levy-Tzedek et al.'s experiments to 'give strong support to the hypothesis that neural representations of motor control are sensory-modality-independent' isn't premature merely because it relies on too small a data set (p. 2). It is also premature because it underappreciates general difficulties that arise from trying to make inferences about mental representation from behavioural data.

8

Limits of the Classical Functionalist Perspective on Sensory Substitution

MAURICE PTITO, KATRINE IVERSEN, MALIKA AUVRAY,
OPHELIA DEROY AND RON KUPERS

Abstract The tongue display unit (TDU) is a sensory substitution device that translates visual images into electrotactile stimulation that is transmitted to the tongue and leads to new perceptual skills following training. Trained users, including blind individuals, become capable of orientation discrimination, motion detection, shape recognition and they can also successfully use the TDU to navigate in an environment, locate objects and avoid obstacles. Many studies and discussions have focused on the effects of training at the behavioural level, and assumed that the effects shown in training blindfolded sighted individuals are similar to those observed in blind people. In doing so, we argue that behavioural research on sensory substitution shows a functionalist bias. Functionalism claims that mental processes can be individuated by their characteristic inputs and outputs, and that the physical realization of a given function introduces no relevant difference, as long as the function is the same. We emphasize here why this assumption biases the interpretation of sensory substitution devices.

8.1 Sensory Substitution: Why Cross-Modal Plasticity Matters

THE LOSS OR ABSENCE of vision is probably one of the most incapacitating events that can befall a human being. The importance of vision for humans is also reflected in brain anatomy as approximately one-third of the human brain is devoted to vision (Kupers and Ptito 2014). It is therefore not surprising that throughout history many attempts have been undertaken to develop devices aimed at substituting for a missing visual capacity. Sensory substitution devices (SSDs) are based on the principle that information from one sensory modality can be used to replace information

Proceedings of the British Academy, **219**, 130–149. © The British Academy 2018.

from a relevant missing sensory modality. Most of the SSD devices designed to date attempt to substitute vision by touch or audition—a hope sparked by Bach-y-Rita's initial ideas (e.g. Bach-y-Rita 1972; Bach-y-Rita et al. 1969). In recent years, the ideal of giving full vision back to blind people by using SSDs has been put under strong pressure as the performance level acquired through training with such devices is nowhere near that experienced by sighted individuals (see Deroy and Auvray 2012, 2014, for a review). In addition, the percept experienced by blind SSD users cannot univocally be assimilated to a visual percept (Arnold et al. 2017; Auvray et al. 2007a, 2007b; Auvray and Farina 2017). In other words, the output can be considered as novel, but not as straightforwardly visual.

Looking only at the level of outputs, for a given input, might however offer only a limited perspective on the acquisition of a novel skill. In neuroscience, the importance of computational models encourages the view that mental processes can be understood in terms of the computational input-output function. Processes that fit the same model are considered of the same type. In philosophy, the rise of computationalism and the importance of artificial intelligence tend to coincide with a broader family of views known as functionalism (see Polger 2004 for an overview; see also Piccinini 2010 for differences between those views). According to this widespread view, mental states or processes can be individuated according to their function, and not according to their physical properties. If different physical substrates (for instance, neurons or computer chips) realize the same input-output function, they should both be counted as carrying the same mental process. Both computational models and functionalist theories have led to the view that the study of the physical realization of mental processes—notably their embodied or neurological basis—would not reveal anything substantial about these mental states, beyond what the input-output relation says. At best, the study of the physical realization of a given mental process could be of local interest: it could help for instance to 'repair' the physical damage causing a loss of function, but would be of limited relevance to larger theories of the mind. Physical differences between species or individuals in the way a given function is carried out can be interesting, but, as long as the same function is carried out, these differences only show that there are different physical tokens for the same mental kind. Even when a certain mental kind is always tokened in the same way, the same kind of argument prevails. If studies show that a certain mental process is de facto always acquired or realized in the same way by our brains or bodies, this is taken to demonstrate—at best—that brains and bodies cause the mental process, but not that they are constitutive of that mental process (e.g. Putnam 1967; Shapiro 2000). After all, any empirical study will fall short of ruling out that the same mental process could possibly be realized in other physical systems: other brains, other bodies or even in physical systems very different from brains and bodies (see Godfrey-Smith 2016 and Deroy 2016 for a case study and discussion). The logical possibility of multiple realizations, stressing that it makes no difference, is then supposed to make the empirical investigation of the embodied and neurological basis of mental processes non-directly relevant for their understanding.

We generally disagree with a method that places our limited capacity to imagine what is possible over and above what the facts may tell us. More importantly here, we argue that sensory substitution offers a potential counter-argument to this line of thought. Understanding (and improving) sensory substitution devices requires taking into account more than just the inputs and outputs of the new skills acquired by trained users. Though we will not insist on this point here, we need to take into account facts about the development of the new function, such as the capacity to develop distal attribution with these devices (O'Brien and Auvray 2014) or the extent to which the code they use is based on pre-existing cross-modal correspondences (Deroy et al. 2016). What we wish to highlight here is why we need to take into account the neurological changes induced by training, especially those documented in congenitally blind people, and recognize that the use of SSDs in blind vs. non-blind users, though functionally comparable, deserves to be considered as two distinct processes. As a result, generalizations across blind and non-blind users, when it comes to sensory substitutions, are weak and, at best, analogies.

The results of our studies, detailed below, successfully demonstrate the occurrence of training-induced plasticity in congenitally blind users of a visual-to-tactile SSD, something that does not occur in equally trained sighted users. In other words, sensory substitution devices trigger our brain's remarkable capacity for reorganizing/rewiring the neural network of the sensory systems that are deprived of their normal input, a process more specifically known as cross-modal plasticity (Frost et al. 2000; Bavelier and Neville 2002). Most importantly, the neurological changes studied in the blind show the recruitment of the same cortical network used for visual tasks in sighted people. This neurological specificity, we argue, is essential to the proper understanding of sensory substitution, and in this respect, it challenges the functionalist indifference to physical realizations.

As the present chapter focuses on a tactile vision SSD, known as the tongue display unit (TDU), we will first locate it in terms of the history and among the variety of SSDs.

8.2 Sensory Substitution Devices for the Blind

Braille reading was one of the first sensory substitution techniques conceived and today it is still the most popular. Braille reading was developed in 1829 by Louis Braille (1809–1852), who himself lost his vision in early childhood; it helps blind individuals to read by replacing visual information by touch. This has led to the development of other blindness aids such as the mechanical Braille printer and typewriter (Brailler). It was not until the early 1960s that the first technical sensory substitution device was developed, the Elektroftalm (Starkiewicz and

Kuliszewski 1963). Originally, the Elektroftalm was an 80-channel photocell array for mechanically producing images on the forehead, designed for spatial orientation and deciphering of large letters or figures against a dark background. However, the real breakthrough in the field of SSD came soon after with Paul Bach-y-Rita who developed a tactile vision substitution system (TVSS) that uses the skin as a substrate for transmitting pictorial information (Bach-y-Rita et al. 1969). The basic idea was to translate in real time images from a video camera into electro- or vibrotactile stimulation that is applied to the skin. The first version of the TVSS transmitted camera signals to an array of 20 × 20 vibrotactile stimulators that were mounted in the back of a dentist's chair. The blind participant was seated in the chair with his back pressed against the array, and was allowed to manipulate a video camera that captured an object that was placed in front of him, thereby redrawing a point-by-point vibrotactile version of the object on the back. With training, blind participants learned to identify simple objects that were presented to them with the TVSS (Figure 8.1a). However, this early prototype was bulky and could therefore only be used inside a laboratory setting. Later on, Bach-y-Rita and co-workers designed a portable TVSS whereby the lens of a lightweight camera was mounted on a pair of eyeglasses. The information captured by the camera was translated into electrotactile stimuli that were relayed in a point-by-point manner to the abdominal skin via a flexible electrode matrix. Case report studies with this device demonstrated that participants could make distance discriminations and even catch objects in motion (Jansson 1983). This new portable TVSS system revolutionized the work done on sensory substitution and has inspired the development of many devices, some of which are described in the next section. These modern TVSS devices have become much smaller, more energy-efficient, and are relatively low-cost to produce. These devices use activators such as solenoids, eccentric inertial motors and voice-coil piezo-electric transducers as means for stimulation.

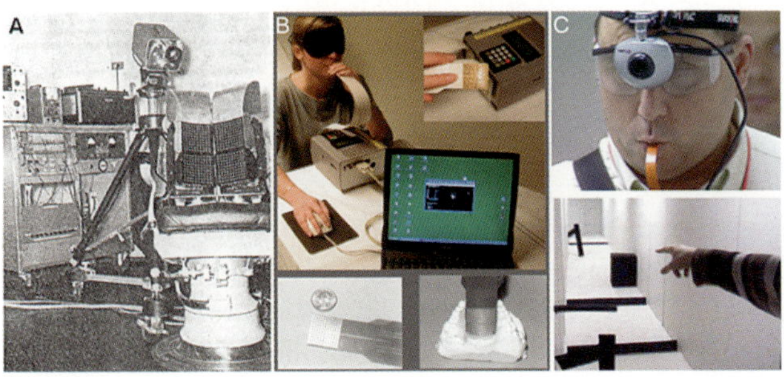

Figure 8.1 Examples of tactile vision sensory substitution devices. A. First TVSS device developed by Paul Bach-y-Rita in which pneumatic stimulation was delivered to the back of the blind subject who was seated in a dental chair; B. Early version of the tongue display unit (TDU); C. An actual version of the TDU model. The system has become completely portable and can be used for navigational purposes.

These more recent devices have become more popular as they are more suitable for daily use and have a rapid and high-quality translation of visual into tactile or auditory information; some of them also do not interfere with audition.

8.2.1 Tactile to Vision Sensory Substitution Systems (TVSS)

The tongue display unit (TDU)

In the late 1990s, Paul Bach-y-Rita developed the tongue display unit (TDU), a sensory substitution device that translates visual images into electrotactile stimuli that are transmitted to the tongue via a flexible electrode array. Compared to earlier TVSS systems that used the abdomen as a substrate for stimulation, the new device was much reduced in size. One of the main reasons for stimulating the tongue is its high spatial tactile acuity (Weinstein 1968; Chebat et al. 2007) that may be explained by the large representation of the tongue in the primary somatosensory cortex (Picard and Olivier 1983). An additional advantage is that stimulation of the tongue only requires a fraction of the voltage needed for stimulation of the skin (abdomen, fingers). The TDU comprises a camera, a control box with micro-controllers, electrode drivers and communication circuits, a laptop computer with custom-made software, and a small electrode array consisting of 144 small gold-plated contacts arranged in a 12 × 12 matrix (Figure 8.1b). The device has an update rate of 14–20 frames per second. An electrical pulse (40 us positive pulse) is generated when a stimulus is presented in the field-of-view of the camera.

The TDU was recently adapted for navigational purposes (Brainport, WICAB Inc., Wisconsin, USA) (Figure 8.1c). The new portable system consists of a web-cam connected to a laptop and a tongue stimulator array of 100 small circular contacts, spaced 1 mm apart and arranged in a 10 × 10 matrix. The entire tongue array measures 2 × 2 cm, and can be comfortably placed on the tongue due to its smooth and soft silicone mouthpiece, which rests on the roof of the mouth. This model has the advantage of being smaller than previous versions of the TDU, thereby enabling the user true mobility for navigating and exploring his/her surroundings.

FLIPPS

FLIPPS is another sensory substitution device for the blind that uses a tactile display. A more minimalistic version was initially developed by Lenay (Lenay and Steiner 2007). Al-Hamdani (2010) further perfected the device by simultaneously stimulating several fingers. This reduces scanning time of the object and provides better spatial information. FLIPPS is a light-sensitive glove with a stimulator at the tip of each finger and a photodiode sensor attached that is activated when light illumination exceeds a certain threshold. FLIPPS can be used to distinguish between light and dark environment or objects, and objects with different illumination.

The EyeCane

The EyeCane, developed at Amedi's laboratory at the Hebrew University of Jerusalem, is a tiny virtual cane that operates as a kind of virtual flashlight, replacing or strengthening the 'classic' walking stick (Maidenbaum et al. 2013). The device comprises sensors that estimate the distance between the user and the object at which it is pointing. This information is transformed into complex vibrations, allowing the blind person to identify obstacles of different heights, understand the distance to objects, and create a spatial picture in order to allow safer navigation.

8.2.2 Auditory-to-Vision Sensory Substitution (AVSS) Systems

A number of sensory substitution devices use auditory information to replace vision. Hence, these systems are often referred to as auditory-to-vision sensory substitution (AVSS) devices. The most popular AVSS systems are the vOICe, the PSVA and EyeMusic. In the following, we will briefly describe these devices.

The vOICe

Peter Meijer (Philips Research, Eindhoven, The Netherlands) developed a device that maps grey-scale video images into corresponding soundscapes. The device, nicknamed 'the vOICe', substitutes visual input with audio output. Like the TDU, the system uses a video camera that captures grey-scale images with a resolution of 64 x 64 pixels. The image is scanned from left to right over one second, one column at a time, converting the image into multi-complex signals that are presented through a headset (Meijer 1992). The user of the vOICe learns to associate brightness with loudness, and height with pitch. To begin with, the soundwaves sound very complex and rather meaningless, but with time the user learns to memorize the wave complexes and to relate them to the objects (Auvray et al. 2007a; Brown et al. 2011; Haigh et al. 2013; Striem-Amit et al. 2012).

The Prosthesis for Substitution of Vision with Audition (PSVA)

In the late 1990s, Veraart and colleagues, at the University of Louvain in Brussels, developed an AVSS prosthesis, called the PSVA (Capelle et al. 1998). Like the vOICe, the PVSA is a head-worn camera that conveys live visual information through complex sounds.

If we compare the two AVSS devices, there are some differences, such as the image-to-sound use. The vOICe exploits an approximate inverse spectrographic mapping involving a scanning approach, whereas the PSVA uses a direct non-scanning mapping. The vOICe technically offers a soundscape image resolution in the order of 4000 pixels for a one-second sound scan of a given camera view, while the PSVA offers up to a 124-pixel resolution for a given view. In addition, in order to better simulate the human visual system, the receptive field of the PSVA has a higher resolution in the centre of the picture. To compensate for the PSVA's lower spatial resolution, manually scanning is required by the user for further details. Consequently, even though the PSVA in a sense gives a more direct real-time feedback, the actual time needed for fully analysing an image or a scene can be significantly longer compared to that for the vOICe.

EyeMusic

The EyeMusic technology has been developed in Amedi's laboratory at the Hebrew University of Jerusalem. EyeMusic uses pleasant musical scales to convey visual information. The system consists of a pair of glasses with attached headphones and a webcam mounted on the nose bridge. The camera scans the scene from left to right; as the camera moves, the earphones play sounds corresponding to the height, colour, and brightness of what the camera records. Several studies have shown that the device can be used after a short period of training to guide movements similar to visually guided movements (Abboud et al. 2014).

Note that two additional devices that function with the similar principle of using musical notes were recently developed: the Vibe, developed by Hanneton and his colleagues (Hanneton et al. 2010), and the system developed by Cronly-Dillon and colleagues (Cronly-Dillon et al. 1999).

8.3 Behavioural and Brain Imaging Studies with the TDU

Over the years, we have conducted a series of studies in which congenitally blind and blindfolded sighted control subjects were trained to use the TDU to resolve a number of visual tasks such as orientation discrimination, motion detection, shape discrimination and spatial navigation. Thereby, we have used a variety of techniques such as positron emission tomography (PET), functional magnetic resonance imaging (fMRI) and transcranial magnetic stimulation (TMS) to examine which brain structures mediate these cross-modal functions.

8.3.1 Orientation processing

In a first experiment, we trained congenitally blind and normal blindfolded participants to use the TDU to determine the orientation of the letter T that was presented in four different orientations (Ptito et al. 2005). Participants were trained in the discrimination task until they reached the learning criterion of 85 per cent or more on two consecutive days. Participants were scanned before and after training with the TDU, using the same orientation task. Behavioural results showed that blind and control subjects learned the task at the same speed. The results of our PET

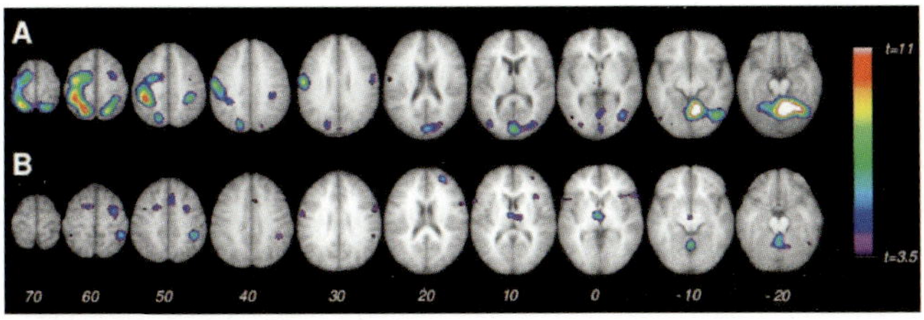

Figure 8.2 Results of the orientation discrimination task. Note the activation of the visual cortex in the blind after training (upper row). In contrast, trained blindfolded control subjects did not activate their occipital cortex (lower row), despite equal task performance (adapted after Ptito et al. 2005).

study indicated that congenitally blind subjects trained to resolve an orientation discrimination task activated their visual cortex, whereas control subjects did not, despite equal task performance (Figure 8.2). Importantly, blind participants did not activate their visual cortex before training with the TDU. This study was the first demonstration that the recruitment of the occipital cortex via the tongue in congenitally blind individuals is training-induced, and the results support the notion of cross-modal plasticity.

8.3.2 Motion and shape processing

The visual system is classically divided into a dorsal and a ventral stream, involved in motion and object recognition, respectively (Ungerleider and Mishkin 1982) (Figure 8.3A). Interestingly, in the sighted brain, motion and shape selective areas in the dorsal and ventral visual stream are not only activated by appropriate visual input, but also when motion and shape information is conveyed haptically or auditorily (Amedi et al. 2001, 2002; Pietrini et al. 2004; Poirier et al. 2006; Renier et al. 2009, 2010; Ricciardi et al. 2007; Strnad et al. 2013). Using the TDU, we addressed the question of whether the functional segregation of the visual cortical system into a dorsal and a ventral stream is preserved in the absence of vision.

In a first study we used fMRI to determine whether motion-sensitive area hMT+ responds to non-haptically conveyed motion information. We trained a group of congenitally blind and sighted control subjects to resolve a tactile motion discrimination task using the TDU (Matteau et al. 2010). Stimuli consisted of either static dots, dots moving coherently or dots moving in random directions. Both groups learned the task at the same rate in fewer than ten 30-minute training sessions. The fMRI data revealed that both groups activated the hMT+ complex during tactile motion discrimination, although at different anatomical locations (Figure 8.3B). The congenitally blind subjects showed additional activations within the dorsal extrastriate cortical pathway. These results extend previous data in support of the supramodal functional organization of the hMT+ complex (Poirier et al. 2006;

Renier et al. 2009; Ricciardi et al. 2007) by showing that this cortical area processes motion-related information per se, that is, motion stimuli that are not visual in nature and that are administered to a body structure that is not primarily devoted to movement perception. In line with previous studies, the differential activations between sighted and congenitally blind individuals indicate that the lack of vision leads to functional rearrangements of these supramodal cortical areas.

In a subsequent study, we tested whether shape recognition using the TDU activates the ventral visual stream in congenitally blind subjects (Ptito et al. 2012). Blind and blindfolded sighted control subjects were trained to use the TDU to distinguish various shapes (squares, rectangles, letter E, etc.). In line with the behavioural results described above, we found no group differences in task performance. Also in agreement with our earlier brain imaging studies, the fMRI data showed a clear difference in brain activation patterns. Whereas the blind subjects activated large portions of the ventral visual stream, including the cuneus, precuneus, inferotemporal cortex, lateral occipital tactile vision area (LOtv), and fusiform gyrus, control subjects activated only LOtv and none of the other parts of the ventral visual stream (Figure 8.3C). These results indicate that congenitally blind subjects recruit key regions in the ventral visual pathway during non-haptic tactile shape discrimination. The activation of LOtv by non-haptic tactile shape processing in blind and sighted subjects adds further support to the notion that this area subserves an abstract or supramodal representation of shape.

Taken together with findings from other laboratories (Amedi et al. 2001, 2002; James et al. 2002; Pietrini et al. 2004, 2009; Renier et al. 2009), the results of our TDU studies suggest that the segregation of the efferent projections of the primary visual cortex into a dorsal and ventral visual stream is preserved in congenitally blind individuals.

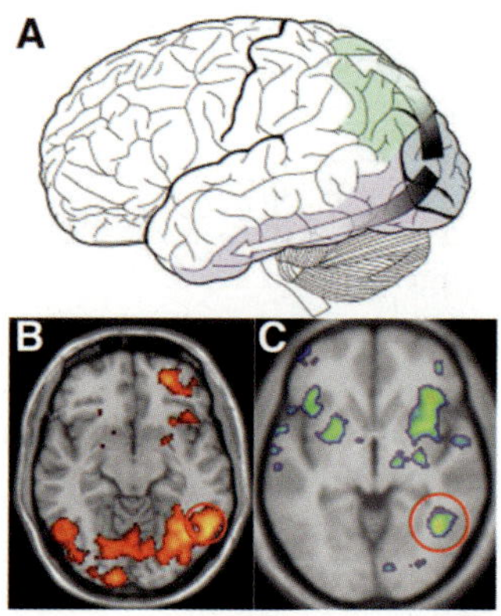

Figure 8.3 A. The two visual streams. B. Motion discrimination activated area hMT+ (red circle) and other parts of the dorsal stream in trained congenitally blind individuals with the TDU. C. Results of the shape discrimination task. Trained congenitally blind individuals activate area LOtv (red circle) and other parts of the ventral stream using the TDU (adapted after Matteau et al. 2010; Ptito et al. 2012).

8.3.3 Navigational skills in the blind

As shown in the first section, many tools have been developed to allow blind subjects to detect, correctly identify and avoid obstacles. However, the classical white cane still remains the most frequently used tool by blind and low-vision adults to provide ground-level information on the location and textural quality of obstacles. An important limitation of the cane is that it does not provide information about obstacles located outside the egocentric space or above waist level. We therefore conducted a series of experiments aimed at testing the efficiency of the TDU in detecting and avoiding obstacles of various sizes and shapes that were placed in a human-sized obstacle course. Wearing a camera mounted on a pair of eyeglasses that was connected to a TDU, participants' task was to detect the obstacles and negotiate a path around them. We used several types of obstacles to simulate an ecological environment and the kinds of obstacles that can be encountered on a typical city sidewalk. Both blind and sighted participants learned the task and we did not find significant differences between sighted and blind subjects in their ability to detect and avoid the obstacles. With training, subjects were able to detect obstacles up to nine metres away, which is largely above the distance they could detect with a cane. Trained participants were also able to navigate in another corridor with a novel configuration of obstacles with the same accuracy as they did in the practised one (Chebat et al. 2011). This implies that the skill they had learned was transferable to a new set of obstacles. These results are encouraging regarding the efficiency of the TDU as a navigational tool for the visually impaired.

Next, we studied the cerebral correlates of spatial navigation in congenitally blind individuals. Thereto, we designed a navigational task in such a way that participants could use the TDU while inside an MRI scanner (Kupers et al. 2010). In brief, a group of congenitally blind and matched blindfolded sighted control subjects were trained to navigate throughout two virtual routes that were presented

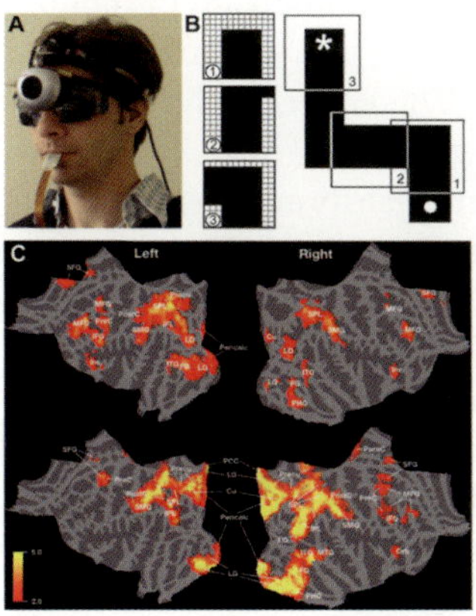

Figure 8.4 Navigation in the blind using the TDU. A. A subject equipped with the TDU and a head-worn camera. B. Navigational route that participants had to navigate through by using the TDU in the scanner. C. Brain activation patterns in trained blindfolded sighted controls (upper row) and congenitally blind individuals (lower row) during spatial navigation. Results are shown on cortical flatmaps. Blind but not sighted controls activated their visual cortex and right parahippocampus (adapted after Kupers et al. 2010).

via the TDU. Once fully learned, participants performed the same task during fMRI. Although both groups learned the task at the same pace, the fMRI data showed again important group differences in activated brain areas. During navigation, congenitally blind individuals recruited several parts of their occipital cortex and the right parahippocampal area, a brain structure devoted to the formation of cognitive maps of the environment in sighted individuals (Figure 8.4). In sharp contrast, blindfolded sighted control individuals did not activate their occipital cortex or parahippocampal area; instead they recruited more frontal areas during the spatial navigation task. In a subsequent experiment, we presented the same navigational task under full vision (and not via the TDU) to a new group of sighted individuals. A conjunction analysis of the results obtained in congenitally blind individuals with the TDU and the sighted individuals performing the same task visually, showed a strong overlap of activation of the occipital cortex and the right parahippocampus.

These data suggest that in the absence of vision, cross-modal plasticity permits the recruitment of the same cortical network used for visual tasks in sighted subjects.

8.3.4 Functional implication of the reorganized visual cortex

The above clearly demonstrates that congenitally blind individuals trained to resolve so-called 'visual' tasks with the TDU activate their occipital cortex. However, this is by itself no proof that the occipital cortex is functionally involved in task performance. In order to have a more direct proof for the functional involvement of the occipital cortex in cross-modal plasticity, we used transcranial magnetic stimulation (TMS), a technique that allows us to temporarily block a brain region (Cowey and Walsh 2001). We used repetitive TMS (rTMS) to study the functional role of area hMT+ in motion processing. We trained a group of congenitally blind and age- and sex-matched blindfolded control subjects to use the TDU to resolve a motion discrimination task. Patterns of random dots were moving to the left or right and subjects had to indicate as fast as possible the direction of motion. Following training, subjects participated in a TMS study. First, we presented two baseline motion discrimination series without TMS. Thereafter, we repeated the same stimuli but during rTMS of right area hMT+ or sham rTMS. All subjects learned the orientation discrimination task and baseline performance did not differ between the groups of blind and sighted subjects. During rTMS of right area hMT+, reaction times became significantly longer in the congenitally blind but not in the sighted control subjects (Kupers and Ptito 2014). Five minutes post-rTMS, reaction times were back to baseline levels. In contrast, rTMS of right area hMT+ had no significant effect on the percentage of correct responses although there was a non-significant trend towards lower values in both groups. In summary, these data indicate a functional role of area hMT+ in the non-haptic detection of tactile motion in congenitally blind but not in sighted control subjects.

8.4 Cross-Modal Plasticity in the Blind Brain

The first experimental demonstration of cross-modal plasticity comes from experiments whereby animals were visually deprived at birth (for reviews see Ptito and Desgent 2006; Desgent and Ptito 2012). These studies showed that the occipital cortex of these animals responds to various forms of non-visual stimulation. This raised the important question of whether similar cross-modal recruitment of the occipital cortex also occurs in humans who are born blind. Ensuing studies conducted in congenitally blind subjects responded positively to this question. Indeed, there is now ample evidence that when deprived of vision at birth, the human visual cortex is recruited by a wide variety of non-visual sensory modalities such as touch, smell or audition, and even by cognitive and language-related tasks (Kupers and Ptito 2014; Pietrini et al. 2009).

We have done a series of studies on the reorganization of the congenitally blind brain. In a first study, we used voxel-based morphometry (VBM) to examine differences in grey matter and white matter between a group of congenitally blind subjects and age-matched blindfolded controls (Figure 8.5A). Our VBM results revealed that all components of the retinofugal visual system of the blind brain undergo strong volumetric reductions. Indeed, we observed atrophic changes of the optic nerve and optic chiasm, lateral geniculate nucleus of the thalamus, optic radiations, and striate and extrastriate cortices (Ptito et al. 2008b; Cecchetti et al. 2016). Interestingly, the volumetric reduction of the striate cortex is associated

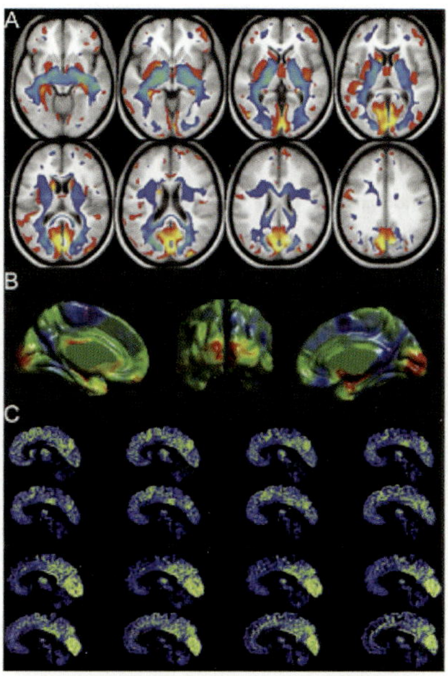

Figure 8.5 Anatomical and metabolic changes in the congenitally blind brain: A. Reductions in grey matter (indicated in hot colours) and white matter (indicated in cold colours) in congenitally blind compared to normal sighted controls. Note the widespread reductions in grey and white matter volume throughout the whole extent of the visual system. B. Increases in cortical thickness in the occipital cortex in congenitally blind individuals. C. Increased resting-state metabolism in the congenitally blind brain as measured with FDG/PET (adapted after Ptito et al. 2008b and Kupers and Ptito 2014).

with an increase in cortical thickness of this area (Jiang et al. 2009; Qin et al. 2013; Voss and Zatorre 2012; Kupers and Ptito 2014). In addition, PET-FDG studies further revealed that the occipital cortex of congenitally blind individuals has a supra-normal metabolism at rest (De Volder et al. 1997; Kupers and Ptito 2014). The data are illustrated in Figure 8.5B and 8.5C respectively. We explain the volume reduction of the striate and extrastriate visual areas by the abnormal development of the brain due to lack of visual input. The absence of retinal input indeed leads to a massive degeneration of the upstream projections to the occipital lobe. However, visual cortical areas deprived of their normal visual input become invaded by other (auditory and tactile) sensory modalities that maintain neuronal activity within the occipital cortex, preventing further atrophy. This absence of visual input may cause an abnormal reduction in synaptic pruning that could explain both the increase in cortical thickness and the abnormal supra-metabolic activation at rest in this cortical area.

The question of through which pathways non-visual information is funnelled to the occipital cortex in the congenitally blind remains a matter of debate. In order to answer this question, we performed electrophysiological measurements, first by classical recordings of somatosensory evoked potentials (SEPs) over the visual cortex (Kupers et al. 2006), and more recently using magnetoencephalography (MEG) (Ioannides et al. 2013). The results of both studies indicate that tactile information is routed from the primary somatosensory cortex (S1) first to the posterior parietal cortex (BA 7/BA 40), and then further to the occipital visual areas V5 and V3, and eventually also to V1 (Ioannides et al. 2013). A time-frequency analysis further revealed a strong gamma band activity at latencies of 20–50 ms in S1, and posterior parietal cortex (BA7 and 40), that was substantially more

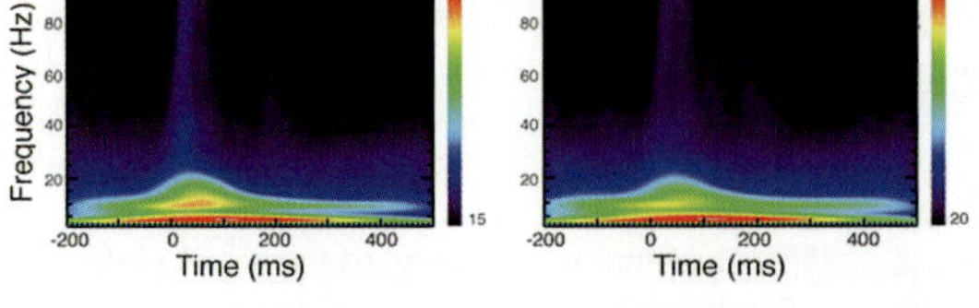

Figure 8.6 Results of an MEG study in congenital blindness. Time frequency analysis of regional activations for motor threshold stimulation in a typical congenitally blind (upper row) and sighted control subject (lower row). Note the increased activity in the gamma band range in the blind subject in somatosensory cortex and posterior parietal areas (adapted after Ioannides et al. 2013).

pronounced in the blind than in the sighted subjects (Figure 8.6). These electrophysiological results lend support to the assumption that non-visual information reaches the occipital cortex via strengthening of existing corticocortical pathways (Kupers et al. 2006), although a faster thalamocortical route cannot be ruled out.

8.5 General Discussion

This review has focused on our recent work on cross-modal plasticity in the blind. The review highlights two important points. First, neuronal cross-modal plasticity underlies the training effects with the TDU in congenitally blind individuals but not in sighted individuals. The extent to which this claim can be generalized to all visually deprived individuals, including late blind and temporarily visually deprived sighted individuals, is a topic of ongoing investigation. Our prediction is that the degree of cross-modal plasticity induced by training is likely to increase with the duration and earlier onset time of the loss of vision (Burton et al. 2003; Noppeney et al. 2005). The distinctive recruitment of occipital areas in congenitally blind individuals after training with the TDU for a relatively short time demonstrates the strength of training to induce the reorganization of the blind brain's neural network. Second, the effects of cross-modal plasticity exhibit a degree of specificity. Our studies have shown that the cross-modal effects are task- or function-related, that is, the reorganization in the occipital areas follows the functions served by the visual areas in sighted individuals. The same area that is activated during a given task performed through vision by sighted individuals can be activated in congenitally blind individuals when performing an analogous task through the use of a visuo-tactile sensory substitution device. In other words, even in the absence of any visual input, the brain is predisposed to implement a function originating, let's say, from tactile inputs into areas phylogenetically specialized to mediate vision.

These results clearly demonstrate the extraordinary potential to study congenital blindness with SSDs in order to understand how the brain's functional architecture is programmed. Moreover, they encourage us to take a step back from a series of claims that minimize the importance of the study of the physical realization of a given mental process. Ultimately, we want to argue that brain plasticity is so instrumental for the understanding of a mental function that we should abandon the functionalist idea whereby only input-output functions matter. If one only considers input and outputs, no differences are observed between trained users of the TDU, be they congenitally blind or sighted. From the functionalist perspective, there is no difference that should surface in our theories of the cognitive process at stake. The only thing to argue about is whether this TDU input-output function is similar to vision or not (a debate which we consider as misplaced; see Arnold et al. 2017; Deroy and Auvray 2014).

However, the neuroscientific investigation of the effects of training with the TDU suggests a totally different lesson: differences in the neurological underpinnings of the same function do matter. The recruitment of occipital areas in congenitally blind individuals, more especially of areas predisposed to implement certain functions, illustrates two important points. First, training-induced plasticity shows that functional differentiation pre-exists the specification of an input-output function. There can be a sense in which a function is implemented in our brains, or pre-disposed to be, before it gets any input. Before the rewiring induced by training, occipital areas are anatomically and functionally differentiated, and they have not yet acquired a certain function. This functional differentiation—although latent—cannot be accounted for as a mere predisposition to realize a given input-output function. As shown in our studies, these areas can be recruited for a variety of inputs (tactile or visual) and lead to generic kinds of outputs. It is here important to underscore that, if the occipital areas of the blind respond to tactile inputs through training-induced plasticity, the kind of subjective sensations associated with such occipital activation in blind individuals are not un-ambivalently visual. For instance, we showed that TMS over the occipital cortex evoked tingling sensations (paresthesiae) that were referred to the tongue in congenitally blind individuals who were highly trained with the TDU (Kupers et al. 2006). These results are consistent with those of a later study in which we showed that TMS of the occipital cortex in proficient blind Braille readers produced tactile sensations referred to the fingers used for Braille reading (Ptito et al. 2008a). It thus seems that the 'occipital cortex' of the congenitally blind shows various degrees of visual and tactile functions. The limits of training-induced cross-modal plasticity remain to be further explored, but the existing results are sufficient to show that we need to consider functional differentiation as a property of the brain, and not only as an input-output function. The second lesson is that, after training, the difference in neurological realization is likely to introduce differences in the way the function is carried out. Following training, blind users of the TDU will recruit striate and extrastriate visual cortex to perform a given task, whereas sighted subjects won't, relying still on higher cognitive areas. We can therefore expect that the same task will generate a lesser cognitive load and highlight a higher degree of automatization in trained blind individuals. This might not affect the visible output and the degree of performance, but is potentially crucial to understand other features of SSD use, for instance, that the motivation for the blind to wear the device relates to the progressive reduction of cognitive load induced by plasticity, but will remain low in sighted users even after training. Similarly, the lack of automation might explain the lack of affective reactions to objects sensed through the SSD (Bach-y-Rita and Kercel 2003).

8.6 Conclusion

A number of studies dealing with the tactile modality agree on the recruitment of the occipital areas (corresponding to the visual cortex in sighted individuals) of the blind in various experimental conditions either through stimulation of the tongue or the fingers. Moreover, the efferent streams of the visual cortex, namely the dorsal and ventral pathways, involved in motion detection and shape recognition respectively, are still functional although they show some alterations in their microstructural organization. Effects of training, such as the ones reviewed above, suggest that a proper understanding of sensory substitution should build on studies of the blind brain.

Acknowledgements

Maurice Ptito and Ron Kupers are supported by the Lundbeck Foundation (Denmark), the Danish Medical Research Council (FSS) and the Harland Sanders Foundation (Canada); Malika Auvray is supported by the ANR grant FRESCO (ANR-11-JSH2-003-1); Ophelia Deroy is supported by the AHRC grant 'Re-thinking the Senses' (AH/L007053/1). Katrine Iversen received a student fellowship from the Lundbeck Foundation (Denmark).

References

Abboud, S., Hanassy, S., Levy-Tzedek, S., Maidenbaum, S. and Amedi, A. (2014) EyeMusic: introducing a 'visual' colorful experience for the blind using auditory sensory substitution. *Restorative Neurology Neuroscience* 32: 247–257.

Al-Hamdani, S. (2010) FLIPPS for the blind. A new device for medium distance object detection by multiple fingertip stimulation. Unpublished Master's thesis, Danish Technical University.

Amedi, A., Malach, R., Hendler, T., Peled, S. and Zohary, E. (2001) Visuo-haptic object-related activation in the ventral visual pathway. *Nature Neuroscience* 4: 324–330.

Amedi, A., Jacobson, G., Hendler, T., Malach, R. and Zohary, E. (2002) Convergence of visual and tactile shape processing in the human lateral occipital complex. *Cerebral Cortex* 12: 1202–1212.

Arnold, G., Pesnot-Lerousseau, J. and Auvray, M. (2017) Individual differences in sensory substitution. *Multisensory Research* 6: 579–600.

Auvray, M. and Farina, M. (2017) Patrolling the boundaries of synaethesia: a critical appraisal of transient and artificially-acquired forms of synaesthetic experiences. In O. Deroy (ed.) *Synaesthesia: Philosophical and Psychological Challenges.* Oxford: Oxford University Press, 248–274.

Auvray, M., Hanneton, S. and O'Regan, J. K. (2007a) Learning to perceive with a visuo-auditory substitution system: localisation and object recognition with 'the vOICe'. *Perception* 36: 416–430.

Auvray, M., Philipona, D., O'Regan, J. K. and Spence, C. (2007b) The perception of space and form recognition in a simulated environment: the case of minimalist sensory-substitution devices. *Perception* 36: 1736–1751.

Bach-y-Rita, P. (1972) *Brain Mechanisms in Sensory Substitution*. New York: Academic Press.

Bach-y-Rita, P. (2002) Sensory substitution and qualia. In A. Noë and E. Thompson (eds) *Vision and Mind*. Cambridge, MA: MIT Press, 497–514.

Bach-y-Rita, P. and Kercel, S. (2003) Sensory substitution and the human-machine interface. *Trends in Cognitive Sciences* 7: 541–546.

Bach-y-Rita, P., Collins, C. C., Saunders, F. A., White, B. and Scadden, L. (1969) Vision substitution by tactile image projection. *Nature* 221: 963–964.

Bavelier, D. and Neville, H. J. (2002) Cross-modal plasticity: where and how? *Nature Review Neuroscience* 3: 443–452.

Brown, D., Macpherson, T. and Ward, J. (2011) Seeing with sound? Exploring different characteristics of a visual-to-auditory sensory substitution device. *Perception* 40: 1120–1135.

Burton, H., Diamond, J. B. and McDermott, K. B. (2003) Dissociating cortical regions activated by semantic and phonological tasks: a fMRI study in blind and sighted people. *Journal of Neurophysiology* 90: 1965–1982.

Capelle, C., Trullemans, C., Arno, P. and Veraart, C. (1998) A real-time experimental prototype for enhancement of vision rehabilitation using auditory substitution. *IEEE Transactions on Biomedical Engineering* 45: 1279–1293.

Cecchetti, L., Ricciardi, E., Handjaras, G., Kupers, R., Ptito, M. and Pietrini, P. (2016) Congenital blindness affects diencephalic but not mesencephalic structures in the human brain. *Brain Structure and Function* 221: 1465–1480.

Chebat, D. R., Rainville, C., Kupers, R. and Ptito, M. (2007) Tactile-'visual' acuity of the tongue in early blind individuals. *Neuroreport* 18: 1901–1904.

Chebat, D. R., Schneider, F. C., Kupers, R. and Ptito, M. (2011) Navigation with a sensory substitution device in congenitally blind individuals. *Neuroreport* 22: 342–347.

Cowey, A. and Walsh, V. (2001) Tickling the brain: studying visual sensation, perception and cognition by transcranial magnetic stimulation. *Progress in Brain Research* 134: 411–425.

Cronly-Dillon, J., Persaud, K. and Gregory, R. P. F. (1999) The perception of visual images encoded in musical form: a study in cross modality information transfer. *Proceedings of Royal Society of London* 266: 2427–2433.

Deroy, O. (2016) The intelligent invertebrate. *Science* 354(6316): 1110.

Deroy, O. and Auvray, M. (2012) Reading the world through the skin and ears: a new perspective on sensory substitution. *Frontiers in Psychology* 3: 457. doi: 10.3389/fpsyg.2012.00457.

Deroy, O. and Auvray, M. (2014) A crossmodal perspective on sensory substitution. In S. Biggs, M. Matthen, and D. Stokes (eds) *The Senses*. Oxford: Oxford University Press, 327–349.

Deroy, O., Fasiello, I., Hayward, V. and Auvray, M. (2016) Differentiated audio-tactile correspondences in sighted and blind individuals. *Journal of Experimental Psychology: Human Perception and Performance* 42: 1204–1214.

Desgent, S. and Ptito, M. (2012) Cortical GABAergic interneurons in cross-modal plasticity following early blindness. *Neural Plasticity* 590725. doi: 10.1155/2012/590725.

De Volder, A. G., Bol, A., Blin, J. et al. (1997) Brain energy metabolism in early blind subjects: neural activity in the visual cortex. *Brain Research* 750: 235–244.

Frost, D. O., Boire, D., Gingras, G. and Ptito, M. (2000) Surgically created neural pathways mediate visual pattern discrimination. *Proceedings of the National Academy of Sciences USA* 97: 11068–11073.

Godfrey-Smith, P. (2016) *The Octopus, the Sea, and the Deep Origins of Consciousness*. New York: Farrar, Straus and Giroux.

Haigh, A., Brown, D. J., Meijer, P. and Proulx, M. J. (2013) How well do you see what you hear? The acuity of visual-to-auditory sensory substitution. *Frontiers of Psychology* 4: 330. doi: 10.3389/fpsyg.2013.00330.

Hanneton, S., Auvray, M. and Durette, B. (2010) The Vibe: a versatile vision-to-audition sensory substitution device. *Applied Bionics and Biomechanics* 7: 269–276.

Ioannides, A., Liu, L., Poghosyan, V., Saridis, G. A., Gjedde, A., Ptito, M. and Kupers, R. (2013) MEG reveals a fast pathway from somatosensory cortex to occipital areas via posterior parietal cortex in a blind subject. *Frontiers of Human Neuroscience* 7: 429. doi: 10.3389/fnhum.2013.00429.

James, T. W., Humphrey, G. K., Gati, J. S., Servos, P., Menon, R. S. and Goodale, M. A. (2002) Haptic study of three-dimensional objects activates extrastriate visual areas. *Neuropsychologia* 40: 1706–1714.

Jansson, G. (1983) Tactile guidance of movement. *International Journal of Neuroscience* 19: 37–46.

Jiang, J., Zhu, W., Shi, F., Liu, Y., Li, J., Qin, W., Li, K., Yu, C. and Jiang, T. (2009) Thick visual cortex in the early blind. *Journal of Neuroscience* 29(7): 2205–2211.

Kupers, R. and Ptito, M. (2014) Compensatory plasticity and cross-modal reorganization following early visual deprivation. *Neuroscience and Biobehavoral Reviews* 41: 36–52.

Kupers, R., Fumal, A., de Noordhout, A. M., Gjedde, A., Schoenen, J. and Ptito, M. (2006) Transcranial magnetic stimulation of the visual cortex induces somatotopically organized qualia in blind subjects. *Proceedings of the National Academy of Sciences USA* 103: 13256–13260.

Kupers, R., Chebat, D. R., Madsen, K. H., Paulson, O. B. and Ptito, M. (2010) Neural correlates of virtual route recognition in congenital blindness. *Proceedings of the National Academy of Sciences USA* 107: 12716–12721.

Lenay, C. and Steiner, P. (2007) Externalism and enaction. 4th International Conference on Enactive Interfaces, 1–4.

Maidenbaum, S., Levy-Tzedek, S., Chebat, D. R. and Amedi, A. (2013) Increasing accessibility to the blind of virtual environments, using a virtual mobility aid based on the 'EyeCane': feasibility study. *PLoS One* 8(8): e72555. doi: 10.1371/journal.pone.0072555.

Matteau, I., Kupers, R., Ricciardi, E., Pietrini, P. and Ptito, M. (2010) Beyond visual, aural and haptic movement perception: hMT+ is activated by electrotactile motion stimulation of the tongue in sighted and in congenitally blind individuals. *Brain Research Bulletin* 82: 264–270.

Meijer, P. B. (1992) An experimental system for auditory image representations. *IEEE Transactions on Biomedical Engineering* 39: 112–121.

Noppeney, U., Friston, K. J., Ashburner, J., Frackowiak, R. and Price, C. J. (2005) Early visual deprivation induces structural plasticity in gray and white matter. *Current Biology* 15: 488–490.

O'Brien, J. and Auvray, M. (2014) The process of distal attribution illuminated through studies of sensory substitution. *Multisensory Research* 27: 421–441.

Picard, C. and Olivier, A. (1983) Sensory cortical tongue representation in man. *Journal of Neurosurgery* 59: 781–789.

Piccinini, G. (2010) The mind as neural software? Understanding functionalism, computationalism, and computational functionalism. *Philosophy and Phenomenological Research* 81(2): 269–311.

Pietrini, P., Furey, M. L., Ricciardi, E., Gobbini, M. I., Wu, W. H., Cohen, L., Guazzelli, M. and Haxby, J. V. (2004) Beyond sensory images: object-based representation in the human ventral pathway. *Proceedings of the National Academy of Sciences USA* 101: 5658–5663.

Pietrini, P., Ptito, M. and Kupers, R. (2009) Blindness and consciousness: new lights from the dark. In S. Laureys and G. Tononi (eds) *The Neurology of Consciousness*. London: Elsevier, 360–374.

Poirier, C., Collignon, O., Scheiber, C., Renier, L., Vanlierde, A., Tranduy, D., Veraart, C. and De Volder, A. G. (2006) Auditory motion perception activates visual motion areas in early blind subjects. *NeuroImage* 31: 279–285.

Polger, T. (2004) *Natural Minds*. Cambridge, MA: MIT Press.

Ptito, M. and Desgent, S. (2006) Sensory input-based adaptation and brain architecture. In P. Baltes, P. Reuter-Lorenz and F. Rosler (eds) *Lifespan Development and the Brain*. Cambridge: Cambridge University Press, 111–133.

Ptito, M., Moesgaard, S., Gjedde, A. and Kupers, R. (2005) Cross-modal plasticity revealed by electrotactile stimulation in the congenitally blind. *Brain* 128: 606–614.

Ptito, M., Fumal, A., de Noordhout, A. M., Schoenen, J., Gjedde, A. and Kupers, R. (2008a) TMS of the occipital cortex induces tactile sensations in the fingers of blind Braille readers. *Experimental Brain Research* 184: 193–200.

Ptito, M., Schneider, F. C. G., Paulson, O. B. and Kupers, R. (2008b) Alterations of the visual pathways in congenital blindness. *Experimental Brain Research* 187(1): 41–49.

Ptito, M., Matteau, I., Zhi Wang, A., Paulson, O. B., Siebner, H. R. and Kupers, R. (2012) Crossmodal recruitment of the ventral visual stream in congenital blindness. *Neural Plasticity* 304045. doi: 10.1155/2012/304045.

Putnam, H. (1967) Psychological predicates. In W. H. Capitan and D. D. Merrill (eds) *Art, Mind, and Religion*. Pittsburgh: University of Pittsburgh Press, 37–48.

Qin, W., Liu, Y., Jiang, T. and Yu, C. (2013) The development of visual areas depends differently on visual experience. *PLoS One* 8: e53784.

Renier, L. A., Anurova, I., De Volder, A. G., Carlson, S., VanMeter, J. and Rauschecker, J. P. (2009) Multisensory integration of sounds and vibrotactile stimuli in processing streams for 'what' and 'where'. *Journal of Neuroscience* 29: 10950–10960.

Renier, L. A., Anurova, I., De Volder, A. G., Carlson, S., VanMeter, J. and Rauschecker, J. P. (2010) Preserved functional specialization for spatial processing in the middle occipital gyrus of the early blind. *Neuron* 68: 138–148.

Ricciardi, E., Vanello, N., Sani, L., Gentili, C., Scilingo, E. P., Landini, L., Guazzelli, M., Bicchi, A., Haxby, J. V. and Pietrini, P. (2007) The effect of visual experience on the development of functional architecture in hMT+. *Cerebral Cortex* 17: 2933–2939.

Shapiro, L. (2000) Multiple realizations. *Journal of Philosophy* 97: 635–654.

Starkiewicz W. and Kuliszewski, W. (1963) The 80-channel elektroftalm. *Proceedings of the International Congress on Technology and Blindness*, American Foundation for the Blind, New York.

Striem-Amit, E., Guendelman, M. and Amedi, A. (2012) 'Visual' acuity of the congenitally blind using visual-to-auditory sensory substitution. *PLoS One* 7(3): e33136. doi: 10.1371/journal.pone.0033136.

Strnad, L., Peelen, M. V., Bedny, M. and Caramazza, A. (2013) Multivoxel pattern analysis reveals auditory motion information in MT+ of both congenitally blind and sighted individuals. *PLoS One* 8: e63198.

Ungerleider, L. G. and Mishkin, M. (1982) Two cortical visual systems. In D. J. Ingle, M. A. Goodale and R. J. W. Mansfield (eds) *Analysis of Visual Behavior*. Cambridge, MA: MIT Press, 549–586.

Voss, P. and Zatorre, R. J. (2012) Occipital cortical thickness predicts performance on pitch and musical tasks in blind individuals. *Cerebral Cortex* 22: 2455–2465.

Weinstein, S. (1968) Intensive and extensive aspects of tactile sensitivity as a function of body part, sex and laterality. In D. R. Kenshalo (ed.) *The Skin Senses*. Springfield, IL: Thomas, 195–222.

9

The Processing of What, Where, and How

Insights from Spatial Navigation via Sensory Substitution

MICHAEL J. PROULX, DAVID J. BROWN AND ACHILLE PASQUALOTTO

Abstract Vision is the default sensory modality for normal spatial navigation in humans. Touch is restricted to providing information about peripersonal space, whereas detecting and avoiding obstacles in extrapersonal space is key for efficient navigation. Hearing is restricted to the detection of objects that emit noise, yet many obstacles such as walls are silent. Sensory substitution devices provide a means of translating distal visual information into a form that visually impaired individuals can process through either touch or hearing. Here we will review findings from various sensory substitution systems for the processing of visual information that can be classified as what (object recognition), where (localization), and how (perception for action) processing. Different forms of sensory substitution excel at some tasks more than others. Spatial navigation brings together these different forms of information and provides a useful model for comparing sensory substitution systems, with important implications for rehabilitation, neuroanatomy, and theories of cognition.

VISION HAS MANY FORMS and behaviours. It is much more complex than first meets the eye—our visual abilities are so rapid and seemingly effortless that they belie the underlying complex mechanisms required. Fortunately we have a fantastic computational machine to solve this task for us—the brain. Sensory substitution devices aim to provide vision in many of its forms and definitions to the visually impaired. The devices do so by translating visual information into tactile or auditory information (Bach-y-Rita and Kercel 2003). What appears to be a simple question, 'What does it mean, to see?', is more complicated than was first considered.

Proceedings of the British Academy, **219**, 150–166.

Marr provides a useful, functional definition as a starting point: 'The plain man's answer (and Aristotle's, too) would be, to know what is where by looking' (Marr 1982). If we unpack this, it is clear that this overlaps with the idea of two processing streams in the visual brain: 'where' information in a dorsal stream and 'what' information in a ventral stream (Mishkin and Ungerleider 1982). There have been suggested modifications to these categories, in particular that the 'where' aspects be considered in terms of perception versus action, and thus 'how' rather than just 'where' (Milner and Goodale 2008). Although overly simplistic—the idea of seeing for pleasure, aesthetics, and such are missing (Ishizu and Zeki 2011)—these divisions of what, where and how are useful starting points in considering how to restore vision (Proulx et al. 2016).

Spatial navigation provides an important practical and theoretical topic to consider for vision and its substitution. Navigation is a task that is made up of all aspects of vision noted above, and more (Maguire et al. 1999). For example, if you were to visit a city for the first time and needed to have your smartphone looked at, you would need to find the appropriate shop. Doing this would first require accessible information in a database, to find out the location and opening hours. Then a survey representation, such as a map, would often be assessed in some way to determine a route from a starting location to the end point at the shop. Once the general location of the shop is reached, then visual-like behaviours would be of particular use. The 'what' information might be the icon for the shop's logo. Then one must localize 'where' it is and, with an assessment of the potential path to it, determine 'how' to get there. This level of spatial navigation that integrates information on multiple scales of representation is computationally diverse and challenging. However the components involved have been assessed by different sensory substitution devices, and we can build up an understanding of the strengths, and weaknesses, of different approaches to restoring vision through the other sensory modalities for navigation.

Vision might have some special properties that are challenging to convey to the other senses. A substantial body of work, much of it inspired by Treisman's Feature Integration Theory (Treisman and Gelade 1980), has established the role of parallel processing in vision. That is, multiple features, and even multiple objects, can be processed simultaneously to a certain extent in vision. The non-visual modalities, in particular haptics, are instead often characterized by sequential or serial processing (Henriques and Soechting 2005; Hsiao et al. 2002). This contrast was made clear in an experiment that tested sighted participants by reducing the visual field with tunnel vision. This forced the serial acquisition of information and thus made visual object recognition performance equivalent to haptic object recognition (Loomis et al. 1991; Rieser et al. 1992). In a recent review, we concluded that developmental vision has a special role in conveying information in parallel (Pasqualotto and Proulx 2012; see also Brown and Proulx 2016). This is a key ability that is crucial for multisensory integration of stimulation that occurs within the same spatial and temporal window vital for perception and learning (Proulx et al. 2014). Visual perception thus provides the necessary high level of spatial acuity and throughput to bind together the multisensory experience of the environment.

In this essay we will build up to spatial navigation through a consideration of the evidence for what, where and how forms of information. We will highlight examples from the literature and in particular from our research on some of these topics. We will then return to the larger problem of spatial navigation. We will end with a review of our recent work examining the ways visual experience affects cognition, and suggest further research that builds upon knowledge of multisensory cognition in the visually impaired, and that takes advantage of the strengths of different forms of sensory substitution.

9.1 What: Image Resolution and Object Recognition

Knowing 'what' an object is has focused on two general issues in sensory substitution research: image resolution and object recognition. In examining the literature on object recognition and resolution from the perspective of sensory substitution, it appears that visual-to-auditory devices have an advantage. There appear to be two potential reasons for this: the nature of the sensory modality used to substitute for vision, and the capacity of the devices. First, the auditory modality is considered a higher-resolution sensory modality. Second, the extant devices provide a higher theoretical translation of information, and have a higher resolution, in auditory rather than tactile devices.

Vision has the highest capacity for conveying information, even in just the phenomenological sense, well captured by the saying that a picture is worth a thousand words. A sighted person would also likely describe more attributes of a sound (such as music) than of an object only known through touch. Kokjer (1987) estimated the informational capacity of the human fingertip to be in the order of 100 bits per second (bps). The eye, by comparison, has been estimated to deliver around 4.3×10^6 bps (Jacobson 1951), some four orders of magnitude greater bandwidth. The ear falls between these two limits: its capacity has been estimated at around 10^4 bps (Jacobson 1950).

Do the levels of magnitude that separate the modalities in terms of information-processing capacity imply that the auditory and tactile modalities cannot possibly capture the full experience of vision? Not necessarily. Total information processing in terms of bits per second might allow much more unconscious processing in vision than in the other modalities, as seen by the capability for parallel processing in vision yet serial processing in tactile perception (Pasqualotto and Proulx 2012). This suggests that many aspects of perception for action (Proulx et al. 2016), normally unconscious in vision, might require intentional processing in another modality such as through touch. However the phenomenological experience of vision might be within the processing capabilities of the other sensory modalities. It is well known that visual information is selectively reduced at all levels of processing due to the limits of the cones and rods in the retina and onward due to the receptive field properties of neurons through the thalamus and cortex. Raichle (2010) summarizes research findings that demonstrate that only 10^{10} bps of the potentially unlimited (or with a very high limit) information from the environment is processed at the retina, with a further reduction to 6×10^6 bps leaving the retina via a reduced number of axons in the optic nerve. Further, this is narrowed to 10^4 bps that reaches V1. Conscious processing of visual information is further restricted to just 100 bps, or perhaps less. Therefore even the bandwidth of visual consciousness is reduced to the information-processing capacity of touch (though perhaps the bandwidth of tactile consciousness is similarly reduced).

The visual acuity, or functional resolution, possible with sensory substitution devices is an important aspect for ascertaining both 'what' and 'where' information. Visual acuity provides a measure of the distance at which two points are resolvable. Traditionally, optotypes in the form of letters or shapes are presented with decreasing size to determine acuity expressed as a Snellen fraction. The Snellen fraction is the ratio of the testing distance to the distance at which the smallest recognizable optotype subtends 5 arc-minutes, or 0.083 degrees. We noted in our recent work on visual acuity with visual-to-auditory sensory substitution (Haigh et al. 2013) that measuring visual acuity with sensory substitution must consider additional variables taken for granted in normal acuity testing, such as the field of view provided by the device. Vision with normal acuity achieved using a sensory substitution device that employs telescopic techniques would still be classified as visually impaired if restricted by severe tunnel vision (these issues are further explained here: www.seeingwithsound.com/acuity.htm). It is important to note that there are currently physical limitations on the best visual acuity possible through extant sensory substitution devices. A visual-to-auditory sensory substitution device used in our research, the vOICe (Meijer 1992), has a maximum visual acuity in the range 20/160 to 20/240 with a 60° field of view.

The first studies to assess visual acuity with sensory substitution used touch with the 'tongue display unit' or TDU (Chebat et al. 2007; Sampaio et al. 2001). Both studies employed the Snellen tumbling E paradigm to test participants' performance. Sampaio et al. (2001) used a 3 cm^2 12×12 electrotactile array and a camera with a 54° horizontal and 40° vertical field of view. The 280×180 pixel frames were down-sampled to the 12×12 tactile display resolution by averaging adjacent pixels with an image converted to black and white only (the vOICe uses grey-scale images). Because the device provided a resolution of 12 pixels horizontally, we estimated that the functional acuity might have a maximum acuity of 20/2160 when calculated for the camera's 54° field of view. Chebat et al. (2011) used a 4 cm^2 10×10 array TDU. We estimated that the maximum theoretical acuity for a 10-pixel device such as this would be 20/1392 when calculated for the 29° field of view.

More recent studies have found higher levels of acuity using hearing as the substituting modality. Acuity using the vOICe was reported by Striem-Amit et al. (2012) and by Haigh et al. (2013). The study by Haigh et al. (2013) in particular found that very little training or explanation was required to find high levels of visual acuity in the participants. The final acuity category of 20/408 in this study represented the upper limit of performance for all participants; this corresponded to optotypes reduced to 5 pixels in width. This limitation was perhaps due to the physical representation of the optotype provided being a sub-sampling of the original image. This suggested that participants were able to discriminate the orientation of the optotype with two vertical pixels representing the letter *E* when a minimum of five should be necessary for accurate discrimination. The expert blind participants in the Striem-Amit et al. (2012) study may have performed even better (in the range of 20/600 to 20/200) due to multisensory perceptual learning processes (Proulx et al. 2014). Also, all of their participants were blind, all but one of them congenitally, and this may have been a factor in their high performance (Chebat et al. 2007).

So although parallels between the auditory and visual systems are not obvious in the way that the skin/retina analogue is (which was the inspiration for Bach-y-Rita's original tactile sensory substitution device), the ear has the potential to provide a higher-throughput means of directing visual information to the brain than the skin. Moreover, even though the visual system might have the greatest information-processing capacity and spatial acuity, the auditory system is also a high-resolution sensory modality in the temporal sense. An experiment that assessed acuity in this domain used temporal order judgements to assess the temporal acuity of the senses and found there were 141 ms for tactile stimulation, 21.5 ms for auditory, and 29 ms for visual stimulation (Laasonen et al. 2001). Thus the auditory system excels at temporal processing, and a system that draws on this capacity for the translation of visuospatial information might be best placed to provide high-resolution sensory substitution (however, see also Brown et al. 2015). Indeed the superior visual acuity performance found with the vOICe might be due not only to the number of pixels that can be translated by the device but also to the higher information-processing capacity of hearing versus touch (Brown et al. 2014).

Ultimately, a decent level of acuity will allow one to recognize objects with some level of accuracy and, ideally, speed. Perhaps not coincidentally, most research on the recognition of natural objects with sensory substitution has focused on hearing as the substituting sense. For example, Auvray et al. (2007) found that participants using the vOICe were able to discriminate among natural, three-dimensional objects belonging to the same category and identify object categories as well (see also Pasqualotto and Esenkaya 2016). Pollok et al. (2005), with the same participants as Proulx et al. (2008), found that training with three-dimensional objects at home and in the lab generalized to two-dimensional object recognition presented via images sonified with the vOICe. Another visual-to-auditory device, the PSVA, has been used to demonstrate the recognition of visual patterns, though not the complex objects used in the other work described here (Arno et al. 1999). Tactile-based substitution has not been used for object recognition beyond that of the pattern recognition necessary for testing visual acuity. More recent work has examined the learning and transfer of novel, natural, three-dimensional objects in greater detail. For example, Stoerig and Proulx (2008) required participants learning to use the vOICe to specifically identify objects seen through sound, including details to verify object recognition. All participants exceeded chance levels within the first few hours of training, reaching an average of over 60 per cent correct after 15 hours of training, with some reaching perfect performance. Of course the experimental conditions were much simpler than normal natural scenes, and reducing the amount of clutter that is normally presented to the eye allowed the focus to be on purely identifying the objects rather than having to also perform scene segregation (see also Brown and Proulx 2016).

9.2 Where and How: Localization for Action

The superior resolution available currently with visual-to-auditory sensory substitution might also be of use for fine-grained spatial localization. However the method of sonifying spatial locations and the use of active motion might also be crucial. Due to the potential applications of sensory substitution in the daily lives of visually impaired persons, many tests require active localization via pointing or grasping; thus this work provides both 'where' and 'how' forms of information; the need to not only perceive objects, but to act in response to them, is a key component of this work, consistent with the perspective of Milner and Goodale (2008) on the primacy of perception for action, rather than perception alone (Proulx et al. 2016).

Auditory localization of objects has been extensively studied in human and non-human participants (Konishi 2000). The type of localization task that is crucial for sensory substitution is distinct from normal auditory localization, even if hearing is the substituting modality. Instead of relying upon a distal source of sound (such as a person's footsteps), a user must rely upon the conversion system generating sound representations of silent, distal and immobile objects. Lateral auditory localization normally depends on two input properties known as interaural loudness difference (ILD) and interaural time difference (ITD); for a review see Moore (1982). In general, the human system for horizontal auditory localization can take advantage of both of these types of information, or each one separately if they are not both present (Middlebrooks and Green 1991). Performance is best when all forms of information are present, providing a rich signal to localize a sound source. Behavioural cost in terms of response time and accuracy results when only one type of information is supplied (Schroger 1996), and has also been observed with neurophysiological methods (Palomaki et al. 2005). Vertical (elevation) auditory localization primarily depends on the spectrum of the sound cue, as created by the shape of the pinna, or outer ear (Middlebrooks and Green 1991). The pinna amplifies some frequencies and weakens others, resulting in a specific spectral tuning that is unique for each person (Hofman et al. 1998).

The perceptual learning of sound localization in humans has been examined with other objectives and methods. For example, Hofman et al. (1998) modified the outer ears of human subjects with a mould, and examined the sound localization of the subjects over time. They found that their subjects could indeed learn to hear with their newly-shaped ears, but proposed that this was only because of the richness of the auditory cues, perhaps consistent with multisensory perceptual learning (Proulx et al. 2014), and the use of the new ears in daily life. Like Hofman and colleagues, Proulx et al. (2008) provided daily experience with a novel auditory input to participants, although for less time than in Hofman's study (10 or 21 days for Proulx et al. versus 39 days in Hofman et al.'s study). In further contrast, the participants had two artificial signals provided by the vOICe for object position: laterality was coded by stereo panning and the time provided by the left-to-right scanning transformation of each image, and elevation by frequency, so that up was represented by high frequencies and down by low frequencies. Pixel brightness was coded by loudness. Images were taken by a small video camera hidden in sunglasses and converted into the sound patterns that the subjects heard through stereo headphones. The object's horizontal location in the image is coded by time and stereo panning, so that the sound pertaining to an object on the right of the image will be heard late in the scan and predominantly through the right ear, using both ILD and ITD. Whether it is located higher up or lower down in the image is expressed by frequency, so that an object in the upper part of the image is heard in higher tones than one in the lower part. Together this provided the 'where' information.

The first experiment by Proulx et al. (2008) assessed localization with a perimetry device that was constructed with an array of LEDs for a manual search task. One LED would light up and would be accompanied by a tone until pressed, when the light and tone were extinguished. Over a three-week period, those participants using the vOICe in daily practice with natural objects in natural environments (their own homes) were able to generalize that experience to the lab test with significant improvements in speed and accuracy. A second experiment examined the localization and grasping of natural objects placed on a large table (Auvray et al. 2007). Again we found successful transfer of experience in the home to the lab, where those trained to use the vOICe had significant improvement in not only locating the objects, but reaching with grasp-appropriate hand configurations. This suggested that they not only understood 'where' the objects were, but had access to features related to 'what' the objects were, too: size, shape, and orientation.

More recent work by Brown et al. (2011) found that the location of the camera providing visual input interacted with the goal of the task. For example, while Proulx et al. (2008) used a head-mounted camera to mimic eyesight, Auvray et al. (2007) used a handheld camera for their tasks. Brown and colleagues compared the performance for tasks requiring either object identification or localization with both camera positions. They reported an interesting dissociation: object identification was better with the handheld camera and localization was better with the head-mounted camera. This suggests that the ability to sample many viewpoints of the object via the hand is particularly useful for identifying it, and also that mimicking the perceptual-motor contingencies used in normal localization can improve performance as well, with the viewpoint near the eyes.

The ability to correct fast reaching movements has been assessed with a device that is similar to the vOICe in its basic structure, except with the addition of timbre as a feature to code for colour in EyeMusic (Levy-Tzedek et al. 2012). The tasks required rapid reaching to a target, and with little training participants were able to perform the task nearly as accurately with the device as with seeing. One problem for interpreting the results, however, is that the amount of time allowed to listen to the object location was, potentially, unlimited before the fast reaching movement was required. That period of time is crucial for real-world navigational needs, and for making crucial comparisons with vision. If visual perception is thought of as 'unconscious inference' in the ways proposed by Von Helmholtz (2005), with some requirement for rapid processing that would go beyond conscious, effortful inference, then the current state of sensory substitution would require extensive training and experience before that threshold is reached. This and a number of visual-to-tactile studies often report either accuracy or time as the primary measure of performance; it is challenging to benchmark the relative costs and benefits of different devices and sensory modalities in the absence of all the necessary data to consider their use.

Another visual-to-auditory sensory substitution device has been used for studies of localization: the PSVA or prosthesis for substitution of vision by audition (Capelle et al. 1998). Unlike the vOICe, which sweeps the image from left to right to create the sonification, the PSVA provides a simultaneous sonification of the entire image and thus requires manual movement (either by the participant or the camera) to make sense of the image, similar to the concept of using eye movements to perceive a scene. While the studies described above that employed the vOICe implicitly required the perception of depth for the accurate localization and grasping of objects, a study with the PSVA explicitly examined the problem of depth. Both devices use a single camera, thus depth must be inferred from monocular cues rather than stereopsis. Renier et al. (2005) examined the ability of participants to locate items in depth using cues similar to those present in a natural corridor (and consequently the same cues that can create compelling corridor illusions). Although reaching and grasping were not employed, the participants were able to perceive and report the depth relations between the objects in the display.

The qualitative debriefings reported by Renier et al. (2005) provide interesting observations about the learning process, and how depth was understood by the participants. Those participants who were blind from birth or in early childhood had to first learn the basics of vision that a sighted person can take for granted: shape, size constancy, depth information, occlusion, perspective, and other ways in which the brain has learned, through development, to 'correct' for distortions in the two-dimensional image that are simply due to the viewing perspective rather than revealing changes in the object itself (Proulx and Harder 2008). It was noteworthy that all early blind participants were aware that relative size was a depth cue on the basis of hearing how sighted persons described the world. This is crucial because the acquisition of object information through haptics is size-invariant of course; a far-off object is out of reach, and any object that can be touched is perceived as its unchanging three-dimensional size. Similar findings have been reported for visual-to-tactile sensory substitution (Segond et al. 2013). Even with this top-down knowledge of how distance impacts the perception of size, the early blind participants still had more difficulty correcting for that than those who were sighted (but blindfolded) and those who became blind later in life. Thus learning the vocabulary of vision through sensory substitution (Deroy and Auvray 2012) might require not only active experience (Proulx 2010), but perhaps visual experience as well for full functioning (Pasqualotto and Proulx 2012).

9.3 Spatial Navigation as the Processing of What, Where and How

Given the superiority of auditory perception in the domain of temporal processing, most studies have focused on the performance of visual-to-auditory sensory substitution for representing object information with high fidelity and acuity. However one study has also examined the use of the vOICe for spatial navigation. One challenge for using the vOICe for navigation is that such a task requires online perception and correction to avoid stationary obstructions, much less moving ones. The vOICe only samples the environment with an image every 1–2 seconds (even though it can be set at much higher refresh rates, no studies have examined the ability of users to function at those sampling rates). Brown et al. (2011) had participants walk a short route that contained four obstacles using the vOICe. It took them over five minutes to complete the task, though they demonstrated improvement of over one minute with eight trials of practice. Certainly real-world navigation would introduce challenges that would make it practically unfeasible in its current form. However navigation in vision takes advantage of peripheral vision with its lower resolution; perhaps a simpler representation is better for such a task. One auditory example might be the simplified auditory input that can be provided by learned echolocation in some blind humans (Thaler et al. 2011).

Representing spatial information in an online manner might instead provide a task for which visual-to-tactile sensory substitution would excel. Devices like the TDU provide constant stimulation of the environment and as a result require movement for accurate localization and identification of objects (Matteau et al. 2010). As noted previously, the resolution of such devices is lower than that of an auditory device like the vOICe. This might not be a drawback for a task like navigation. Normal obstacle avoidance utilizes peripheral vision, which provides lower-resolution information compared to the fovea due to a combination of having fewer cone cells and the cortical magnification factor that favours foveal vision (Loschky et al. 2005). Peripheral vision is also a primary contributor to magnocellular processing which, like the representation provided by the TDU, is selective for contrast (the TDU only has black and white representation) and motion (Livingstone and Hubel 1988).

The methods of assessing spatial navigation with tactile vision substitution systems have been creative. Segond et al. (2005) created a semi-passive paradigm where the participants using the TDU remained still, but operated a camera-carrying robot with a remote control. The robot was placed in a three-dimensional maze. The accuracy and speed of the maze completion were assessed and demonstrated success from the very first attempt. Again it is challenging to generalize from this experience directly to real-world navigation. A more recent study with the TDU (Chebat et al. 2011) used a real course in a corridor with obstacles, similar to that tested with the vOICe (Brown et al. 2011). Not only were participants able to successfully navigate the course with few errors, but it was also found that congenitally blind individuals were able to out-perform sighted participants. This is interesting because it further suggests that route or egocentric spatial knowledge is preserved even in the absence of visual experience (Pasqualotto and Proulx 2012; Pasqualotto et al. 2013b), although allocentric spatial knowledge might be affected. Although the participants were successful in terms of accuracy, this study, like others in the literature, did not provide as much information about the time required to complete the task, and thus it is difficult to fully assess the use of the TDU and tactile perception rather than the vOICe and auditory perception for such a task.

Real-world navigation requires a combination of cognitive skills such as object recognition (what), localization (where) and obstacle avoidance (how). Furthermore it would be beneficial to have access to allocentric, map-like representations and perhaps even some knowledge of cardinal directions, such as that provided by sensory augmentation devices like vibrotactile belts (Karcher et al. 2012; Nagel et al. 2005). One solution that has yet to be tested is the use of more than one device at once. For example, integrating a smartphone for address and route information, a belt for cardinal directions, a tactile device for obstacle avoidance, and an auditory device for high-resolution shape recognition and localization might be ideal. In fact, this might best represent how human spatial navigation normally works; yet the challenge to monitor and incorporate input from such a plethora of devices might be beyond current human capacities.

9.4 Cross-Modal Correspondences

The basic idea of creating a sensory substitution device is predicated on the utility of translating information from that normally sensed by one modality to a format that can be sensed by another modality. Although humans might be able to learn any arbitrary association between two sensory modalities, it would seem sensible to base the conversion principles upon any natural cross-modal correspondences that humans have. There is increasing evidence that a task that targets one sense can be affected by the stimulation of the other senses, even if such stimulation is task-irrelevant and below the threshold of awareness (Evans and Treisman 2010; Mondloch and Maurer 2004). The vOICe takes its basic conversion principle from experiments that have shown that the perception of high or low frequency (pitch) affects lexical decision tasks, such as deciding one read the word 'down' at the same time as hearing a tone of low frequency (Walker and Smith 1984). Thus stating that an auditory pitch is high or low is not just metaphorical, but directly affects one's perception of the world. Similarly, auditory and vibrotactile stimuli are known to share similar temporal patterns, and research has shown that this similarity can also lead to perceptual bias (Schurmann et al. 2004). Moreover, developmental research shows that cross-modal interaction occurs from an early age (Mondloch and Maurer 2004).

As useful as such studies might be for designing a sensory substitution device, they all have one drawback: each used sighted participants exclusively. Thus, the use of such mappings assumes, as some have proposed, that these cross-modal correspondences are hard-wired or otherwise are based on experience that does not require visual perception (Spence and Deroy 2012). Whether this assumption is correct is currently unknown (however, see also Hamilton-Fletcher et al. 2018), and thus it may be necessary to establish whether the mappings reported in the cross-modal interaction literature apply to individuals with congenital visual impairment. In fact, evidence from research on accessible technology suggests that some visually impaired users have inverse polarity for mapping data values, such as temperature, to acoustic parameters, such as pitch (Walker and Mauney 2001).

We have found other differences between congenitally blind individuals on the one hand, and those with visual experience such as the late blind and sighted, on the other hand. In particular it appears that visual experience is necessary for the normal neural development that underlies spatial cognition (Pasqualotto and Proulx 2012). For example, sighted and late blind participants prefer an allocentric representation to remember the spatial locations of aligned objects in extrapersonal space (outside of arm's reach), even if such a representation requires a form of mental rotation to recode the locations of the objects in relation to one another. Congenitally blind individuals, though, prefer an egocentric representation based on the starting location used for acquiring knowledge of the location of the objects (Pasqualotto et al. 2013b). Visual experience also impacts semantic processing in memory (Amedi et al. 2003; Bedny et al. 2011; Pasqualotto et al. 2013a). Given the role of visual experience for cognitive processing in the sighted, there is certainly a possibility that the cross-modal mappings used by extant sensory substitution devices can stand to be improved, or tailored for users with different amounts of visual experience. Of course, the brain plasticity observed in many studies suggests that almost any arbitrary algorithm can be learned; however, perhaps that arbitrariness is what makes learning so challenging and unappealing to potential users.

9.5 Opportunities of Sensory Substitution

There are many dimensions of the psychology of sensory substitution that are open to active investigation. The current limits on the functionality of devices arise from multiple domains: technological, such as device resolution limit; modality, such as the resolution or nature of the sensory system substituting for vision; mapping algorithm, based upon cross-modal correspondences; and learning and plasticity, such as the optimal training required for multisensory perceptual learning (Proulx et al. 2014) and generalization (Brown and Proulx 2013). There are certainly reasons to be optimistic for the future of sensory substitution. First, naïve users are able to perform not only above chance with minimal training, but even to near ceiling degrees of visual acuity; moreover, even a little bit of training improves performance (Haigh et al. 2013) and that improvement can be maintained over several months and be generalized beyond that specifically practised during training (Brown and Proulx 2013). These points are crucial and should be considered in the context of the development of normal vision; certainly human infants do not learn to see as adults in merely one day. The current state of the art also suggests that different devices and modalities might be advantageous for different tasks, though it is unclear at the present time whether this is due to the nature of the devices or the substituting modalities.

There are also many other unanswered questions of central importance for both basic and applied research in psychology, neuroscience and philosophy. We have noted elsewhere that it appears active sensorimotor expertise and experience might be necessary for full mastery of a sensory substitution device, and to a much lesser extent the experience of visual qualia through these means (Proulx 2010; Proulx and Stoerig 2006). It is therefore an open question whether something like visual qualia is possible in a congenitally blind user who has not had the visual experience necessary to store visual images that can be linked with the device output. This brings up the definition of vision once again. Is vision defined by what one does with it, or the experience of it? A proficient user of a sensory substitution device might appear to see from the perspective of an independent user, even though only some users might have visual qualia evoked by the experience. On the applied side, creating a multimodal device that incorporates the best of the extant devices might be of interest; combining perhaps an auditory device for high-resolution object recognition and a tactile device for navigation, for example. Such a device would require a greater understanding of the attentional demands that would be imposed, not only in attending to the two devices at once, but the ambient environment as well. Although current sensory substitution devices appear to be limited in being adopted universally for use, the potential for using sensory substitution as a tool to better understand basic cognition is clear. Such fundamental investigations should in turn provide opportunities to improve the viability of sensory substitution in the future and overcome the present limitations.

References

Amedi, A., Raz, N., Pianka, P., Malach, R. and Zohary, E. (2003) Early 'visual' cortex activation correlates with superior verbal memory performance in the blind. *Nature Neuroscience* 6(7): 758–766. doi: 10.1038/nn1072.

Arno, P., Capelle, C., Wanet-Defalque, M. C., Catalan-Ahumada, M. and Veraart, C. (1999) Auditory coding of visual patterns for the blind. *Perception* 28(8): 1013–1029.

Auvray, M., Hanneton, S. and O'Regan, J. K. (2007) Learning to perceive with a visuo-auditory substitution system: localisation and object recognition with 'the vOICe'. *Perception* 36(3): 416–430.

Bach-y-Rita, P. and Kercel, S. W. (2003) Sensory substitution and the human-machine interface. *Trends in Cognitive Science* 7(12): 541–546. doi: S1364661303002900 [pii].

Bedny, M., Pascual-Leone, A., Dodell-Feder, D., Fedorenko, E. and Saxe, R. (2011) Language processing in the occipital cortex of congenitally blind adults. *Proceedings of the National Academy of Sciences* 108(11): 4429–4434.

Brown, D., Macpherson, T. and Ward, J. (2011) Seeing with sound? Exploring different characteristics of a visual-to-auditory sensory substitution device. *Perception* 40(9): 1120–1135.

Brown, D. J. and Proulx, M. J. (2013) Increased signal complexity improves the breadth of generalization in auditory perceptual learning. *Neural Plasticity* 9. doi: 10.1155/2013/879047.

Brown, D. J. and Proulx, M. J. (2016) Audio-vision substitution for blind individuals: addressing human information processing capacity limitations. *IEEE Journal of Selected Topics in Signal Processing* 10, 924–931.

Brown, D. J., Simpson, A. J. R. and Proulx, M. J. (2014) Visual objects in the auditory system via sensory substitution: how much information do we need? *Multisensory Research* 27, 337–357. doi: 10.1163/22134808-00002462.

Brown, D. J., Simpson, A. J. R. and Proulx, M. J. (2015) Auditory Scene Analysis and sonified visual images: does consonance negatively impact on object formation when using complex sonified stimuli? *Frontiers in Psychology* 6. doi: 10.3389/fpsyg.2015.01522.

Capelle, C., Trullemans, C., Arno, P. and Veraart, C. (1998) A real-time experimental prototype for enhancement of vision rehabilitation using auditory substitution. *IEEE Transactions on Biomedical Engineering* 45(10): 1279–1293. doi: 10.1109/10.720206.

Chebat, D. R., Rainville, C., Kupers, R. and Ptito, M. (2007) Tactile-'visual' acuity of the tongue in early blind individuals. *Neuroreport* 18(18): 1901–1904. doi: 10.1097/WNR.0b013e3282f2a63.

Chebat, D. R., Schneider, F. C., Kupers, R. and Ptito, M. (2011) Navigation with a sensory substitution device in congenitally blind individuals. *Neuroreport* 22(7): 342–347. doi: 10.1097/WNR.0b013e3283462def.

Deroy, O. and Auvray, M. (2012) Reading the world through the skin and ears: a new perspective on sensory substitution. *Frontiers in Psychology* 3: 457. doi: 10.3389/fpsyg.2012.00457.

Evans, K. K. and Treisman, A. (2010) Natural cross-modal mappings between visual and auditory features. *Journal of Vision* 10(1). doi: 10.1167/10.1.6.

Haigh, A., Brown, D. J., Meijer, P. and Proulx, M. J. (2013) How well do you see what you hear? The acuity of visual-to-auditory sensory substitution. *Frontiers in Psychology* 4. doi: 10.3389/fpsyg.2013.00330.

Hamilton-Fletcher, G., Pisanski, K., Reby, D., Stefańczyk, M., Ward, J. and Sorokowska, A. (2018) The role of visual experience in the emergence of cross-modal correspondences. *Cognition* 175, 114–121.

Henriques, D. Y. and Soechting, J. F. (2005) Approaches to the study of haptic sensing. *Journal of Neurophysiology* 93(6): 3036–3043. doi: 10.1152/jn.00010.2005.

Hofman, P. M., Van Riswick, J. G. and Van Opstal, A. J. (1998) Relearning sound localization with new ears. *Nature Neuroscience* 1(5): 417–421. doi: 10.1038/1633.

Hsiao, S. S., Lane, J. and Fitzgerald, P. (2002) Representation of orientation in the somatosensory system. *Behavioural Brain Research* 135(1–2H): 93–103.

Ishizu, T. and Zeki, S. (2011) Toward a brain-based theory of beauty. *PLoS One* 6(7): e21852. doi: 10.1371/journal.pone.0021852.

Jacobson, H. (1950) The informational capacity of the human ear. *Science* 112(2901): 143–144.

Jacobson, H. (1951) The informational capacity of the human eye. *Science* 113(2933): 292–293.

Karcher, S. M., Fenzlaff, S., Hartmann, D., Nagel, S. K. and Konig, P. (2012) Sensory augmentation for the blind. *Frontiers in Human Neuroscience* 6: 37. doi: 10.3389/fnhum.2012.00037.

Kokjer, K. J. (1987) The information capacity of the human fingertip. *IEEE Transactions on Systems, Man and Cybernetics* 17(1): 100–102. doi: 10.1109/TSMC.1987.289337.

Konishi, M. (2000) Study of sound localization by owls and its relevance to humans. *Comparative Biochemistry and Physiology Part A: Molecular and Integrative Physiology* 126(4): 459–469. doi: http://dx.doi.org/10.1016/S1095-6433(00)00232-4.

Laasonen, M., Service, E. and Virsu, V. (2001) Temporal order and processing acuity of visual, auditory, and tactile perception in developmentally dyslexic young adults. *Cognitive, Affective, and Behavioral Neuroscience* 1(4): 394–410.

Levy-Tzedek, S., Hanassy, S., Abboud, S., Maidenbaum, S. and Amedi, A. (2012) Fast, accurate reaching movements with a visual-to-auditory sensory substitution device. *Restorative Neurology and Neuroscience* 30(4): 313–323. doi: 10.3233/RNN-2012-110219.

Livingstone, M. and Hubel, D. (1988) Segregation of form, color, movement, and depth: anatomy, physiology, and perception. *Science* 240(4853): 740–749. doi: 10.1126/science.3283936.

Loomis, J. M., Klatzky, R. L. and Lederman, S. J. (1991) Similarity of tactual and visual picture recognition with limited field of view. *Perception* 20(2): 167–177.

Loschky, L., McConkie, G., Yang, J. and Miller, M. (2005) The limits of visual resolution in natural scene viewing. *Visual Cognition* 12(6): 1057–1092. doi: 10.1080/13506280444000652.

Maguire, E. A., Burgess, N. and O'Keefe, J. (1999) Human spatial navigation: cognitive maps, sexual dimorphism, and neural substrates. *Current Opinion in Neurobiology* 9(2): 171–177.

Meijer, P. B. L. (1992) An experimental system for auditory image representations. *IEEE Transactions on Biomedical Engineering* 39: 112–121.

Marr, D. (1982) *Vision: A Computational Investigation into the Human Representation and Processing of Visual Information*. San Francisco: W. H. Freeman.

Matteau, I., Kupers, R., Ricciardi, E., Pietrini, P. and Ptito, M. (2010) Beyond visual, aural and haptic movement perception: hMT+ is activated by electrotactile motion stimulation of the tongue in sighted and in congenitally blind individuals. *Brain Research Bulletin* 82(5–6): 264–270. doi: 10.1016/j.brainresbull.2010.05.001.

Middlebrooks, J. C. and Green, D. M. (1991) Sound localization by human listeners. *Annual Review of Psychology* 42: 135–159. doi: 10.1146/annurev.ps.42.020191.001031.

Milner, A. D. and Goodale, M. A. (2008) Two visual systems re-viewed. *Neuropsychologia* 46(3): 774–785. doi: 10.1016/j.neuropsychologia.2007.10.005.

Mishkin, M. and Ungerleider, L. G. (1982) Contribution of striate inputs to the visuospatial functions of parieto-preoccipital cortex in monkeys. *Behavioural Brain Research* 6(1): 57–77.

Mondloch, C. J. and Maurer, D. (2004) Do small white balls squeak? Pitch-object correspondences in young children. *Cognitive, Affective, and Behavioral Neuroscience* 4(2): 133–136.

Moore, B. C. J. (1982) *An Introduction to the Psychology of Hearing*. London: Academic Press.

Nagel, S. K., Carl, C., Kringe, T., Martin, R. and Konig, P. (2005) Beyond sensory substitution—learning the sixth sense. *Journal of Neural Engineering* 2(4): R13–26. doi: 10.1088/1741-2560/2/4/R02.

Palomaki, K. J., Tiitinen, H., Makinen, V., May, P. J. and Alku, P. (2005) Spatial processing in human auditory cortex: the effects of 3D, ITD, and ILD stimulation techniques. *Brain Research. Cognitive Brain Research* 24(3): 364–379. doi: 10.1016/j.cogbrainres.2005.02.013.

Pasqualotto, A. and Esenkaya, T. (2016) Sensory substitution: the spatial updating of auditory scenes 'mimics' the spatial updating of visual scenes. *Frontiers in Behavioral Neuroscience* 10: 79.

Pasqualotto, A. and Proulx, M. J. (2012) The role of visual experience for the neural basis of spatial cognition. *Neuroscience and Biobehavioral Reviews* 36(4): 1179–1187. doi: 10.1016/j.neubiorev.2012.01.008.

Pasqualotto, A., Lam, J. S. and Proulx, M. J. (2013a) Congenital blindness improves semantic and episodic memory. *Behavioural Brain Research* 244: 162–165. doi: 10.1016/j.bbr.2013.02.005.

Pasqualotto, A., Spiller, M. J., Jansari, A. S. and Proulx, M. J. (2013b) Visual experience facilitates allocentric spatial representation. *Behavioural Brain Research* 236(1): 175–179. doi: 10.1016/j.bbr.2012.08.042.

Pollok, B., Schnitzler, I., Stoerig, P., Mierdorf, T. and Schnitzler, A. (2005) Image-to-sound conversion: experience-induced plasticity in auditory cortex of blindfolded adults. *Experimental Brain Research* 167(2): 287–291. doi: 10.1007/s00221-005-0060-8.

Proulx, M. J. (2010) Synthetic synaesthesia and sensory substitution. *Consciousness and Cognition* 19(1): 501–503. doi: 10.1016/j.concog.2009.12.005.

Proulx, M. J. and Harder, A. (2008) Sensory substitution. Visual-to-auditory sensory substitution devices for the blind. *Dutch Journal of Ergonomics/Tijdschrift voor Ergonomie* 33: 20–22.

Proulx, M. J. and Stoerig, P. (2006) Seeing sounds and tingling tongues: qualia in synaesthesia and sensory substitution. *Anthropology and Philosophy* 7: 135–151.

Proulx, M. J., Stoerig, P., Ludowig, E. and Knoll, I. (2008) Seeing 'where' through the ears: effects of learning-by-doing and long-term sensory deprivation on localization based on image-to-sound substitution. *PLoS One* 3(3): e1840. doi: 10.1371/journal.pone.0001840.

Proulx, M. J., Brown, D. J., Pasqualotto, A. and Meijer, P. (2012) Multisensory perceptual learning and sensory substitution. *Neuroscience and Biobehavioral Reviews* 41: 16–25. doi: 10.1016/j.neubiorev.2012.11.017.

Proulx, M. J., Brown, D., Pasqualotto, A. and Meijer, P. (2014) Multisensory perceptual learning and sensory substitution. *Neuroscience and Biobehavioral Reviews* 41, 16–25. doi: 10.1016/j.neubiorev.2012.11.017.

Proulx, M. J., Gwinnutt, J., Dell'Erba, S., Levy-Tzedek, S., de Sousa, A. A. and Brown, D. J. (2016) Other ways of seeing: from behavior to neural mechanisms in the online 'visual' control of action with sensory substitution. *Restorative Neurology and Neuroscience* 34, 29–44.

Raichle, M. E. (2010) Two views of brain function. *Trends in Cognitive Science* 14(4): 180–190. doi: 10.1016/j.tics.2010.01.008.

Renier, L., Collignon, O., Poirier, C., Tranduy, D., Vanlierde, A., Bol, A., et al. (2005) Cross-modal activation of visual cortex during depth perception using auditory substitution of vision. *NeuroImage* 26(2): 573–580. doi: 10.1016/j.neuroimage.2005.01.047.

Rieser, J. J., Hill, E. W., Talor, C. R., Bradfield, A. and Rosen, S. (1992) Visual experience, visual field size, and the development of nonvisual sensitivity to the spatial structure of outdoor neighborhoods explored by walking. *Journal of Experimental Psychology: General* 121(2): 210–221.

Sampaio, E., Maris, S. and Bach-y-Rita, P. (2001) Brain plasticity: 'visual' acuity of blind persons via the tongue. *Brain Research* 908(2): 204–207. doi: S0006-8993(01)02667-1 [pii].

Schroger, E. (1996) Interaural time and level differences: integrated or separated processing? *Hearing Research* 96(1–2): 191–198.

Schurmann, M., Caetano, G., Jousmaki, V. and Hari, R. (2004) Hands help hearing: facilitatory audiotactile interaction at low sound-intensity levels. *The Journal of the Acoustical Society of America* 115(2): 830–832.

Segond, H., Weiss, D. and Sampaio, E. (2005) Human spatial navigation via a visuo-tactile sensory substitution system. *Perception* 34(10): 1231–1249.

Segond, H., Weiss, D., Kawalec, M. and Sampaio, E. (2013) Perceiving space and optical cues via a visuo-tactile sensory substitution system: a methodological approach for training of blind subjects for navigation. *Perception* 42(5): 508–528.

Spence, C. and Deroy, O. (2012) Crossmodal correspondences: innate or learned? *i-Perception* 3(5): 316–318. doi: 10.1068/i0526ic.

Stoerig, P. and Proulx, M. J. (2008) Learning to recognize objects with an image-to-sound conversion-based sensory system. Paper presented at the Volkswagen Foundation status symposium on 'Dynamics and adaptivity of neuronal systems', Tübingen, Germany.

Striem-Amit, E., Guendelman, M. and Amedi, A. (2012) 'Visual' acuity of the congenitally blind using visual-to-auditory sensory substitution. *PLoS One* 7(3): e33136. doi: 10.1371/journal.pone.0033136.

Thaler, L., Arnott, S. R. and Goodale, M. A. (2011) Neural correlates of natural human echolocation in early and late blind echolocation experts. *PLoS One* 6(5): e20162. doi: 10.1371/journal.pone.0020162.

Treisman, A. M. and Gelade, G. (1980) A feature-integration theory of attention. *Cognitive Psychology* 12(1): 97–136. doi: 0010-0285(80)90005-5 [pii].

Von Helmholtz, H. (2005) *Treatise on Physiological Optics*, vol. 3. Mineola, NY: Dover Publications.

Walker, B. N. and Mauney, L. M. (2001) Psychophysical scaling of sonification mappings: a comparison of visually impaired and sighted listeners. *Proceedings of the 2001 International Conference on Auditory Display*, Espoo, Finland, 29 July–1 August.

Walker, P. and Smith, S. (1984) Stroop interference based on the synaesthetic qualities of auditory pitch. *Perception* 13(1): 75–81.

10

Rewired Animals and Sensory Substitution: The Cause Is Not Cortical Plasticity

J. KEVIN O'REGAN

Abstract Cortical plasticity is often invoked to explain changes in the quality or location of experience observed in rewired animals, in sensory substitution, in extension of the body through tool use, and in the rubber hand illusion. However this appeal to cortical plasticity may be misleading, because it suggests that the cortical areas that are plastic are themselves the loci of generation of experience. This would be an error, I claim, since cortical areas do not generate experience. Cortical areas participate in enabling the interaction of an agent with its environment, and the quality of this interaction constitutes the quality of experience. Thus it is not plasticity in itself, but the change in modes of interaction which plasticity allows, which gives rise to the change of experience observed in these studies.

William James said that if we were able to re-direct nerves from the eye so that they connected to the brain centres concerned with hearing, and vice versa, then we would 'hear the lightning and see the thunder' (James 1890).

Underlying this statement is the idea that what determines the quality of sensations is the particular brain area that processes the neural influx. Since James' time, an enormous literature has lent support to this idea, including several iconic results. Among these is Penfield's demonstration that tactile sensations in different body locations can be elicited by stimulation of corresponding areas of a somatosensory map or 'Penfield homunculus', and that stimulation of other areas can actually generate visual or auditory experiences (Penfield 1958).

Since those days the idea of 'localization of function' in the brain has become a doctrine (cf. Phillips et al. 1984), with a large portion of neuroscience research devoted to determining the particular functions of the different brain areas.

Applied to perception, the localization of function doctrine is often taken to suggest that there is something special about each kind of cortex that underlies

Proceedings of the British Academy, **219**, 167–173.

the particular quality of sensations that that kind of cortex allows. Just as there is something special about Penfield's somatosensory cortex which allows it to generate tactile sensations, there is something special about visual, auditory, etc., cortices which allows them to generate visual, auditory, etc., sensations.

Within this way of thinking, the studies of 'rewired' animals and visual cortex in blind individuals have added an interesting twist, which reveals a subtle issue concerning the causal status of the notion of cortical plasticity.

10.1 Rewired Animals and Visual Cortex in Blind Persons

The studies of rewired animals investigate what happens when animals are surgically rewired at birth in such a way that information from the eyes, usually transmitted to visual cortex, is re-routed so that it projects into auditory cortex (Frost et al. 2000; Pallas et al. 1990; Pallas and Sur 1993; Sharma et al. 2000). The results show that when mature, the rewired animals are able to perform visual behaviours almost as efficiently as normal animals using their visual cortex. Furthermore, the rewired auditory cortex reorganizes and displays a two-dimensional orientation-sensitive structure similar to that observed in normal visual cortex.

Of particular interest is one very ingenious study which was able to approach an answer to the question of whether the quality of the sensations experienced by such rewired animals via their auditory cortex was actually visual rather than auditory (Von Melchner et al. 2000). The authors used ferrets that were only rewired in one hemisphere. They first trained these animals to distinguish between sounds and lights that were presented in such a way as to be processed only by the normal hemisphere. When completely trained, the animals were tested with lights that were processed only by the rewired hemisphere, that is, through auditory cortex. The animals invariably turned in a way suggesting that they perceived the lights visually, even though the perception occurred via their auditory cortex. When the auditory cortex was removed, the animals behaved as though they were blind.

Note that the authors did not observe any lateral connections between the 'converted' auditory cortex and existing visual cortex. Thus it truly appears that the visual sensations were related to the presence of the auditory cortex, and not to stimulation spreading to visual cortex. We thus seem to have a case in which, contrary to William James' prediction, it seems that the animals end up 'seeing the lightning rather than hearing it'.

Another well-publicized result showing adaptation of sensation generated in cortical areas has emerged recently in studies on blind people. For such persons it has been shown that visual cortex can rewire itself so as to participate in other functions, including language processing, memory, motion detection and navigation. The results are particularly strong in the congenitally blind, where visual cortex has never been exposed to visual stimulation. Of interest as regards the question of the experienced quality of sensations are the results of Kupers et al. (2006) and Ptito et al. (2008). They trained subjects to use a sensory substitution device called the 'tongue display unit', which converts visual stimuli captured by a video camera into tactile stimulation on the tongue. After learning to do orientation, form or motion discrimination tasks with the device, early blind subjects given transcranial magnetic stimulation (TMS) directed onto their visual cortex felt tingling sensations on their tongue. Visual cortex thus seems now to underlie the generation of tactile sensations on the tongue.

10.2 Cortical Plasticity

All these results show that whatever it is about a particular cortical area that gives rise to a particular quality of sensation (e.g. visual, auditory, tactile), it does not lie in the specific cortical area or type of neurons, but in something that can be modified as a function of adaptation to extrinsic stimulation. As noted by Hurley and Noë (2003), the cortex 'defers' to the particular sensory input channel.

Such a modification is generally referred to as being an instance of 'cortical plasticity'. Researchers will tend to say that cortical plasticity has allowed auditory cortex to change its function, going from generating auditory sensations to generating visual sensations. The implicit underlying assumption is that cortex generates sensations, and so to have different sensations, cortex must change its mode of functioning.

But to say this is to fall into a 'category mistake' (Ryle 1949). For suppose it made sense to say that different cortical areas 'generated' different types of sensations. Then we would be faced with the problem of explaining exactly how this came about. Exactly what is it about the different areas that allows them to generate the particular sensations they provide? This is the vexed problem of 'qualia', for which a variety of esoteric hypotheses have been advanced, going from quantum gravity effects in microtubules, through synchronous oscillations in widespread cortical areas, to cortico-thalamic reverberations—see the list provided by Chalmers (1997). For any such hypothesis, as noted by Dennett (1991), an infinite regress of questions ('And *then* what happens?') can always be asked about what exactly it is about these mechanisms that produces feel rather than no feel. And why are the feels the way they are, rather than some other way? Any explanation for similarities and differences in feels that is made in terms of physico-chemical mechanisms requires making a link between the language of neural processes and the language of sensations: and there is no non-arbitrary way to make that link.

For that reason the sensorimotor approach (O'Regan and Noë 2001; O'Regan 2011) proposes to reject the notion that sensations are the kinds of things that can be generated. The sensorimotor approach proposes instead that it is scientifically more fruitful to consider the qualities of sensations as *laws of interaction with the world*. For example the sensation of softness consists in the law that links the sensory inputs you receive from your fingers with the pressure you exert on the sponge. The sponge is soft if it squishes under your fingers. Taking this stance is not just a philosophical trick, it actually leads to scientific predictions and paradigms, like the work on change blindness, inattentional blindness, sensory substitution and colour psychophysics.

In conclusion, if the sensorimotor approach is correct, then it is misleading to say that in rewired animals cortical plasticity has allowed 'auditory cortex to change its function, going from generating auditory sensations to generating visual sensations'.

10.3 The Real Cause

What then is the correct thing to say about what happens with rewired animals?

We must say that the animal has become able to use its auditory cortex instead of its visual cortex in overseeing the sensorimotor interactions it has with the world using its eyes. Initially it tries to react appropriately to input from the eyes, but because at first auditory cortex is not wired up to do the task efficiently, the animal does not process the input or react quite as efficiently as if it were using visual cortex. But gradually there is learning, and auditory cortex reorganizes itself to do the task more efficiently. When things stabilize, however, it would be a mistake to say that auditory cortex is 'generating' visual qualia. No: auditory cortex is now participating in visual-type interactions in a way that is almost as efficient as visual cortex usually would be. Such a situation is called 'seeing'.

Of course we could call the change from inefficient to efficient use of the auditory cortex 'cortical plasticity'. But it is important to be aware that this 'plasticity' is not *in itself* what is causing the transition to seeing with the auditory cortex. The plasticity is allowing the animal to interact in a visual fashion, but it is not effecting a magical transition from generating auditory to generating visual qualia.

Indeed there is another argument supporting the view that cortical plasticity is not the cause of the radical changes in sensory quality observed in rewired animals. It comes from other phenomena where drastic changes in the locus, modality or nature of sensations can occur in a very short time, making cortical plasticity, which is presumably a fairly slow process, a highly unlikely cause.

One such phenomenon is the feeling of 'projecting' your tactile sensation onto the tip of a tool: for example, when you write, you feel the roughness of the paper *at the tip of the pen*; and this happens even though you may hold the pen in any number of ways, and even though the vibrations from the paper are transmitted to widely different areas of your hand. The effect is immediate on setting pen to paper, and is thus presumably not the product of cortical plasticity. A similar example is the feeling you get immediately after learning to drive, of the tyres touching the road or the curb when you park your car. The rapidity of these adaptations argues against cortical plasticity as an explanation.

On the other hand, cortical plasticity does of course occur. As has been shown by an extensive literature, cortical changes occur when you use a tool: receptive fields normally situated at the hand can extend to the end of the tool (cf. Maravita and Iriki 2004). This cortical plasticity, which may take weeks to set up in a macaque monkey, participates in improving the monkey's ability to move objects with a rake. But it is not this cortical plasticity which is the original cause of a change in felt location of touch. On the contrary, the felt location of touch is the brain's way of best accounting for the currently occurring sensorimotor contingencies. Cortical plasticity may improve this estimation, but it is not itself the cause of the change in sensation.

The rubber hand illusion is another example: in this illusion, which takes only minutes to establish, touch actually occurs on the observer's arm, but is perceived as occurring on the rubber arm (Botvinick and Cohen 1998). This is not because of cortical plasticity, but because the sensorimotor contingencies established artificially by the experimental manipulation can best be interpreted by the brain in terms of touch on the rubber arm rather than on the observer's arm.

Finally sensory substitution, though often 'explained' in terms of cortical plasticity (Bach-y-Rita et al. 2005; Bach-y-Rita 1972), is in fact also not essentially caused by cortical plasticity. People using the TVSS or the vOICe report after only a few hours, if not within minutes, that they are getting 'something like' a visual sensation. Of course the sensation can only be visual to the extent that the apparatus, and the observer's motor, sensory and cognitive faculties allow the interaction to approximate visual-type interactions with the world. But the effect occurs almost immediately, and is thus presumably not caused by cortical plasticity.

Again, it is of course the case that over time, when a person becomes experienced with sensory substitution devices, cortical changes will occur. Brain structures will adapt so as to more efficiently do the processing involved in entertaining interaction with the world corresponding to the perceived modality. The experienced sensation will then more accurately approximate the normal sensation in that modality. But again, the cause for the experienced sensations lies not in the plasticity itself, but in the fact that the plasticity has enabled a mode of interaction with the environment which better approximates the new sensory modality.

10.4 Conclusion

It seems that the notion of cortical plasticity that researchers often refer to in the context of rewiring and sensory substitution may be somewhat misleading. Whereas the dramatic changes in experienced sensations seem to warrant appeal to some equally significant cortical modifications, I claim that taking this view would be to fall into Ryle's category mistake of thinking that sensations are the kinds of things that can be generated in the brain.

In fact, if we admit that the quality of sensory experiences is constituted by the modes of interaction with the environment that they involve, then we see that the real cause of modification of sensations in cases like rewired animals and sensory substitution will necessarily lie in changes in the modes of interaction which are involved. These changes in modes of interaction can be enabled, or favoured, by cortical plasticity, but cortical plasticity is not in itself what causes the changes. What causes the modification in sensory experience is just the fact that, through the use of special instrumentation or interfaces, a person or an animal interacts with the world in a way which approximates a sensory modality that involves cortical areas or sensory apparatus usually used for other modalities.

References

Bach-y-Rita, P. (1972) *Brain Mechanisms in Sensory Substitution*. New York: Academic Press.

Bach-y-Rita, P., Danilov, Y., Tyler, M. E. and Grimm, R. J. (2005) Late human brain plasticity: vestibular substitution with a tongue BrainPort human-machine interface. *Intellectica* 40: 115–122.

Botvinick, M. and Cohen, J. (1998) Rubber hands 'feel' touch that eyes see. *Nature* 391(6669): 756. doi:10.1038/35784.

Chalmers, D. J. (1997) *The Conscious Mind: In Search of a Fundamental Theory*. New York: Oxford University Press.

Dennett, D. C. (1991) *Consciousness Explained*. Boston: Little, Brown & Co.

Frost, D. O., Boire, D., Gingras, G. and Ptito, M. (2000) Surgically created neural pathways mediate visual pattern discrimination. *Proceedings of the National Academy of Sciences USA* 97(20): 11068–11073. doi:VL-97.

Hurley, S. and Noë, A. (2003) Neural plasticity and consciousness. *Biology and Philosophy* 18(1): 131–168.

James, W. (1890) *The Principles of Psychology*. New York: Dover Publications.

Kupers, R., Fumal, A., de Noordhout, A. M., Gjedde, A., Schoenen, J. and Ptito, M. (2006) Transcranial magnetic stimulation of the visual cortex induces somatotopically organized qualia in blind subjects. *Proceedings of the National Academy of Sciences USA* 103(35): 13256–13260.

Maravita, A. and Iriki, A. (2004) Tools for the body (schema). *Trends in Cognitive Sciences* 8(2): 79–86. doi:10.1016/j.tics.2003.12.008.

O'Regan, J. K. (2011) *Why Red Doesn't Sound Like a Bell: Understanding the Feel of Consciousness*. New York: Oxford University Press.

O'Regan, J. K. and Noë, A. (2001) A sensorimotor account of vision and visual consciousness. *Behavioral and Brain Sciences* 24(5): 883–917.

Pallas, S. L. and Sur, M. (1993) Visual projections induced into the auditory pathway of ferrets: II. Corticocortical connections of primary auditory cortex. *Journal of Comparative Neurology* 337(2): 317–333. doi:10.1002/cne.903370212.

Pallas, S. L., Roe, A. W. and Sur, M. (1990) Visual projections induced into the auditory pathway of ferrets. I. Novel inputs to primary auditory cortex (AI) from the LP/pulvinar complex and the topography of the MGN-AI projection. *Journal of Comparative Neurology* 298(1): 50–68. doi:10.1002/cne.902980105.

Penfield, W. (1958) Some mechanisms of consciousness discovered during electrical stimulation of the brain. *Proceedings of the National Academy of Sciences USA* 44(2): 51–66.

Phillips, C. G., Zeki, S. and Barlow, H. B. (1984) Localization of function in the cerebral cortex: past, present and future. *Brain* 107(1): 328–361. doi:10.1093/brain/107.1.328.

Ptito, M., Schneider, F. C. G., Paulson, O. B. and Kupers, R. (2008) Alterations of the visual pathways in congenital blindness. *Experimental Brain Research* 187(1): 41–49. doi:10.1007/s00221-008-1273-4.

Ryle, G. (1949) *The Concept of Mind*. Chicago: University of Chicago Press.

Sharma, J., Angelucci, A. and Sur, M. (2000) Induction of visual orientation modules in auditory cortex. *Nature* 404(6780): 841–847.

Von Melchner, L., Pallas, S. L. and Sur, M. (2000) Visual behaviour mediated by retinal projections directed to the auditory pathway. *Nature* 404(6780): 871–876. doi:10.1038/35009102.

11

Bodily Action and Distal Attribution in Sensory Substitution

ROBERT BRISCOE

Abstract According to proponents of the sensorimotor contingency theory of perception (Hurley and Noë 2003; Noë 2004; O'Regan 2011), active control of camera movement is necessary for the emergence of distal attribution in tactile-visual sensory substitution (TVSS) because it enables the subject to acquire knowledge of the way stimulation in the substituting modality varies as a function of self-initiated, bodily action. This chapter, by contrast, approaches distal attribution as a solution to a *causal inference* problem faced by the subject's perceptual systems. Given all of the endogenous and exogenous evidence available to those systems, what is the most probable source of stimulation in the substituting modality? From this perspective, active control over the camera's movements matters for rather different reasons. Most importantly, it generates proprioceptive and efference-copy based information about the camera's body-relative position necessary to make use of the spatial cues present in the stimulation that the subject receives for purposes of egocentric object localization.

11.1 Two Questions about Sensory Substitution

SENSORY SUBSTITUTION DEVICES (SSDs) convert images from a video camera into patterns of vibrotactile stimulation (White et al. 1970; Bach-y-Rita 1972, 2004), electrotactile stimulation (Sampaio et al. 2001; Ptito et al. 2005; Chebat et al. 2011), or auditory stimulation (Meijer 1992; Capelle et al. 1998; Renier et al. 2005; Amedi et al. 2007; Kim and Zatorre 2008) that visually-impaired individuals can use to perform tasks ordinarily guided by non-prosthetic vision. An adequate account of how SSDs enable trained users to interact with the environment in an adaptive manner must answer two main questions. The first question concerns the end-product of the learning process in sensory substitution. What kind (or kinds) of representational states do properly trained subjects form in response to stimulation in the substituting perceptual modality? There are at least five possibilities:

Proceedings of the British Academy, **219**, 174–187.

(a) The SSD extends the range of properties represented by the *substituting* modality. The device, for example, enables trained users to perceive the shapes and sizes of objects at a distance from their body by means of touch.
(b) The SSD enables trained subjects to perceive properties of the distal environment via the *substituted* modality, i.e. the device to a certain extent restores the sense of sight.
(c) The SSD enables trained subjects to perceive properties of the distal environment via a *new* prosthetic modality, i.e. the subject enjoys experiences that are not straightforwardly in the substituting or substituted modality.
(d) Trained subjects transform stimulation in the substituting modality into accurate visual and/or spatial *mental images* of surrounding objects and their properties.
(e) Trained subjects perform quick *cognitive inferences* from stimulation in the substituting modality to properties of the distal environment.

The second question, by contrast, concerns the nature of the learning process itself. How do blindfolded, late blind, and early blind subjects respectively learn to use the stimulations provided by a given type of SSD for such purposes as object-directed motor control, wayfinding, or object recognition? It is on this second question that I shall focus primarily in this chapter.

Before proceeding, it should be emphasized that both questions need to be relativized not only to the specific type of SSD being deployed, but also to subjects' history of visual impairment, if any. Effective visualization strategies, for example, may be available to blindfolded and late blind subjects, but not to subjects who have been blind since birth (Poirier et al. 2007). It is also important to keep in mind findings concerning the cross-modal plasticity of the visually deafferentated brain. In particular, there is extensive evidence that occipital cortex is recruited for tactile and auditory processing when it is deprived of its standard sources of retinal input (Pascual-Leone and Hamilton 2001; Proulx et al. 2014; Kupers et al. 2011). This means that subjects who are blind or undergo prolonged visual deprivation may make rather different use of the information conveyed by stimulation in the substituting modality than normally sighted subjects. Contrary to possibility (b), but in keeping with (a), Kupers et al. (2006) found that, after one week of training with an electrotactile tongue display unit, transcranial magnetic stimulation (TMS) of occipital cortex evoked tactile sensations on the tongues of one late blind and three early blind subjects—'short-lasting experiences of distinct tingling, varying in intensity, extent, and topography depending on the locus of the occipital cortex that was stimulated' (Kupers et al. 2006: 13257)—but only phosphenes in blindfolded subjects.[1]

[1] This result is consistent with the finding that TMS applied to occipital cortex induces experiences of touch that are referred to the fingertips in blind Braille readers (Ptito et al. 2008). See Ortiz et al. 2011, however, for evidence that tactile stimulation elicits phosphenes in some late blind subjects.

Whether or not subjects have previously enjoyed visual experience seems also likely to affect how they learn to detect and disambiguate the spatial information present in SSD-mediated sensory stimulation. Unlike early blind subjects, blindfolded and late blind subjects may be able to exploit various cross-modal correspondences that obtain between the substituting modality and vision, for example, the link between tactile and visual shape or between auditory frequency and elevation in the visual field (Evans and Treisman 2010; Spence 2011). Consistent with this, studies by Kim and Zatorre (2008) have found that, prior to any training, blindfolded subjects can perform image identification tasks using the vOICe at an above-chance level so long as they are given an explicit explanation of the image-to-sound conversion rules.

11.2 Action Movement in Sensory Substitution

In tactile-visual sensory substitution (TVSS), low-resolution, grey-scale images from a video camera are converted by a human–machine interface (HMI), pixel by pixel, into vibrotactile stimulations on the skin of one's back. A main finding in early experiments conducted by Paul Bach-y-Rita and colleagues was that subjects learned to discriminate the spatial layout of the scene in front of them via TVSS only when they had active control over movement of the video camera (White et al. 1970; Bach-y-Rita 1972). Subjects who received visual input passively experienced only a changing pattern of tactile stimulation:

> When asked to identify static forms with the camera fixed, subjects have a very difficult time; but when they are free to turn the camera to explore the figures, the discrimination is quickly established. With fixed camera, subjects report experiences in terms of feelings on their backs, but when they move the camera over the displays, they give reports in terms of externally localized objects in front of them.
>
> (White et al. 1970: 25)

Motivated by this finding, proponents of the sensorimotor contingency theory of perception have maintained that passively stimulated subjects do not learn to localize objects in surrounding space by means of TVSS because they are unable to master the sensorimotor contingencies that govern use of the device. '[A]ctive movement', Susan Hurley and Alva Noë write, 'is required in order for the subject to acquire practical knowledge of the change from sensorimotor contingencies characteristic of touch to those characteristic of vision and the ability to exploit this change skillfully' (2003: 145; also see Noë 2004; Kiverstein 2010; O'Regan 2011).[2]

[2] Sensorimotor contingencies are regularities that govern the way moving in relation to the surrounding environment gives rise to changes in proximal sensory stimulation. Approaching an object, for example, causes its retinal image to undergo expansion, which, in turn, causes a corresponding change in the pattern of retinal stimulation. Moving away from the object has the opposite effect. In the modality

Hurley and Noë make two main claims about TVSS. The first claim is an answer to the question concerning the end-product of learning in sensory substitution. They argue that TVSS is best understood as a case of cortical deference in which activity in a blind subject's somatosensory cortex takes its 'qualitative expression' from the character of the externally rerouted *visual input* that it receives. TVSS, in other words, enables blind subjects to perceive the spatial layout of the distal environment in a phenomenologically vision-like manner—possibility (b) above. The second claim is an answer to the question concerning the nature of the learning process in sensory substitution. Subjects learn to make efficient use of TVSS only by acquiring knowledge of the sensorimotor contingencies associated with the prosthetic modality. 'The distinctively visual character of TVSS-perception stems from the way perceivers can acquire and use practical knowledge of the common laws of sensorimotor contingency that vision and TVSS-perception share' (Hurley and Noë 2003: 145).

It seems clear that there is significant overlap between the sensorimotor contingencies that respectively characterize ordinary, non-prosthetic vision and TVSS. This is because the HMI systematically converts the two-dimensional image produced by the video camera, pixel by pixel, into a corresponding two-dimensional array of vibrotactile stimulation on the skin. In consequence, the effects of camera movements on the structure of the former are mirrored by changes in the structure of the latter. Approaching an object, for example, causes its image in the camera to loom, which, in turn, causes its size in the vibrotactile array (functionally, the prosthetic retina) to increase. Retreating from the object causes its image to shrink, which, in turn, causes its size in the vibrotactile array to decrease. Panning to the right causes the object's image to shift to the left, which, in turn, causes a structurally similar change in the pattern of vibrotactile stimulation on the skin. And so on.

Psychological and neuroscientific investigations of sensory substitution undertaken in the last decade provide reasons to be sceptical about Hurley and Noë's account. According to Hurley and Noë, activity in somatosensory cortex takes its 'qualitative expression' in TVSS from the character of the externally rerouted visual input that it receives. In other words, TVSS-perception is a case of somatosensory cortical deference. The TMS studies by Kupers et al. (2006), mentioned above, as well as brain imaging studies of cortical activation during visual-to-tactile sensory substitution tasks (for reviews, see Kupers et al. 2011, Kupers and Ptito 2014) present a different picture. In particular, they suggest, first, that in blind subjects occipital cortex is recruited to process the somatosensory inputs produced by a visual-to-tactile SSD and, second, that the resulting experience is, in at least some respects, phenomenologically touch-like in character (Kupers and Ptito 2014: 44). As most researchers would readily acknowledge, however, there are also salient contrasts between the representational content of TVSS-perception

of touch, squeezing a soft sponge produces a distinctive pattern of tactile stimulations in one's hand. Squeezing a clod of dry clay produces quite another.

and the representational content of ordinary touch. Proficient users of TVSS, in particular, acquire the ability to discern the geometrical properties and locations of objects at a distance from the body in space. In this respect, the representational content of TVSS-perception is akin to that of vision in normally sighted subjects.

11.3 Distal Attribution and Causal Inference

There are also reasons to be sceptical that passively stimulated subjects fail to discriminate spatial layout via TVSS because they lack the opportunity to learn the sensorimotor contingencies that govern use of the device. An alternative explanation is that subjects who do not control the camera's movement—and who are not otherwise attuned to its current position—are simply unable to detect and make effective use of the *spatial information* present in the vibrotactile stimulations that they receive. In consequence they do not engage in 'distal attribution' (Loomis 1982; Epstein et al. 1986): they do not attribute the cause of those stimulations to a three-dimensional scene in the external world.

Evidence that subjects with active control over camera movement do engage in distal attribution comes from the earliest experiments on TVSS by Bach-y-Rita and colleagues. Trained subjects, for example, exhibited defensive, startle responses when objects loomed in the tactile array (Bach-y-Rita 1972: 98–99) and were spontaneously able to make sense of kinetic depth displays:

> A modified version of the Metzger apparatus was used, consisting of a turntable on which two vertical white rods were mounted. This was rotated slowly before the camera and the subjects were asked to describe what they 'saw.' Some sighted subjects, upon first tactile presentation of this moving display, have spontaneously described it as moving in depth. Several blind subjects were given experience with a yoked pair of turntables. On one of these, an object was placed within view of the camera, while the subject turned the other freely, experiencing the transformations that the object underwent with the rotation. After an hour's experience with this equipment, they could report accurately the eccentric placement of two and three objects on the turntable, and could also experience rotation in depth with the Metzger display.
>
> (White et al. 1970: 25)

In keeping with a recently influential Bayesian approach to perception in cognitive science (Mamassian et al. 2002; Kersten and Yuille 2003; Shams and Beierholm 2010; Clark 2013; Hohwy 2013; Rescorla 2015), it is helpful, I would suggest, to think of distal attribution as the solution to a *causal inference* problem faced by the subject's perceptual systems. Patterns of proximal sensory stimulation significantly underdetermine their causal antecedents in the environment (hence, the so-called 'inverse optics' problem for vision). The central challenge faced by any perceptual system, on Bayesian models of perception, is to infer the most probable cause of a given pattern of proximal sensory stimulation on the basis of (1) the low-level cues present in the pattern itself, i.e. properties of the pattern that are predictive of properties in the environment, and (2) pre-wired or learned assumptions about the environment's statistical structure (the perceptual system's 'prior knowledge' about the world).[3] The cues constrain the inference process from the bottom up, while the assumptions constrain the process by, among other things, determining which way of integrating cues, in context, is statistically optimal (Knill 2007). The content of the perceptual state formed in response to a particular pattern of stimulation—the brain's operative 'hypothesis' about the structure of the impinging environment—is the cause to which the highest probability is assigned given all the available endogenous and exogenous evidence. In the case of vision, this will normally be one of indefinitely many possible three-dimensional scenes.[4] The default hypothesis space for causal inference in everyday vision (the space of world states over which the posterior distribution is computed) is a *distant scene space*, in which different hypotheses correspond to different possible arrays of objects at a distance from the perceiver's eyes. (One such hypothesis picks out the very scene present in front of the reader now.) By contrast, the default hypothesis space for causal inference in everyday touch is a *contacting object space*, in which different hypotheses correspond to different possible objects in contact with the surface of the perceiver's body. Distal attribution in visual-to-tactile sensory substitution can be predicted to occur, when, from the standpoint of the perceiver's perceptual systems, the most likely environmental cause of incoming vibrotactile or electrotactile stimulation—contrary to the default haptic interpretation—is a distant scene rather than an object of some sort touching the surface of her body.

The question to ask now is: What role does active control of camera movement play in enabling such radical re-shaping of the hypothesis space for touch in TVSS?

It is easiest to explain why such re-shaping is unlikely to occur when the subject is passively stimulated. When a subject outfitted with a TVSS device lacks control of the camera's movements and is not otherwise able to register its position, all of the available endogenous and exogenous evidence is consistent with the default haptic interpretation of incoming sensory stimulation: the most likely cause of that stimulation is direct, bodily contact with an object of some kind. From a causal

[3]This is a simplification. Bayesian models often incorporate other kinds of prior world knowledge. For discussion, see Geisler 2008. Two further points are important. First, perceptual inference is a non-conscious, subpersonal process. It is the perceiver's brain rather than the perceiver herself that is confronting the causal inference problem described here. Second, Bayesian models do not assume that perceptual systems explicitly represent either the norms of Bayesian decision making or the various forms of prior knowledge imputed to them for purposes of explaining the formation of perceptual mental states. Bayesian models only assume that perceptual processes typically proceed in *accordance* with the principles of Bayesian decision making (see Burge 2010: 95–97; Rescorla 2015).

[4]Although multistable perceptual experiences can occur in which the selected hypothesis alternates from one moment to the next, depending on the allocation of attention and other factors. Examples include the flip in depth assignments when viewing a drawing of a Necker cube or the reversal in the perceived direction of rotation in the silhouette illusion.

inference perspective, it is thus unsurprising that she does not learn to perceive spatially remote objects and features by means of TVSS. There is simply no reason for her perceptual systems to shift away from the hypothesis that the tactile stimulations she is receiving have an ordinary tactile cause. In consequence, although multiple sources of information about the visible scene are *present* in those stimulations—these derive from monocular cues in the two-dimensional image such as height in the visual field, relative size, familiar size, linear perspective, motion parallax, shape-from-motion, and looming (White et al. 1970; Bach-y-Rita 1972)—the subject's perceptual systems are unable to detect and exploit them.

By contrast, when the subject has the ability to guide and keep track of the camera's movement, she also has a significant amount of voluntary control over whether and how the vibrotactile stimulation she experiences undergoes change. In consequence, the situation is now one that conflicts with the default haptic interpretation: it is not typically possible to modify tactile stimulation on the surface of one's back by moving a camera mounted on a tripod or on one's head! The observed coupling between camera movement and vibrotactile stimulation is evidence that the latter's cause resides outside of the hypothesis space for everyday touch.

In addition to evidence against the default haptic interpretation, there is now also evidence required for inference to a spatial layout in the hypothesis space of vision (or rather what constitutes the hypothesis space of vision in normally sighted subjects). To begin with, there are the aforementioned spatial cues present in the pattern of vibrotactile stimulation produced by the HMI. In addition, because the subject has control over how the camera moves she now also has access to real-time information about its body-relative position. This is important because the spatial cues present in the vibrotactile stimulation the subject is receiving are sources of information about the way objects fill out three-dimensional space *in front of the camera*. Height in the visual field, relative size, motion parallax, looming, etc. are all variations in image structure that are predictive of the distances of objects that reflect light to the camera's lens. The HMI in TVSS works by converting these variations in image structure into corresponding variations in the structure of the vibrotactile array. To engage in causal inference to the way objects fill out space in front of her own body—to make use of the cues contained in the stimulation that she receives from the HMI as sources of *egocentric* spatial information—the subject thus needs to be able to keep track of the camera's body-relative position, where it is located, for example, relative to her head, or torso, or hand. As Bach-y-Rita writes, 'In the absence of motor control over the orientation of the sensory input, a person may have no idea from where the information is coming, and thus no ability to locate [its source] in space' (2004: 90). Another key reason, then, that active control over the movements of the camera matters is that it generates information about the camera's body-relative position necessary for causal inference to the way objects are arrayed in space at distance from the subject's body. Such causal inference, on the present interpretation, is the essence of distal attribution.

I should emphasize that it is the availability of up-to-date and accurate information about how the camera is positioned in relation to the body that is important here, rather than the particular *way* in which the information is generated. In the case of the subject who actively controls the camera's movements, the information is presumably based on proprioceptive signals and efference copy of motor commands to move the head or hand (depending, respectively, on whether the camera is mounted on a pair of eyeglasses or, as in the earliest experiments, on a tripod). But reliable information about body-relative camera position could, in principle, be made available in other ways to passively stimulated subjects.[5]

Siegle and Warren (2010) offer a similar interpretation of the role of self-produced arm movements in learning to make distance judgements using a simple visual-to-tactile SSD (Figure 11.1). The device in their experiments consisted of a single photodiode mounted on the index finger linked to a vibrating motor worn on the back. The motor was active when a subject pointed the photodiode in the direction of a light source and inactive otherwise. Subjects fitted with the device were trained to sweep their arm back and forth in order to estimate the egocentric distance of a target light, which could be stationed at various locations along a 193-cm track in front of them. On Siegle and Warren's preferred Gibsonian interpretation, action is necessary for subjects to perform this task successfully not because it enables them to learn the sensorimotor contingencies associated with use of the SSD, but rather 'to reveal invariant information about the distal layout and to dissociate it from varying stimulation that depends on self-movement' (2010: 221). According to this 'invariance hypothesis', action generates proprioceptive information about pointing direction (generated by changes in the orientation of the torso and the joint angles of the shoulder and elbow), which, when combined with the motor signal, is sufficient to triangulate the body-relative position of the distal target. Such triangulation, whether undertaken explicitly or implicitly, is clearly also available to subjects who control camera movement when using more sophisticated visual-to-tactile SSDs. They can use information about the camera's changing, body-relative orientation together with concurrent tactile stimulations to confirm that an object is 'out there' at a certain egocentrically defined distance and direction in space.

The interpretation of the role of active camera control in learning to make use of TVSS offered above is a version of the invariance hypothesis. A main reason that subjects who control the camera's movements engage in distal attribution, I have argued, is that such control generates reliable information about the camera's body-relative position needed to exploit the spatial cues in incoming vibrotactile stimulations for purposes of egocentric object localization. Subjects do not need to acquire knowledge of the relevant sensorimotor contingencies.

[5] I am grateful to Fiona Macpherson and David Pence for discussion of this point.

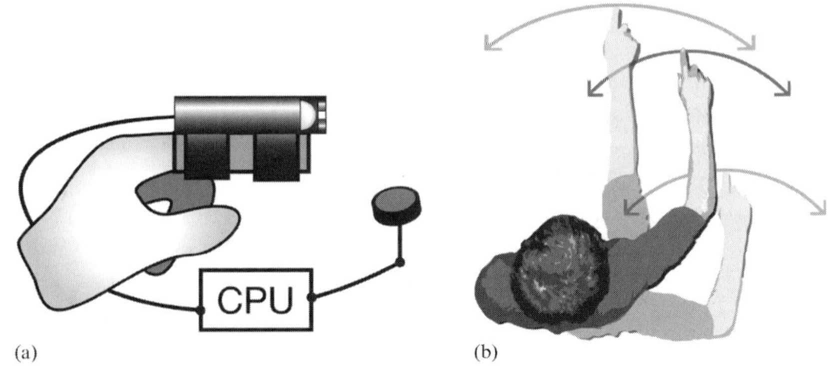

Figure 11.1 (a) The sensory substitution device used by Siegle and Warren (2010). A photodiode on the index finger responds to light from the target, driving a vibrating motor on the subject's back. (b) Pattern of arm movements participants were instructed to make when exploring the target. From Siegle and Warren 2010 by permission of Pion Ltd (www.pion.co.uk).

11.4 Bodily Action and Prism Adaptation

The discussion in the last section suggests that we cannot straightforwardly infer from the apparent dependence of a given form of perceptual learning on self-produced bodily movement to the dependence of that form of learning on knowledge of sensorimotor contingencies, i.e. knowledge of the sensory consequences of action. Otherwise, we may overlook the Gibsonian possibility that it is not self-produced movement *per se* that makes the crucial difference to the learning process, but rather the perceptual or proprioceptive information to which such movement gives rise.[6]

A final example illustrating this point comes from studies of how subjects adapt to prisms that reverse, invert, or laterally displace the retinal image (for overviews, see Rock 1966; Welch 1978; Briscoe and Grush 2017). Richard Held and Alan Hein conducted an influential series of experiments in which participants wore laterally displacing prisms during either active or passive movement conditions (Held and Hein 1958; Hein and Held 1962; Held 1965). In the active movement condition, the subject moved her visible hand back and forth along a fixed arc in synchrony with a metronome. In the passive movement condition, the subject's hand was passively moved at the same rate by the experimenters. Although the overall pattern of visual stimulation was identical in both conditions, adaptation was reported only when subjects engaged in self-produced movement. Held and Hein used these findings to defend what in the literature has come to be known as

[6] For useful discussions of this point, see the commentaries in Gyr et al. 1979 and Campos et al. 2000.

the 'reafference theory' of adaptation. According to the reafference theory, subjects exhibit stable adaptation to optical rearrangement only when they receive visual feedback from self-produced bodily movement, i.e. reafferent visual stimulation.

Contrary to reafference theory, subsequent experiments in the 1960s found that adaptation to lateral displacement is not restricted to situations in which subjects engage in movements that generate reafferent visual feedback, but can also take place when subjects receive visual feedback generated by passive effector or whole-body movements (Singer and Day 1966; Templeton et al. 1966; Fishkin 1969). Evidence was even garnered that prism adaptation is possible in the complete absence of motor action (Howard et al. 1965; Kravitz and Wallach 1966). In general, the extent to which adaptation occurs seems to depend not on the availability of reafferent stimulation from motor actions, as Held proposed, but rather on the presence of either of two related kinds of information concerning 'the presence and nature of the optical rearrangement' (Welch 1978: 24). Following Welch, I shall refer to this alternative to the reafference theory as the *information hypothesis*.

One source of such information concerns the veridical directions of objects from the observer (Rock 1966: chs 2–4). Normally, when engaging in forward locomotion, the apparent radial direction of an object straight ahead of the body remains constant, while the apparent radial directions of objects to either side undergo change. This pattern also obtains when the observer wears prisms that displace the retinal image to the side. Hence, as Rock writes, 'an object seen through prisms which retains the same radial direction as we approach must be seen to be moving in toward the sagittal plane' (1966: 105). On Rock's view, at least some forms of prism adaptation can be explained by our ability to detect and exploit such stable sources of spatial information in locomotion-generated patterns of optic flow.

Another more effective source of information for prism adaptation is the registered discrepancy between seen and proprioceptively experienced limb position (Wallach 1968). Proponents of the information hypothesis have found that, when this conflict is made conspicuous, passively moved (Melamed et al. 1973), involuntarily moved (Mather and Lackner 1975), and even immobile subjects (Kravitz and Wallach 1966) exhibit significant adaptation. Although active bodily movement is unnecessary for adaptation to occur, it provides subjects with especially salient and precise information about the discrepancy between sight and touch (Moulden 1971): subjects are able proprioceptively to determine the location of a moving limb much more accurately than a stationary or passively moved limb.

11.5 Conclusion

Sources of evidence for the information hypothesis discussed above indicate that adaptation to displacing prisms can occur in the absence of self-produced movement.

The information hypothesis, however, predicts that action will *facilitate* adaptation when it generates information either about the world (in particular, the real radial directions of objects from the perceiver) or about the perceiver's body (in particular, the real positions of her limbs) that conflicts with the way things look as a result of prismatic displacement. 'According to this view', Rock writes, '[active] movement is important only because it allows for certain kinds of information to be registered, not because movement *per* se is necessary' (1966: 42).

In this chapter, my aim has been to show that something analogous holds true of the learning process in tactile-visual sensory substitution. In particular, I have argued that active control over camera movement facilitates distal attribution in TVSS not because it enables subjects to master the laws of sensorimotor contingency governing use of the device, but rather because it generates proprioceptive and efference-copy-based information about the camera's changing body-relative position. Such information is important to the emergence of distal attribution for two main reasons. First, without knowledge that the vibrotactile stimulations she is receiving can be modified by camera movement, the subject's perceptual systems have no reason to budge from the default haptic interpretation of those stimulations. The coupling between changes in camera position and changes in sensory stimulation is evidence that the cause of the latter resides outside the ordinary hypothesis space for touch. Second, having the ability to keep track of the camera's body-relative position enables the subject to exploit the spatial cues present in vibrotactile stimulation for causal inference to the egocentrically specified distances and directions of objects in space around her. Such causal inference, on the interpretation I have defended here, is the basis of distal attribution.[7]

References

Amedi A., Stern, W., Camprodon, J., Bermpohl, F., Merabet, L. and Rotman, S. (2007) Shape conveyed by visual-to-auditory sensory substitution activates the lateral occipital complex. *Nature Neuroscience* 10: 687–689.

Bach-y-Rita, P. (1972) *Brain Mechanisms in Sensory Substitution.* New York: Academic Press.

Bach-y-Rita, P. (2004) Tactile sensory substitution studies. *Annals of the New York Academy of Sciences* 1013: 83–91.

Briscoe, R. and Grush, R. (2017) Action-based theories of perception. In E. N. Zalta (ed.) *The Stanford Encyclopedia of Philosophy* (Spring 2017 edn). Retrieved from https://plato.stanford.edu/archives/spr2017/entries/action-perception.

[7] For helpful discussions, I am grateful to Amir Amedi, Derek Brown, Jonathan Cohen, Joshua Downing, Julian Kiverstein, Fiona Macpherson, Mohan Matthen, Paul Noordhof, Kevin O'Regan, David Pence, Michael Proulx, and Jamie Ward.

Burge, T. (2010) *Origins of Objectivity*. Oxford: Oxford University Press.

Campos, J., Anderson, D., Barbu-Roth, M., Hubbard, E., Hertenstein, M. and Witherington, D. (2000) Travel broadens the mind. *Infancy* 1: 149–219.

Capelle, C., Trullemans, C., Arno, P. and Veraart, C. (1998) A real-time experimental prototype for enhancement of vision rehabilitation using auditory substitution. *IEEE Transaction on Biomedical Engineering* 45: 1279–1293.

Chebat, D., Schneider, F., Kupers, R. and Ptito, M. (2011) Navigation with a sensory substitution device in congenitally blind individuals. *Neuroreport* 22: 342–347.

Clark, A. (2013) Whatever next? Predictive brains, situated agents, and the future of cognitive science. *Behavioral and Brain Sciences* 36: 181–253.

Epstein, W., Hughes, B., Schneider, S. and Bach-y-Rita, P. (1986) Is there anything out there? A study of distal attribution in response to vibrotactile stimulation. *Perception* 15(3): 275–284.

Evans, K. and Treisman, A. (2010) Natural cross-modal mappings between visual and auditory features. *Journal of Vision* 10: 1–12.

Fishkin, S. (1969) Passive vs. active exposure and other variables related to the occurrence of hand adaptation to lateral displacement. *Perceptual and Motor Skills* 29: 291–297.

Geisler, W. (2008) Visual perception and the statistical properties of natural scenes. *Annual Review of Psychology* 59: 167–192.

Gyr, J., Siley, R. and Henry, A. (1979) Motor-sensory feedback and the geometry of visual space. *Behavioral and Brain Sciences* 2: 59–94.

Hein, A. and Held, R. (1962) A neural model for labile sensorimotor coordinations. In E. Bernard and M. Kare (eds) *Biological Prototypes and Synthetic Systems*, vol. 1. New York: Plenum Press, 71–74.

Held, R. (1965) Plasticity in sensory-motor systems. *Scientific American* 213: 84–94.

Held, R. and Hein, A. (1958) Adaptation of disarranged hand-eye coordination contingent upon re-afferent stimulation. *Perceptual and Motor Skills* 8: 87–90.

Hohwy, J. (2013) *The Predictive Brain*. Oxford: Oxford University Press.

Howard, I., Craske, B. and Templeton, W. (1965) Visuomotor adaptation to discordant exafferent stimulation. *Journal of Experimental Psychology* 70: 189–191.

Hurley, S. and Noë, A. (2003) Neural plasticity and consciousness. *Biology and Philosophy* 18: 131–168.

Kersten, D. and Yuille, A. (2003) Bayesian models of object perception. *Current Opinion in Neurobiology* 13: 150–158.

Kim, J. and Zatorre, R. (2008) Generalized learning of visual-to-auditory substitution in sighted individuals. *Brain Research* 1242: 263–275.

Kiverstein, J. (2010) Sensorimotor knowledge and the contents of experience. In N. Gangopadhyay, M. Madary and F. Spicer (eds) *Perception, Action, and Consciousness*. Oxford: Oxford University Press, 257–274.

Knill, D. (2007) Learning Bayesian priors for depth perception. *Journal of Vision* 7: 1–20.

Kravitz, J. and Wallach, H. (1966) Adaptation to displaced vision contingent upon vibrating stimulation. *Psychonomic Science* 6: 465–466.

Kupers, R., Fumal, A., de Noordhout, A., Gjedde, A., Schoenen, J. and Ptito, M. (2006) Transcranial magnetic stimulation of the visual cortex induces somatotopically organized qualia in blind subjects. *Proceedings of the National Academy of Sciences* 103: 13256–13260.

Kupers, R., Pietrini, P., Ricciardi, E. and Ptito, M. (2011) The nature of consciousness in the visually deprived brain. *Frontiers in Psychology* 2.

Loomis, J. (1982) Distal attribution and presence. *Presence* 1: 113–119.

Mamassian, P., Landy, M. and Maloney, L. (2002) Bayesian modeling of visual perception. In R. Rao, B. Olshausen and M. Lewicki (eds) *Probabilistic Models of the Brain.* Cambridge, MA: MIT Press.

Mather, J. and Lackner, J. (1975) Adaptation to visual rearrangement elicited by tonic vibration reflexes. *Experimental Brain Research* 24: 103–105.

Meijer, P. B. L. (1992) An experimental system for auditory image representations. *IEEE Transactions on Biomedical Engineering* 39: 112–121.

Melamed, L., Halay, M. and Gildow, J. (1973) Effect of external target presence on visual adaptation with active and passive movement. *Journal of Experimental Psychology* 98: 125–130.

Moulden, B. (1971) Adaptation to displaced vision: reafference is a special case of the cue-discrepancy hypothesis. *The Quarterly Journal of Experimental Psychology* 23: 113–117.

Noë, A. (2004) *Action in Perception.* Cambridge, MA: MIT Press.

O'Regan, J. (2011) *Why Red Doesn't Sound Like a Bell: Explaining the Feel of Consciousness.* Oxford: Oxford University Press.

Ortiz, T., Poch, J., Santos, J., Requena, C., Martínez, A., et al. (2011) Recruitment of occipital cortex during sensory substitution training linked to subjective experience of seeing in people with blindness. *PLoS One* 6: e23264.

Pascual-Leone, A. and Hamilton, R. (2001) The metamodal organization of the brain. *Progress in Brain Research* 134: 427–445.

Poirier, C., De Volder, A. and Scheiber, C. (2007) What neuroimaging tells us about sensory substitution. *Neuroscience and Biobehavioral Reviews* 31: 1064–1070.

Proulx, M., Brown, D., Pasqualotto, A. and Meijer, P. (2014) Multisensory perceptual learning and sensory substitution. *Neuroscience and Biobehavioral Reviews* 41: 16–25.

Ptito, M., Moesgaard, S., Gjedde, A. and Kupers, R. (2005) Cross-modal plasticity revealed by electrotactile stimulation of the tongue in the congenitally blind. *Brain* 128: 606–614.

Ptito, M., Fumal, A., de Noordhout, A. M., Schoenen, J., Gjedde, A. and Kupers, R. (2008) TMS of the occipital cortex induces tactile sensations in the fingers of blind Braille readers. *Experimental Brain Research* 184: 193–200.

Renier, L., Collignon, O., Poirier, C., Tranduy, D., Vanlierde, A., Bol, A., Veraart, C. and De Volder, A. (2005) Cross-modal activation of visual cortex during depth perception using auditory substitution of vision. *NeuroImage* 26: 573–80.

Rescorla, M. (2015) Bayesian perceptual psychology. In M. Matthen (ed.) *The Oxford Handbook of the Philosophy of Perception.* Oxford: Oxford University Press, 694–716.

Rock, I. (1966) *The Nature of Perceptual Adaptation.* New York: Basic Books.

Sampaio, E., Maris, S. and Bach-y-Rita, P. (2001) Brain plasticity: 'visual' acuity of blind persons via the tongue. *Brain Research* 908: 204–207.

Shams, L. and Beierholm, U. (2010) Causal inference in perception. *Trends in Cognitive Sciences* 14: 425–432.

Siegle, J. and Warren, W. (2010) Distal attribution and distance perception in sensory substitution. *Perception* 39: 208–223.

Singer, G. and Day, R. (1966) Spatial adaptation and aftereffect with optically transformed vision. *Journal of Experimental Psychology* 71: 725–731.

Spence, C. (2011) Crossmodal correspondences: a tutorial review. *Attention, Perception, and Psychophysics* 73: 971–995.

Templeton, W., Howard, I. and Lowman, A. (1966) Passively generated adaptation to prismatic distortion. *Perceptual and Motor Skills* 22: 140–142.

Wallach, H. (1968) Informational discrepancy as a basis of perceptual adaptation. In S. Friedman (ed.) *The Neuropsychology of Spatially Oriented Behaviour*. Homewood, IL: Dorsey Press, 209–230.

Welch, R. (1978) *Perceptual Modification: Adapting to Altered Sensory Environments*. New York: Academic Press.

White, B., Saunders, F., Scadden, L., Bach-y-Rita, P. and Collins, C. (1970) Seeing with the skin. *Perception and Psychophysics* 7: 23–27.

12

Sensory Substitution Devices as Advanced Sensory Tools

THOMAS D. WRIGHT AND JAMIE WARD

Abstract There has been considerable effort devoted towards understanding sensory substitution devices in terms of their relationship to canonical sensory modalities. The approach taken in this essay is rather different, although complementary, in that we seek to define a broad conceptual space of 'sensory tools' in which sensory substitution devices can be situated. Such devices range from telescopes, to cochlear implants, to attempts to create a magnetic sense. One feature of these devices is that they operate at the level of 'raw' sensory information. As such, systems such as Braille which operate at a symbolic/conceptual level do not count as a sensory tool (or a sensory substitution device) and nor would a device such as CCTV which, although capturing raw sensory information, would not meet a conventional definition of a tool. With this approach, we hope to avoid the circularity inherent in previous attempts at defining sensory substitution and provide a better starting point to explore the effects of sensory tools, more generally, on the functioning of the nervous system.

12.1 Sensory Substitution and Sensory Substitution Devices

Sensory substitution is, broadly, a term used to describe the process of conveying information from one sensory modality via another. Typically the motivation is to restore some functionality of a lost or impaired sense. Indeed, since the creation of the first sensory substitution device (SSD) in the 1960s (Bach-y-Rita et al. 1969), sensory substitution has been closely associated with visual impairment: in this first device, and in many of the devices created in the years since, vision is the substituted sense.

Over the past four decades, sensory substitution has been defined primarily by the devices which enable it. Bach-y-Rita's first such system, called the tactile-vision sensory substitution (TVSS) device, conveyed the image captured by

Proceedings of the British Academy, **219**, 188–204. © The British Academy 2018.

camera to a 20 × 20 array of solenoid stimulators arranged on a dentist's chair so as to stimulate the skin on one's back (Bach-y-Rita et al. 1969). Each one of the vibrating solenoids acts as a tactile pixel (or 'taxel') corresponding to the visual pixel occupying the equivalent space in the array from the camera.

Since the TVSS, there have been a number of subsequent systems that have been widely accepted as examples of sensory substitution devices (SSDs). The most direct descendant of the TVSS is the tongue display unit (TDU) developed by Bach-y-Rita's laboratory (Bach-y-Rita et al. 1998). What sets the TDU apart is the fact that it uses electrodes instead of solenoids and stimulates the (highly conductive) surface of the tongue. The TDU has also been used to demonstrate that the substituted sense need not be limited to vision. It was successfully adapted to provide balance information to patients with bilateral vestibular damage (BVD), so as to restore a stable gait and posture (Tyler et al. 2003).

While the TVSS and TDU both use touch as the substituting sense, the vOICe (Meijer 1992) was the first SSD to use audition and operates as a reverse spectrograph. Each image is scanned from left to right over the course of one second. As well as time, horizontal position is also conveyed using stereo panning. Frequencies are assigned along the Y axis, the amplitudes of which are based on the brightness of each pixel. A simple horizontal white line on a black background will therefore be represented as a single continuous tone, whereas a white line crossing a black background diagonally would sound like a single rising (or falling) tone. Subsequent visual-auditory sensory substitution devices include the PVSA (Capelle et al. 1998) and the Vibe (Auvray et al. 2005). As noted by the developers of the PVSA, 'the time-multiplexed system of Meijer can be considered as working in real-time, but the refreshing rate (about one Hz) does not allow rapid sensory–motor interactions, as required in several tasks such as, e.g., mobility or reading' (Capelle et al. 1998). As a result of the implications of time-multiplexing, neither the PVSA nor the Vibe use time to denote any aspect of vision, but instead rely on our natural ability to localize sounds. The PVSA is particularly noteworthy due to its use of a weighted 'foveal' region that gives the centre of the image as much auditory space as the periphery.

In general terms, sensory substitution devices may be defined by a tripartite component model consisting of an artificial sensor, a coupling system (implementing an algorithm) and a stimulator. As described by Veraart (1989: 60): 'artificial systems should include a transducer corresponding to the receptor organ, an encoder corresponding to the sensory processing system, and finally an interpreter corresponding to perceptual functions'. This description appears to have been widely adopted: first in direct relation to Veraart's initial observation (Arno et al. 1999), but later accepted *prima facie* (Lenay et al. 2003; Raj et al. 2011; Ward and Wright 2014). Other accounts broadly agree—one only alludes to the coupling system (Visell 2009) and another refers to the stimulator as the 'human-machine interface' (Bach-y-Rita and Kercel 2003). This general, tripartite model of sensory substitution devices is illustrated in Figure 12.1.

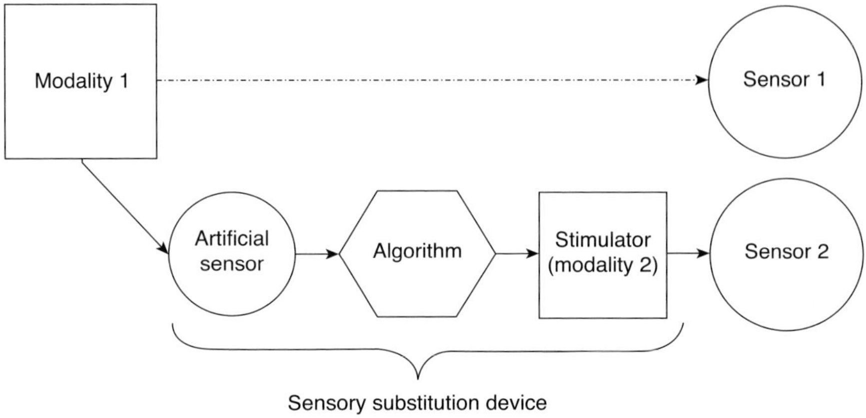

Figure 12.1 General schematic of the components of a sensory substitution device.

The overview presented thus far gives examples of typical sensory substitution devices that are generally accepted as such. Problems arise when one considers other examples that resemble sensory substitution devices either superficially or conceptually. These include examples such as Braille, canes, or devices that convert electricity or magnetism into sound and touch. The primary goal of the current essay is to present a new framework for conceptualizing what we term 'sensory tools', of which sensory substitution devices represent one particular category. In so doing we hope to break the previous circular definitions between the phenomenon of sensory substitution and the devices that afford it.

12.2 Defining Sensory Substitution

Sensory substitution has been operationally defined as 'the use of one human sense to receive information normally received by another sense' (Kaczmarek et al. 1991) and, similarly, sensory substitution devices have been defined as 'systems [that] transform stimuli characteristic of one sensory modality (for example, vision) into stimuli of another sensory modality (for example, touch)' (Lenay et al. 2003). Typically, definitions such as these do not make the crucial distinction between sensory substitution as a *process* (i.e. a series of interactions between user and device, and the ensuing changes in the brain of the user) and the sensory substitution *device* itself.

This point is illustrated well by the controversy surrounding the term 'substitution'. In terms of the device itself, the term substitution is entirely appropriate (at least in the examples introduced thus far). To take the vOICe as an example, signals that would normally be sensed by the eyes get conveyed to the ears. However, in terms of the cognitive process itself it is far less clear whether the term 'substitution' is appropriate or not. Is the auditory signal treated by the user as if it is vision (i.e. substituted) or sound (non-substituted)? Thus, whilst we can say with certainty that the vOICe device converts (or substitutes) vision to sounds, it is not possible to say, from first principles, whether the user of the vOICe converts the sounds back into vision. The evidence on the latter remains keenly debated (e.g. Auvray and Myin 2009; Ward and Wright 2014). The argument ultimately turns on what kind of evidence (neurophysiological, behavioural, phenomenological) one would need to determine that vision was occurring and the extent to which currently available research meets those criteria of proof.

The approach taken in the present essay sidesteps the arguments as to whether the user treats the input modality as if it were the substituted modality, the substituting modality, a new sense, or a combined synaesthetic sense. It instead focuses on the nature of the devices themselves and the nature of the interactions they afford with the user. As such, our primary aim is to offer a new taxonomy of sensory tools (in which sensory substitution devices sit amongst a host of others) rather than provide a new definition of sensory substitution.

12.3 Sensory Substitution Devices as Sensory Tools

We believe that the appropriate context for sensory substitution, and related devices, is that of sensory tools. SSDs are tools in the sense that they are actively employed by a user to perform a task: thus the perceiver is also the agent who manipulates the tool. Unlike more iconic examples of tools (e.g. a hammer), the operation they are used to accomplish is primarily sensory. That is, instead of mediating the way in which the user manipulates their surroundings, these tools mediate how their surroundings are perceived by the user. Accordingly, examples of non-SSD sensory tools include telescopes and cochlear implants.

Some systems, such as closed-circuit television (CCTV), can be classed as sensory tools only when they are used in certain ways. For CCTV to count as a sensory tool, it must be live (i.e. not recorded) and controllable via a joystick or similar. Without these features, the operator is less a user and more a viewer: they retain no agency over the operation of the device.

We have resisted offering a formal definition of 'sensory' but, instead, want to make a few key distinctions. First, we do *not* wish to make a sharp distinction between the classical human senses (vision, hearing, etc.) and the sensing of normally inaccessible physical properties (magneto-reception, electro-reception, etc.). The term sensory tool should be understood to encompass both of these possibilities. Second, we do wish to distinguish between the different levels of abstraction that different devices operate on. Our previous working definition of a sensory substitution device was 'the artificial conveyance of rich, abstract sensory information of one sense via a different modality' (Ward and Wright 2014).

The term 'abstract' refers to the assumption that the device operates on raw sensory information rather than information that is categorized or semanticized. For instance, optical character recognition (OCR) systems that convert printed words into speech would not be considered a 'sensory' tool because the algorithm for converting between characters and speech operates at the symbolic level rather than the sensory level. Similarly, a computer vision system that takes a visual image and produces a label such as 'car' should not be classed as a sensory tool. In both of these examples, the device is not being used as a tool for delivering sensory information.

This preamble brings us to consider a more detailed example: Braille. Bach-y-Rita and Kercel (2003) suggested that Braille is '[t]he most successful sensory substitution system to the present'. More recently others have argued that Braille is 'an obvious and widely used example' of sensory substitution (Haigh et al. 2013). Braille undoubtedly uses one sense to 'receive information normally received by another sense' (and so meets the definition offered by Bach-y-Rita), but it does not seem to resemblc canonical SSDs like the TVSS in any other way. Braille does not meet our definition of a sensory tool (or an SSD) because the relationship between the pattern of raised dots and the printed words is not a sensory one. Consider the written text in Figure 12.2. The letters can be transliterated to Braille cells, but these tell us nothing about the sensory properties of the original letters (e.g. their size or font).

The above argument also applies to sign language which has also been put forward as an example of an SSD (Bach-y-Rita 1983). However, the argument does not apply to attempts to recognize printed letters using systems such as the vOICe (Striem-Amit et al. 2012) or TDU (Sampaio et al. 2001) which are operating at a non-symbolic level. In these examples, the device is translating information at the sensory level (e.g. luminance patterns) and thus acts as a sensory tool. It is the user of the device (rather than the device itself) that converts sensory information into categorical entities such as letters. Other perceptual features of the stimulus (e.g. the size of the letters) are captured too that would be lost by systems operating at the symbolic level.

We can therefore expand our earlier definition to fit sensory tools: sensory tools are devices whose primary function is to manipulate rich, abstract sensory

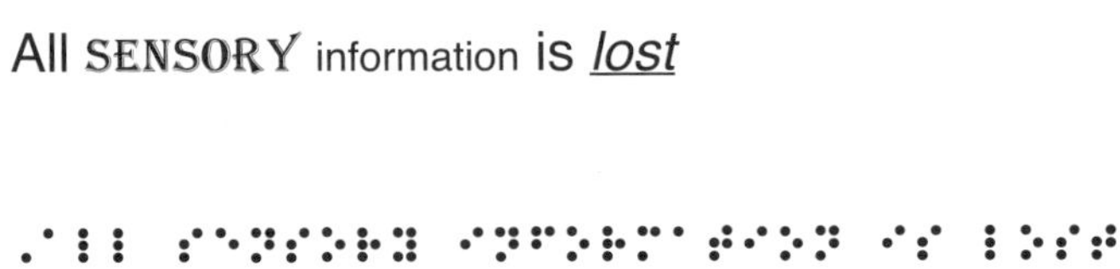

Figure 12.2 A Braille transliteration of printed text operates at a symbolic level that is stripped of sensory information.

information and present the product to a user who retains agency over the sensory experience.

12.4 A Taxonomy for Sensory Tools

In order to meaningfully discuss the relationships, we further propose that most (if not all) sensory tools may be classified on two scales: the nature of the sensory change (having four levels), and advanced/simple, which refers to the presence or absence of a converting algorithm (having two levels). The four categories describing the level of sensory change are:

1. **Compensatory prostheses:** Compensatory prostheses are tools which manipulate sensory information in such a way as to restore some functionality of a sensory organ. This category includes spectacles and hearing aids as well as cochlear and retinal implants. As the name suggests, the aim of these devices is to correct for some deficit, rather than add or change any natural experience.
2. **Within-sense referral (WSR) devices:** These are tools which transform sensory information whilst retaining the modality. This could be to change the effective location of the sensor: examples of this include stethoscopes and mirrors. A WSR device could also act so as to change some other aspect of a sensor, such as its orientation (e.g. prism glasses), its intensity (e.g. night vision goggles), or apparent size (e.g. microscopes, telescopes).
3. **Between-sense referral (BSR) devices:** These include (and are perhaps limited to) sensory substitution devices. These devices include the TVSS and the vOICe.
4. **Novel-sense referral (NSR) devices:** This category consists of tools that convey information from a novel sensory modality via an existing modality; for instance, sensing of magnetic fields by touch or electrical fields by sound, or more commonly used devices such as thermal imaging. These have also been referred to in the literature as 'sensory augmentation' devices.

These four categories can be grouped together in other ways. The most obvious of these is the uni-sensory and bi-sensory split: compensatory prostheses and within-sense referral devices are uni-sensory, but between-sense referral devices and sensory augmentation devices are both bi-sensory. Alternatively, one could contrast the compensatory devices against the transformative devices (i.e. the other three).

The second dimension has just two levels: simple and advanced. The distinction can be represented as in Figure 12.3. This distinction refers specifically to the way the device is implemented rather than the complexity per se: i.e. whether it uses an algorithm as part of its coupling system. A simple sense tool is one that works primarily because of a natural physical or mechanical relationship between

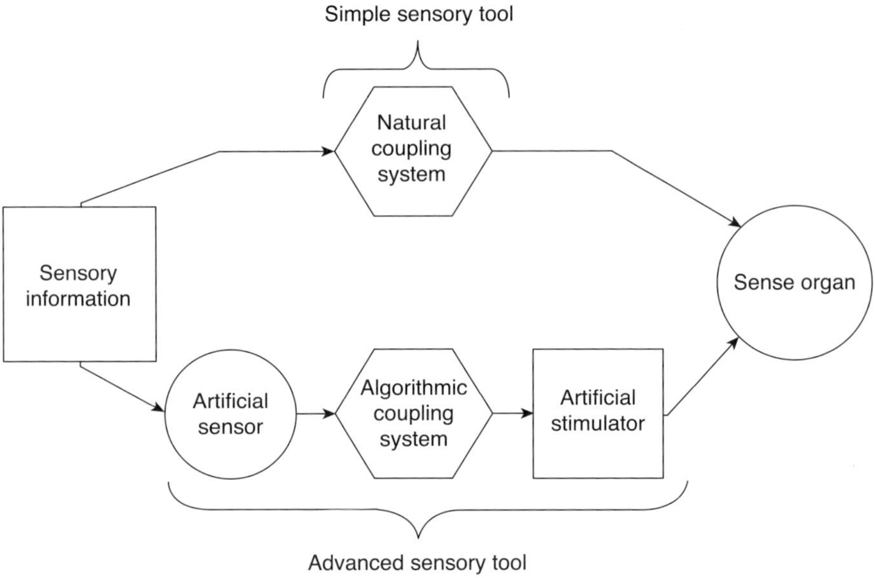

Figure 12.3 Comparison of simple and advanced sensory tools.

the source and target modalities. An advanced sensory tool is one which requires some degree of algorithmic processing in between the sensor and the stimulator. Consider, for instance, the examples of spectacles and cochlear implants. Cochlear implants contain an artificial sensor (a microphone) in addition to a coupling device that converts different frequency components of the signal detected by the sensor in order to stimulate an array of electrodes in the cochlea. In spectacles, the coupling system depends on the natural tendency of lenses to refract light. Both are compensatory prostheses, in our taxonomy, but spectacles are simple and cochlear implants are advanced. Simple sensory tools may afford a quicker path to competent use, but this is not a necessary feature.

Since these two dimensions are orthogonal, there are eight resulting combinations: see Table 12.1 for examples. It is possible to easily classify most (if not all) sensory tools within this framework. Conversely, it is possible to find several good

Table 12.1 A summary of our taxonomy for sensory tools with representative examples

	Simple	Advanced
Compensatory prostheses	Glasses	Cochlear implant
Within-sense referral (WSR)	Periscope	Leprosy glove
Between-sense referral (BSR)	?	The vOICe
Novel-sense referral (NSR)	Magnetic implants	FeelSpace

examples for most of the eight combinations except for one: simple between-sense referral. It is possible that there are no natural physical or mechanical coupling systems between any of our sensory modalities. It would require, for instance, a device for converting light to sound without employing an algorithm or skin-based vibrating sensor that responds to sound (i.e. air-based pressure changes).

12.5 Examples of Different Kinds of Sensory Tools

Having introduced a definition of sensory tools and provided a new taxonomy, this section will discuss specific examples that illustrate our approach.

12.5.1 The long cane

Bach-y-Rita and Kercel (2003) state that '[a] blind person using a cane is exhibiting another very successful simple sensory substitution system'. Whilst it is true that a long cane is used to receive information usually received from sight (relating to distant objects), it is operating within a single sensory modality (touch) and does not use an artificial sensor of any kind. In our taxonomy, the long cane is an example of a simple within-sense referral system. In the neuroscience literature there is evidence that hand-held tools lead to remapping of peri-personal space such that objects normally processed as far (i.e. requiring locomotion to reach) are treated as near (i.e. accessible without locomotion) (Longo and Lourenco 2006). For sighted animals, using a hand-held rake extends the visual receptive fields of visuo-tactile neurons that are centred on the hands to include the ends of the object itself (Iriki et al. 1996). In humans who have used such tools, they are able to integrate tactile signals on the hand with visual signals at the end of the tool (Holmes et al. 2007). Similar effects are found for cane users for whom auditory perception is enhanced at the end of the cane (Serino et al. 2007). Regardless of whether the conveyed sensory modality is visual, tactile or 'spatial', long canes easily meet our definition for being a sensory tool. They are actively employed by a user to perform a primarily sensory task.

12.5.2 The leprosy glove

One sensory tool consists of a glove for people whose extremities have been damaged by leprosy or diabetes. This glove captures tactile sensations via artificial sensors and refers these to tactors typically on the forehead (Pax et al. 1989). It has been suggested that similar technology could be used by astronauts. Not only could a tactile glove compensate for bulky clothing that renders the wearer's hands insensate, but it could also facilitate remote operation of robotic equipment (Sulzman and Wolfe 1991). In a much more clear-cut way than the long cane discussed above, such a glove would not be substituting any modality for another: it would merely refer the tactile information from the glove to the forehead (or wherever the tactors are situated). Clearly then, this device is not a sensory substitution device, but our taxonomy of sensory tools classifies it as an advanced within-sense referral device and consequently situates it close to SSDs.

12.5.3 Oscilloscopes

Oscilloscopes consist of a coupling system that translates electronic signals into a visualized form. Oscilloscopes are often used to examine electronics and, hence, the visualization of electronic waveforms in this manner could be described as an advanced form of novel-sense referral (sensory augmentation).

An alternative source of an electrical signal is a microphone. When an oscilloscope is displaying a visualization of a sound, it acts like a reverse-vOICe and is clearly an example of a between-sense referral system. Others have used the example of a sound-displaying oscilloscope to argue against the notion that this could be related to sensory substitution. For instance, Leon argues: ‘It is not more persuasive than the suggestion that we would hear sounds and various properties by means of the eyes, simply because we observe an optical transformation of an aural input by using, say, an oscilloscope’ (1988: 252). As noted before, it is important not to confuse whether the device is converting one sense to another with the issue as to whether the user performs some kind of back-conversion. In terms of the device itself, an oscilloscope displaying sound should be regarded in the same way as more generally accepted examples of SSDs (e.g. the vOICe). The question of why the user of different devices may treat some, but not other, auditory signals as visual-like is an important issue but it is orthogonal to the categorization of sensory tools per se.

12.5.4 Subdermal magnetic implants

Some electrical engineering researchers have explored the insertion of small rare-earth magnets into their fingertips in order to tangibly perceive magnetic fields (Hameed et al. 2010). When the magnets are stimulated, they move slightly. These subtle movements activate the mechanoreceptors on the overlying skin that normally support the detection of exteroceptive touch. As such, the coupling system is analogous to the lenses in spectacles (it requires no conversion algorithm) and this is a simple sensory tool. However, it is one that refers a novel sense (magnetism) to an existing sense (touch). As one implant recipient explains, even this simple interface between magnetism and touch can give rise to profoundly new experiences:

> Each object has its own unique field, with different strength and 'texture.' I started holding my finger over almost everything that I could, getting a feeling for each object's invisible reach [. . .] It has unlocked an entirely new world for me, one that I can touch and interact with in a very real way. While a magnet implant doesn't technically count as a 'sixth sense' (it's more of an extension of our existing sense of touch), the way that the body internalizes these tiny magnetic vibrations feels truly foreign.
> (Berg 2012)

12.5.5 FeelSpace

The FeelSpace device conveys magnetic north to a belt of vibrating pads attached around the waist (Nagel et al. 2005). This represents an example of advanced novel-sense referral because the direction of the Earth's magnetism is not normally within the repertoire of sensible information, and it is advanced in that the coupling system involves an algorithm for transforming information extracted from an artificial sensor. Sighted participants who used the belt over six weeks improved in blindfolded navigation tasks (finding their way to a starting location), and the use of the belt also interacted with vestibular information (e.g. reducing body sway). Some participants reported novel experiences such as: 'After removing the belt, my living space shrank quickly: the world appeared smaller and more chaotic because relative positions to places beyond the visual horizon were rather unorderly.' More recently, it has been shown that a blind user of the device shows improvement in a wide range of tasks, such as walking in a straight line, pointing and returning to a starting position (Karcher et al. 2012).

12.5.6 The Enactive Torch

The Enactive Torch uses an infrared sensor that detects proximity which is encoded as the intensity of vibration in the hand-held device (Froese et al. 2012). This resembles the example of the long cane except that the coupling system implements an algorithm. However, the information extracted is quite different as the cane senses the presence of obstacles (at a fixed distance) whereas the Enactive Torch senses the distance of the nearest surface/object in the direction of the infrared beam. On this basis, the creators of the device argue that it should be classed as a form of novel-sense referral (or sensory augmentation).

12.5.7 Virtual reality

Virtual reality and augmented reality are not forms of sensory tool, but can certainly act as platforms for the creation of virtual sensory tools. In a typical virtual reality set-up, the user wears at least a set of immersive goggles and a pair of headphones. Accordingly, any sensory tool that targets either vision or audition may be simulated. Similarly, in augmented reality a user will typically view the world through a screen (perhaps mounted in goggles) that adds a computer-generated layer.

This presents some interesting opportunities. Since a simulated world need not follow the physical laws of our universe, it is possible to use virtual sensory augmentation to create entirely novel sensory modalities, devoid of any connection to any natural phenomena. Or, as demonstrated by a recent game produced at MIT, normal physical laws can be altered. 'A Slower Speed of Light' allows the player to experience moving at speeds close to the speed of light by seeing red-shift and blue-shift (Kortemeyer et al. 2013). This manipulation represents virtual visual within-sense referral.

12.6 Discussion: Implications for Neuroscience

The point of forming a structured ontology is not merely to end up with more appropriate names for the different elements, but also allows us to systematically compare and contrast them. By making explicit our understanding of the relationships between sensory substitution and other devices and phenomena, we don't simply give them new labels: we form the basis for testable hypotheses that may further our understanding. In this final section we discuss the implications of our taxonomy for neuroscience research and we relate it to existing theoretical approaches.

All sensory tools will invoke some degree of neural adaptation. What is likely to differ across tools is the extent to which this adaptation is confined to one sensory modality, several sensory modalities, amodal spatial processes, and motor mechanisms.

Compensatory prostheses are likely to elicit neural adaptation primarily in the affected sensory system. However, this may depend on the extent to which the neural resources normally dedicated to that sense have been recruited by other cognitive functions during a sensitive period. For instance, the extent to which the 'auditory' cortex becomes activated by sounds after the introduction of cochlear implants depends on the age of onset of deafness (Lee et al. 2001; Harrison et al. 2005), perhaps because this part of the brain has taken on non-auditory functions (e.g. processing sign language). Tools such as spectacles and cochlear implants do not require learning of novel sensorimotor mappings but instead tap existing contingencies associated with the sensory organs.

Within-sense referral devices may, similarly to compensatory prostheses, be linked to relatively localized changes within the affected sensory modality. Unlike compensatory prostheses, these devices typically involve learning of new sensorimotor contingencies and so are likely to involve plasticity within regions involved in spatial cognition and motor control. To give one example, George Stratton investigated the effects of inverting his visual field by means of a pair of prism-glasses (Stratton 1896, 1897). Adaptation seems to occur primarily in the motor system, despite (or at least in addition to) phenomenological reports of perceptual adaptation (Morton and Bastian 2004). In terms of neural resources, this involves changes in the cerebellum (Morton and Bastian 2004) and the parietal cortex (Pisella et al. 2002). An example of a similar tool in everyday use is the angled mirror used by dentists: as with Stratton's device, there is a mismatch between the location of an object and its visual image. It would be interesting to establish whether the same network is involved in learning to use non-visual within-sense referral tools, such as the leprosy glove. Would the remapping of tactile percepts between hand and forehead occur solely within the somatosensory system, as has been suggested for referred tactile sensations in amputees (Ramachandran et al. 1992), or would it require more general neural resources implicated in amodal spatial cognition and motor control?

To move on to between-sense referral devices (including our canonical examples of sensory substitution), there have been many studies examining the neural basis of these devices and they won't be reviewed in detail here (see Bubic et al. 2010). Far less is known about the neural substrates linked to novel-sense referral devices, or sensory augmentation. In both cases, the input signal to the user is *unimodal*. As such, one might expect that the user's brain should treat these devices in exactly the same way as within-sense referral devices. Specifically, it should involve plasticity within the stimulated sensory modality, and learning of new sensorimotor contingencies and spatial relationships. However, many argue that between-sense referral devices also lead to functional plasticity within the substituted system (e.g. Ptito et al. 2005) and may even lead to phenomenology within the substituted modality (Ward and Meijer 2010). The relevant question then becomes: how does the brain know that, say, a tactile signal should be processed visually in the case of a between-sense referral device (e.g. TVSS) but processed within the tactile system for a within-sense referral device (e.g. long cane, leprosy glove)? The answer, according to some, lies in the nature of the sensorimotor contingencies (e.g. O'Regan and Noë 2001). Specifically, the sensorimotor contingencies of touch-from-vision resemble, in certain ways, those of natural vision (e.g. greater spatial extent with increasing proximity, occluded objects not sensed, shadowing). This depends on appropriate use of the device: for instance a static camera that is not controlled by the user would not be predicted to have the same effect. This also suggests potential differences amongst between-sense referral devices. For instance a sound-to-vision oscilloscope is not normally linked to auditory-like motor behaviour, but such a device could, in principle, be constructed.

It should be pointed out that this view is not universally accepted. For instance, Block (2003) argues that sensory substitution devices only involve creating new spatial mappings (e.g. externalizing touch to in front of the body) rather than involving the substituted sense (e.g. vision). In this view, between-sense referral devices (and presumably novel-sense referral devices) are equivalent both cognitively and neurally to within-sense referral devices. One important line of future research, highlighted as a result of our taxonomy, is to compare directly the functional (or structural) changes in the brain when using between-sense versus within-sense devices.

Not all of the available empirical evidence is consistent with the view that use of visual neural resources stems from visual-like sensorimotor contingencies. Indeed, Ortiz et al. (2011) trained blind participants on a device consisting of an array of tactors felt with the hand. Their task was simply to discriminate line orientation. Over time, the participants improved their ability at orientation detection and, moreover, many of them reported visual phenomenology (e.g. seeing white lines) which was linked to electrical activity in the occipital cortex (measured with EEG). The device itself was referred to in terms of sensory substitution but it doesn't meet any conventional definitions of this and nor was the device linked to visual input or visual sensorimotor contingencies (there was no live camera). Rather, it was a purely tactile discrimination task. It may well be the case that, in certain blind participants, demanding auditory or tactile processing is sufficient to elicit recruitment of the occipital lobes (possibly including visual phenomenology) irrespective of the sensorimotor functionality of the tool.

12.7 Relationship to Other Approaches

We have already discussed one influential approach to sensory substitution: the sensorimotor approach (e.g. O'Regan and Noë 2001). The sensorimotor account of perception maps well onto our proposed ontology of sensory tools. Indeed, the four levels of sense tools described above can be accurately defined in terms of their effect on sensorimotor contingencies. Compensatory prostheses typically alter some physical attribute of the sensory information, whilst preserving the sensorimotor contingencies. Within-sense referral devices preserve the basic structure of the sensorimotor contingencies of the source modality, but do alter specific properties of these contingencies. Inverting prisms, for example, do not change the fact that occlusion is a contingency of vision. Between-sense referral devices can change the sensorimotor contingencies to those more closely resembling a different modality (but they are not obliged to, e.g. an oscilloscope). Novel-sense referral (or sensory augmentation) devices are interesting because they expose the perceiver to entirely novel contingencies. Magnetism is the most obvious example source of entirely novel sensorimotor contingencies. For instance, the FeelSpace belt (Nagel et al. 2005) exposes a set of novel sensorimotor contingencies, such as: changing tactile sensations as the body rotates about an axis perpendicular to the ground; remaining constant through bodily translation; being impervious to occlusion; and so on. Thus, the sensorimotor account of perception is entirely compatible with the taxonomy of sensory tools described in this essay, and offers a new way of thinking about how different tools work and the effects they might have on the brain.

Our approach is also similar to the argument developed by Auvray and Myin (2009) that sensory substitution devices arc mind-enhancing tools. The starting point of their argument is the idea that tools are not merely objects that the cognitive system acts upon but, rather, that the use of tools shapes cognition itself—hence 'mind-expanding' (see also Clark 2003, 2008). They suggest that SSDs transform sensorimotor and perceptual capabilities but argue against the view that this is like any of the naturally occurring senses (e.g. vision). The kinds of non-SSD tools that they consider are very different from the ones considered in our taxonomy. For instance, they discuss how sketchpads are aids for memorizing and calculating. Whilst we agree with the general approach of situating sensory substitution within a framework of tool use, we argue that there is likely to be particular value in thinking of SSDs specifically in the context of other sensory tools.

Auvray and Myin (2009) also argue that learning to use a sensory substitution device is not like the normal development of perception. For instance, they state that 'There is no analog in natural perception to the way the user of an SSD retains explicit and conscious control over it even after having become skilled.' These ideas are expanded upon in a more recent paper by Deroy and Auvray (2012) who suggest that learning to use an SSD is more like learning to read than learning to see. For instance they claim that both reading and using an SSD require some form of training to reach expertise. They also suggest that both involve learning to map perceptual stimuli to meaning, rather than forming correspondences between one sense and another. They argue that the analogy with reading is more useful than attempts to describe sensory substitution in terms of the operation of existing senses. This latter point is clearly at odds with the approach that we have developed. We have argued that we should consider SSDs as an example of sensory tools and that a useful future direction is to consider the general effects that these tools have upon the existing sensory and motor systems of the brain. When SSD users are presented with a sound-based or touch-based representation of an image of a car, they not only extract its meaning ('it is a car'): there is other information that is present, such as whether it is facing left or right, whether it is dark or light, and its location in space. The latter enables actions to be performed. This is completely different from the kind of information that can be extracted from the written word CAR. Although we can determine that the letters are capitalized (etc.), it tells us nothing about our external environment, including how to act upon it. (This is essentially the same point made earlier with respect to Braille's non-status as a sensory tool.) It is for these reasons that we think that it is helpful to regard SSDs as sensory tools.

12.8 Concluding Comments

In this essay we have demonstrated that the term 'sensory substitution' is used too broadly by many researchers but the opposite approach (i.e. a very narrow definition) misses many other devices that are conceptually similar and potentially informative. As noted by many others, the term 'substitution' is potentially misleading and one needs to be careful about whether it is the device or the user's brain that is performing a substitution. We have consequently proposed a novel conceptual framework and nomenclature that sets sensory substitution alongside other sensory tools. We view this as an important step towards a coherent model of sensory tools and the perceptual alterations they afford.

References

Arno, P., Capelle, C., Wanet-Defalque, M. C., Catalan-Ahumada, M. and Veraart, C. (1999) Auditory coding of visual patterns for the blind. *Perception* 28(8): 1013–1029.

Auvray, M., Hanneton, S., Lenay, C. and O'Regan, K. (2005) There is something out there: distal attribution in sensory substitution, twenty years later. *Journal of Integrative Neuroscience* 4(4): 505–521.

Auvray, M. and Myin, E. (2009) Perception with compensatory devices: from sensory substitution to sensorimotor extension. *Cognitive Science* 33(6): 1036–1058.

Bach-y-Rita, P. (1983) Tactile vision substitution: past and future. *International Journal of Neuroscience* 19(1–4): 29–36.

Bach-y-Rita, P. and Kercel, S. W. (2003) Sensory substitution and the human-machine interface. *Trends in Cognitive Sciences* 7: 541–546.

Bach-y-Rita, P., Collins, C. C., Saunders, F. A., White, B. and Scadden, L. (1969) Vision substitution by tactile image projection. *Nature* 221: 963.

Bach-y-Rita, P., Kaczmarek, K. A., Tyler, M. E. and Garcia-Lara, J. (1998) Form perception with a 49-point electrotactile stimulus array on the tongue: a technical note. *Journal of Rehabilitation Research and Development* 35(4): 427–430.

Berg, D. (2012) 'I have a magnet implant in my finger.' 22 March. http://gizmodo.com/5895555/i-have-a-magnet-implant-in-my-finger.

Block, N. (2003) Tactile sensation via spatial perception. *Trends in Cognitive Neurosciences* 7: 285–286.

Bubic, A., Striem-Amit, E. and Amedi, A. (2010) Large-scale brain plasticity following blindness and the use of sensory substitution devices. In M. J. Naumer and J. Kaiser (eds) *Multisensory Object Perception in the Primate Brain*. New York: Springer, 351–380.

Capelle, C., Trullemans, C., Arno, P. and Veraart, C. (1998) A real-time experimental prototype for enhancement of vision rehabilitation using auditory substitution. *IEEE Transactions on Biomedical Engineering* 45(10): 1279–1293.

Clark, A. (2003) *Natural-Born Cyborgs: Minds, Technologies, and the Future of Human Intelligence*. Oxford: Oxford University Press.

Clark, A. (2008) *Supersizing the Mind: Embodiment, Action and Cognitive Extension*. Oxford: Oxford University Press.

Deroy, O. and Auvray, M. (2012) Reading the world through the skin and ears: a new perspective on sensory substitution. *Frontiers in Theoretical and Philosophical Psychology* 3(457).

Froese, T., McGann, M., Bigge, W., Spiers, A. and Seth, A. (2012) The Enactive Torch: a new tool for the science of perception. *IEEE Transactions on Haptics* 5(4): 365–375.

Haigh, A., Meijer, P. and Proulx, M. J. (2013) How well do you see what you hear? The acuity of visual-to-auditory sensory substitution. *Frontiers in Cognitive Science* 4(330).

Hameed, J., Harrison, I., Gasson, M. N. and Warwick, K. (2010) A novel human-machine interface using subdermal magnetic implants. *In IEEE 9th International Conference on Cybernetic Intelligent Systems (CIS)*, 1–2 September, University of Reading, UK, 106–110 (IEEE London). doi: 10.1109/UKRICIS.2010.5898141.

Harrison, R. V., Gordon, K. A. and Mount, R. J. (2005) Is there a critical period for cochlear implantation in congenitally deaf children? Analyses of hearing and speech perception performance after implantation. *Developmental Psychobiology* 46: 252–261. doi: 10.1002/dev.20052.

Holmes, N. P., Calvert, G. A. and Spence, C. (2007) Tool use changes multisensory interactions in seconds: evidence from the crossmodal congruency task. *Experimental Brain Research* 183: 465–476.

Iriki, A., Tanaka, M. and Iwamura, Y. (1996) Coding of modified body schema during tool use by macaque postcentral neurons. *NeuroReport* 7: 2325–2330.

Kaczmarek, K. A., Webster, J. G., Bach-y-Rita, P. and Tompkins, W. J. (1991) Electrotactile and vibrotactile displays for sensory substitution systems. *IEEE Transactions on Biomedical Engineering* 38(1): 1–16. doi: 10.1109/10.68204.

Karcher, S. M., Fenzlaff, S., Hartmann, D., Nagel, S. K. and Konig, P. (2012) Sensory augmentation for the blind. *Frontiers in Human Neuroscience* 6(15).

Kortemeyer, G., Tan, P. and Schirra, S. (2013) *A Slower Speed of Light: Developing Intuition about Special Relativity with Games*. FDG 2013, ACM, New York.

Lee, D. S., Lee, J. S., Oh, S. H., Kim, S. K., Kim, J. W., Chung, J. K., Lee, M. C. and Kim, C. S. (2001) Deafness—cross-modal plasticity and cochlear implants. *Nature* 409(6817): 149–150.

Lenay, C., Gapenne, O., Hanneton, S., Marque, C. and Genouëlle, C. (2003) Sensory substitution: limits and perspectives. In Y. Hatwell, A. Streri and E. Gentaz (eds) *Touching for Knowing: Cognitive Psychology of Haptic Manual Perception*. Amsterdam: John Benjamins Publishing.

Leon, M. (1988) Characterizing the senses. *Mind and Language* 3: 243–270.

Longo, M. R. and Lourenco, S. F. (2006) On the nature of near space: effects of tool use and the transition to far space. *Neuropsychologia* 44(6): 977–981.

Meijer, P. B. L. (1992) An experimental system for auditory image representations. *IEEE Transactions on Biomedical Engineering* 39: 112–121.

Morton, S. M. and Bastian, A. J. (2004) Prism adaptation during walking generalizes to reaching and requires the cerebellum. *Journal of Neurophysiology* 92(4): 2497–2509.

Nagel, S. K., Carl, C., Kringe, T., Martin, R. and Konig, P. (2005) Beyond sensory substitution—learning the sixth sense. *Journal of Neural Engineering* 2(4): R13–26.

O'Regan, J. K. and Noë, A. (2001) A sensorimotor account of vision and visual consciousness. *Behavioral and Brain Sciences* 24: 939–1031.

Ortiz, T., Poch, J., Santos, J. M., Requena, C., Martinez, A. M., Ortiz-Teran, L., Turrero, A., Barcia, J., Nogales, R., Calvo, A., Martinez, J. M., Cordoba, J. L. and Pascual-Leone, A. (2011) Recruitment of occipital cortex during sensory substitution training linked to subjective experience of seeing in people with blindness. *PloS One* 6(8): 11.

Pax, R. A., Webster, J. G. and Radwin, R. G. (1989) A conductive polymer sensor for the measurement of palmar pressures. *Proceedings of the Annual International Conference of the IEEE Engineering* 5: 1483–1484.

Pisella, L., Rode, G., Farnè, A., Boisson, D. and Rossetti, Y. (2002) Dissociated long lasting improvements of straight-ahead pointing and line bisection tasks in two hemineglect patients. *Neuropsychologia* 40(3): 327–334.

Ptito, M., Moesgaard, S. M., Gjedde, A. and Kupers, R. (2005) Cross-modal plasticity revealed by electrotactile stimulation of the tongue in the congenitally blind. *Brain* 128: 606–614.

Raj, A. K., Neuhaus, P. D., Moucheboeuf, A. M., Noorden, J. H. and Lecoutre, D. V. (2011) Mina: a sensorimotor robotic orthosis for mobility assistance. *Journal of Robotics*, Article ID 284352.

Ramachandran, V. S., Stewart, M. and Rogers-Ramachandran, D. C. (1992) Perceptual correlates of massive cortical reorganization. *NeuroReport* 3(7): 583–586.

Sampaio, E., Maris, S. and Bach-y-Rita, P. (2001) Brain plasticity: 'visual' acuity of blind persons via the tongue. *Brain Research* 908: 204–207.

Serino, A., Bassolino, M., Farne, A. and Ladavas, E. (2007) Extended multisensory space in blind cane users. *Psychological Science* 18: 642–648.

Stratton, G. M. (1896) Some preliminary experiments on vision without inversion of the retinal image. *Psychological Review* 3(6): 611–617.

Stratton, G. M. (1897) Vision without inversion of the retinal image. *Psychological Review* 4(4): 341–360.

Striem-Amit, E., Cohen, L., Dehaene, S. and Amedi, A. (2012) Reading with sounds: sensory substitution selectively activates the visual word form area in the blind. *Neuron* 76(3): 640–652.

Sulzman, F. M. and Wolfe, J. W. (1991) Neurosciences research in space: future directions. *Acta Astronautica* 23: 289–293.

Tyler, M., Danilov, Y. and Bach-y-Rita, P. (2003) Closing an open-loop control system: vestibular substitution through the tongue. *Journal of Integrative Neuroscience* 2: 159–164.

Veraart, C. (1989) Neurophysiological approach to the design of visual prostheses: a theoretical discussion. *Journal of Medical Engineering and Technology* 13(1–2): 57–62.

Visell, Y. (2009) Tactile sensory substitution: models for enaction in HCI. *Interacting with Computers* 21(1–2): 38–53.

Ward, J. and Meijer, P. (2010) Visual experiences in the blind induced by an auditory sensory substitution device. *Consciousness and Cognition* 19: 492–500.

Ward, J. and Wright, T. D. (2014) Sensory substitution as an artificially acquired synaesthesia. *Neuroscience and Biobehavioral Review* 41: 26–35.

13

Sensory Substitution and Perceptual Emergence

JONATHAN COHEN

Abstract Designers of sensory substitution devices (SSDs) typically aim to capture a wide representational scope by requiring their devices to present in the substituting modality the full range of basic energy available to the substituted modality, and then using this information to code up any further representations needed. On this view, if we could build a device that represents to touch (say) the distal distribution of light intensity—the basic form of energy to which visual receptors are normally responsive—our device could, in principle, represent everything available to vision: colour, shape, form, motion, and so on. Unfortunately, I will argue, this simple idea fails. For perceptual modalities represent 'emergent' features—i.e. features whose exemplification is not fixed by the representation of the distribution of basic energy. Hence, an SSD whose basic representational vocabulary is limited to the distribution of such basic energy will leave things out. None of this shows that SSDs will inevitably fail to represent what sensory modalities normally represent. It does suggest, however, that if we want them to represent what sensory modalities normally represent, we will have to do more than preserve the representation of basic energy to which the substituted modalities are sensitive.

> The problems with which we are confronted in our strivings for a scientific understanding of mental phenomena are gigantic, and there is little reason to be overenthusiastic about the present state of the field. But one certitude remains: The mental can be driven out of psychology as little as the biological can be driven out of biology or the chemical out of chemistry. Where no psychology is put in, no psychology is put out.
> (Mausfeld 2003: 190)

Sensory substitution devices (ssds) can be thought of as sensory prosthetics—as devices by which information represented by one perceptual modality (the substituted modality) is instead represented by an alternative, non-canonical representational channel involving a second perceptual modality (the substitut-

Proceedings of the British Academy, **219**, 205–235.

ing modality). The hope is that such devices might aid subjects with an impaired perceptual modality in exploiting their unimpaired modalities to connect perceptually with the world in ways that their impairments otherwise make inaccessible. Beginning in the 1960s, researchers have developed and built a range of SSDs, including mainly visual-to-tactile systems (e.g. the Optacon of Linvill and Bliss (1966); the Tactile Visual Substitution System (TVSS) of Bach y Rita et al. (1969)) and visual-to-auditory systems (e.g. the vOICe of Meijer (1992); the Prosthesis Substituting Vision for Audition of Capelle et al. (1998)).

Among the many design challenges that must be met by successful SSDs, one of the most serious is the *scope problem*—that of ensuring that the novel substituting modality has whatever representational resources are required to encode the full range of targets normally covered by the substituted modality. The solution to this problem built into extant SSDs is, roughly, to work bottom up—to preserve the representation of the basic distribution of energy to which the substituted modality is sensitive, and then to hope that all other perceptually relevant representations can be derived therefrom. Unfortunately, I will argue below, this attractively simple solution to the scope problem fails. For there appear to be properties represented by our perceptual modalities whose exemplification is not fixed by the representation of the distribution of (the relevant forms of) basic energy. Hence, an SSD whose basic representational vocabulary is limited to the distribution of such basic energy will inevitably leave things out.

Here is how I will proceed. In section 13.1 I will start from a simple view of perceptual representation, explain how mismatches of representational scope create a serious obstacle for the design of SSDs, and then propose a simple view about how SSDs might solve the scope problem by working bottom up from the representation of the basic energy distribution. Then, in sections 13.2–13.4 I will consider a series of perceptual phenomena that suggest that this bottom-up strategy is inadequate—phenomena suggesting that the representation of the basic energy distribution in a modality is insufficient for fixing representations of all the features made available in that modality. And in section 13.5 I will draw lessons about what this shows about perception and the prospects for SSDs.

13.1 Perception, Substitution, and Scope

On the construal suggested above, sensory substitution amounts to replacing a first suite of representational capacities associated with one perceptual modality—if you like, an informational channel—with a second. I think it is fair to say that this conception of SSDs is reasonably prevalent amongst researchers. Thus, for example, Ward and Meijer write that, 'Sensory substitution devices artificially convert information normally delivered to one sense into a representation that is compatible with an alternative sense' (2010: 492). Or, in the words of Proulx, 'sensory substitution devices for the blind provide the missing visual input by providing information that another sensory modality, such as the tactile or auditory system, can process' (2010: 501).

Of course, as a general matter, it is not always easy or even possible to coerce one informational channel into serving the representational/information-carrying functions of a second. Among many other problems, disparities in carrying capacity, interface properties, or spatiotemporal resolution may render this sort of substitution difficult or impossible. But here I want to focus on an even simpler obstacle to substitution concerning mismatch of scope.

13.1.1 The scope problem

It is hardly earth-shaking news that different modalities ordinarily represent different ranges of properties/events: in the normal run of things (i.e. without special equipment), vision but not audition represents distal shape, touch but not olfaction represents temperature, and so on.[1]

Such mismatches of representational scope create obstacles that successful SSDs must surmount. Obviously, no SSD will count as a fully adequate representational substitute for a modality, considered as a whole, unless it succeeds in representing the full suite of properties normally in that modality's representational scope. This is a highly non-trivial requirement given that modalities have such extensive representational scopes. But even more limited SSDs that aim to replace only a subset of the representational functions of a modality—say, those that attempt to represent through auditory means the normally visually accessible features of size and form, but not colour—face the challenge of taking over those intended representational functions in the wide variety of situations in which the substituted modality normally does its job. Either way, the point is that the design of successful SSDs must, on pain of failing at the task for which they are intended, somehow meet the non-trivial constraint of augmenting the representational scope of the substituting modality so as to make it include some or all of the scope of the substituted modality.

[1] Of course, some properties fall in the representational scope of multiple modalities: thus, for example, some (but not all) shape properties can be represented by both vision and touch. But such properties are isolated exceptions that prove the general rule: the intersection of the representational scopes of two modalities is typically a small subset of both. While we may wish to say that such cases count as a limited, if common, form of sensory substitution, we presumably want our SSDs to be much more general in their operation—we want to build SSDs that represent a much wider range of distal targets. As such, isolated cases of scope overlap won't help with the scope problem we are now considering in anything like its full generality.

13.1.2 Solving the scope problem from the bottom up

There is, however, a way of thinking about perceptual modalities and their operation—one that I suspect underlies the design of many extant SSDs—that suggests a possible (and principled) way forward. This strategy is built from two thoughts.

The first is that each modality is specially connected with one or more types of distal energy to which its proprietary types of transducers are sensitive.[2] Thus, for example, visual (but not auditory, tactile, vestibular, etc.) systems have photoreceptors as their basic transducers, and these transducers are selectively responsive to a particular form of environmental energy—light intensities (or, if you like, light intensities at locations). Likewise, auditory (but not visual, pain, etc.) systems have receptors that are selectively responsive to certain kinds of mechanical pressure waves (possibly at locations). And similarly for the other modalities.[3]

The second is the thought that, though modalities have wide informational scopes, all of the properties that they represent can (in principle) be fixed by their representation of the distribution of whatever types of basic energy to which they are responsive. In other words, the view is that a modality's basic energy distribution forms a computationally sufficient basis for the derivation of its (basic and non-basic) representational scope. So, for example, though vision lacks receptors specifically and selectively sensitive to exemplifications of *squarehood*, vision manages to represent whether there are local squares in the environment because its representation of the array of light intensities (the form of distal energy to which its proprietary receptors are sensitive) is sufficient, given enough computational power, to fix whether or not there is a local instance of *squarehood*. For, the thought goes, if you know where the light is, then you can (given enough computational power) figure out where the edges are, and how long they are, and from this you can figure out where the squares are. And, indeed, though the computational

[2] This idea can perhaps be seen as an expression of the Aristotelian view that individual modalities are particularly, and essentially, bound up with their own proper sensibles/objects.

[3] Heil (1983) defends the related, but stronger view that we can individuate sensory modalities by the distal energy types to which they are responsive; it is also possible to read Keeley (2002: 6) as advocating such a view (though he wants to add further conditions). One problem for the stronger view is that it appears to individuate modalities both too coarsely and too finely. It appears to individuate modalities too coarsely because, for example, it is unobvious that there are indeed distinct distal energy types that correspond to gustatory taste and olfaction. Similarly, the stronger view predicts that thermoregulation and vision in pit vipers comprise a single modality, since both are responsive to wavelength energy (Kardong and Mackessy 1991). On the other hand, the stronger view also appears to individuate modalities too finely: for example, it doesn't allow for a unified modality of touch, since the latter is responsive to several distinct forms of energy including temperature, pressure, and elasticity (Fulkerson 2013).

Crucially, the idea expressed in the main text—to the effect that modalities are specially connected with particular types of distal energy—is unlike the stronger view in not committing to any proposal about the individuation of modalities. Consequently, it is not vulnerable to the problems posed above for the stronger view.

story may be more complicated, we might hope to extend this picture to all of the other features in the representational scope of vision. Thus, perhaps we can derive representations of distal colour by some sorts of complicated comparisons between lightness intensity representations from receptors with different spectral tunings; or perhaps we can derive representations of motion by intertemporal comparisons between representations of the distribution of form (themselves derived ultimately from representations of lightness). Similarly, the thought is that preserving the representations of where the light is would provide for our device a sufficient computational basis for representing, in principle, everything vision can represent. Finally, let us suppose that this thought can be extended to other modalities, so that we would aim to account for the representational scope of each modality in terms of the distribution of energy to which its proprietary receptors are sensitive.

As I suggested above, appeal to these two thoughts offers a hope for a principled approach to the scope problem for SSDs. For even if we can't specify in advance the full representational scope of the modality for which we are attempting to build a representational substitute, it is presumably far easier to determine the form(s) of basic energy to which its receptors are sensitive. And if we can then build an alternative channel that represents those forms of energy—one that preserves in the substituting modality the information about the basic distribution of energy in the substituted modality, we will have in place a computationally sufficient basis for representing all of the properties in the full representational scope we are aiming to capture.

Importantly, on the story we are contemplating, the wide-ranging representational scope of each sensory modality is ultimately constrained by, asymmetrically dependent on, and supervenient on its representation of the distribution of the energy to which its modality-specific transducer types are responsive. Hence it seems reasonable to call the proposal we have been discussing a *bottom-up* strategy for solving the scope problem.

To make clear just what the proposed bottom-up strategy looks like and why it is attractive, it may be helpful to contrast a purely hypothetical approach to the design of a vision-to-audition SSD for shape that does not conform to it. Thus, suppose we somehow build into the device some kind of primitive *squarehood* detector that makes an auditory signal in the presence of local squares, but without doing so by way of representing the distribution of light, or edges, or any other intuitively more basic properties. If we manage to do this, we will have brought the normally visually accessible (but not normally auditorily accessible) property *squarehood* into the representational scope of our system, and so will have made an advance on the scope problem. However, because our imagined system represents *squarehood* without representing the distribution of light, edges, or the like, there is no guarantee that it will have the capacity to represent other normally visually accessible properties, such as texture, depth, illumination, motion, etc. Thus, although our system will have made an advance on a single instance of the scope problem, there are all kinds of other normally visually accessible properties—which are, of course, just other instances of the same problem—about which all bets are off.

In contrast, the bottom-up strategy is one that begins by representing the distribution of light intensity, and from there computing representations of (as it might be) first lightness discontinuities, then edges, then simple shapes, and so on. Crucially, because this style of computational processing works upwards from a representation of the basic energy distribution, and on the assumption that representations of that sort form a computationally sufficient basis for the representation of not only *squarehood* but everything else in the representational scope of vision, we know that our square-detecting system will, by dint of whatever allows it to represent *squarehood*, also (in principle) be capable of representing texture, depth, illumination, motion, and so on. In other words, a system implementing the bottom-up strategy won't find itself stuck with a merely partial solution to the scope problem in the way that the system employing a primitive *squarehood* detector did.

13.1.3 A worry: emergent features?

Near as I can tell, some version of the bottom-up strategy sketched above appears to underlie the design of all extant SSDs. And this fact should come as no surprise if, as I have suggested, that strategy offers a promising, principled, and attractively simple approach to overcoming a problem that any successful SSD must solve (viz., the scope problem).

However, in what follows, I will argue that the bottom-up strategy fails. For there appears to be a range of well-known perceptual phenomena suggesting that, contrary to the explicit assumptions underlying that strategy, there are what I will call *perceptually emergent features*—perceptually represented features for whose representation it turns out that a representation of the basic energy distribution is *not* a sufficient computational basis.[4]

I want to emphasize that the threat about emergent features is not simply about the *de facto* limitations on the stock of available representational vocabulary (as it were, the stock of predicates) that perceptual systems happen to use. To see what that kind of threat would amount to, imagine that we build a representational

[4]The term 'emergence' is intended to suggest a failure of fixity from below. Crucially, the failure of fixity at issue is a relation between representations of properties, rather than properties themselves. To say that *F* is perceptually emergent is to say that representations of *F* are not determined computationally by representations of other (intuitively, lower-level) properties. This claim leaves open the question of whether *F* is *metaphysically* emergent—viz., whether there is a metaphysical failure of determination of *F* by lower-level properties—in the sense discussed by the British Emergentists (e.g. Alexander 1920; Broad 1925), *inter alia*. (Though I won't distinguish explicitly between perceptual and metaphysical notions of emergence in the following, I will always mean the former.)

system that has internal representational states corresponding to the English words for the individual colours 'red', 'green', 'orange', and the rest (viz., states that are selectively responsive to instances of *redness*, *greenness*, *orangeness*, and so on), but that lacks an internal representational state corresponding to the English word 'coloured' (viz., one that is selectively responsive to instances of the relatively determinable property *coloured*). Now, it is a metaphysical fact—one that is independent of the particular features of our imagined representational system—that the extensions of *redness*, *greenness*, *orangeness*, and all the other individual colours collectively fix the extension of *coloured*. *A fortiori*, whatever information comprises a computationally sufficient basis for the representation of the individual colours also comprises a computationally sufficient basis for the representation of *coloured*. Consequently, by fixing the distribution of *redness*, *greenness*, *orangeness*, and all the other individual colours in the scene, our imagined system simultaneously fixes the distribution of *coloured* in the scene. And it does this *even if it lacks a predicate that refers to the latter as such*. Intuitively, the problem for the imagined system we are now considering is a fairly shallow matter of vocabulary limitations. It is not as if there is some extra property about whose distribution our system must remain non-committal. Rather, the problem is only that our system lacks a piece of simple vocabulary for a property about whose distribution it is indeed committal.

In contrast, the challenge emergent features pose to systems implementing the bottom-up approach to the scope problem is deeper. The difficulty about emergent features is that their exemplification is not fixed by the distribution of basic energy, hence that complete representation of the distribution of basic energy is not a sufficient computational basis for deriving representations of them. And this is a problem to which the mere addition of vocabulary is not the answer. For even if a system does contain predicates for such emergent features, representation of the basic energy will, by itself, leave open whether or not these predicates apply.

I hope it is clear that emergent features, if they exist, pose serious threats to the bottom-up solution to the scope problem. For, if they do exist, then this would mean that the representation of the total distribution of basic energy in a modality—what the bottom-up strategy takes to be computationally sufficient for capturing the entire representational scope of its intended target—is not up to the job. And this, of course, would mean that the bottom-up strategy cannot do what it promises.

13.2 Emergent (Visual) Objects

As I say, I believe there are many well-documented and well-known perceptual phenomena that suggest the existence of features that are emergent in the sense just discussed. In this and the next two sections I will present three different representative but not exhaustive clusters of such phenomena, and discuss how they support the existence of emergent features.[5]

I will begin to argue for the existence of emergent features by considering a first cluster of phenomena that involve, in various ways, the notion of visual objecthood. Considerations about visual objecthood seem a good place to begin both because the phenomena are familiar, and because they will suggest morals (which I will draw out below) about where to look for other phenomena germane to our purposes.

The crucial thought behind research on visual objecthood is that the visual system does not just represent (carry information about) an array of exemplified attributes in the local scene. Rather, it parses the scene into individual objects—roughly, bounded and connected things that trace out continuous paths in spacetime (but that needn't retain their kind affiliations to count as persisting over time)[6]—and represents attributes as being exemplified by those objects. That is, the visual system represents not just the content (as it may be) *there is redness*, but *individual a is red*.

Visual objecthood is relevant here because there are a number of (much-studied) configurations in which we have reasons for thinking that the visual system is representing objecthood, but where such representations are not plausibly derived exclusively from information about the distribution of light intensity. In other words, these configurations provide evidence that visual objecthood is an emergent feature.

13.2.1 Apparent motion

A first such configuration involves apparent motion (e.g. Φ- or β-movement).[7] It is well known that, for example, a pair of successively presented static images of a line or other simple figure in different locations (presented within the right spatial and temporal ranges) will be perceived as a single object moving continuously from the first presentation location to the second, rather than as two different objects. Crucially, however, the distribution of light available to vision is by itself insufficient to compel the single object interpretation that is in fact adopted by

[5] The examples below are mostly, though not wholly, taken from vision; hence, standard anti-visuocentric warnings about generalizability to other modalities apply as usual. (I should also mention that Burnston and Cohen (2012) appeal to several of the phenomena about objects discussed below for a different reason—namely, to argue against the view that feature representations are uniformly prior to object representations.)

[6] For one influential account of just what visual objects amount to, see Spelke (1990). What I say below, however, is agnostic about the details of Spelke's view.

[7] Matthen (2005: 278ff.) also discusses apparent motion cases as evidence for something like what I am calling emergent features.

the visual system: the observed light distribution (at the sampling rate available to vision, in any case) is compatible with the presence of either (i) a single object moving through a continuous trajectory, or (ii) a pair of distinct, static, objects presented successively.

It appears that, in such cases, the representation of object identities at work in the visual system commits it to representing the world as per (i). Hence, the visual system *is* representing object identities in a way that results in its choosing between the alternatives (as it happens, it chooses erroneously: the correct description of the world is as per (ii)). The present point is that, because the light distribution caused by situation (i) is identical to the light distribution caused by (ii), its representation of object identities cannot have been fixed by its representation of the light distribution. Since object identity is both represented by the visual system and not fixed by a representation of the complete distribution of light (i.e. that basic form of energy to which visual receptors are sensitive), it is emergent in our sense.

13.2.2 Object tracking through occlusion

A second type of configuration we can use to make the same sort of point arises in experiments involving multiple object tracking. In these experiments, researchers have shown that subjects can successfully track four to five objects as they move randomly and independently among a larger set of qualitatively identical, also randomly and independently moving items.[8] Interestingly, subjects can continue to track objects when, during the motion phase, they appear to move behind and re-emerge smoothly from opaque occluders (and even invisible occluders) on the screen (Scholl and Pylyshyn 1999).

Now, as we remarked about the apparent motion cases, the distribution of light during the temporal interval through which an object appears to move behind and then re-emerge from an occluder is consistent with either of two possibilities. Either (i) there is a single object that is moving behind the occluder, following a continuous trajectory, and then re-emerging, or (ii) a first object moves behind the occluder and stops, at which point a second, distinct object re-emerges.[9] However, and also as in the case of apparent motion, we have reason to believe the representations in the visual system effectively reflect a choice between these open

[8] In a typical setup, the objects are presented before the motion starts, and a subset of them flash briefly to signal that those are the ones the subject should track. All the objects then move randomly and independently around the screen for a while, and then come to a stop, at which point the subject indicates which of them she had been tracking. For an overview of this research, see Scholl et al. (2001) and Pylyshyn (2003, 2004).

[9] It turns out that qualitative identity is not necessary to sustain the single object interpretation in either apparent motion (Kolers and Grunau 1976) or tracking through occlusion (Scholl et al. 1999; Bahrami 2003).

alternatives. For in order to carry out the tracking task successfully (as it does), the visual system must be representing object identities in a way that amounts to a choice in favour of the one-object interpretation, (i). Again, it appears that object identity is both represented by the visual system and not fixed by a representation of the total light distribution: it is emergent.

13.2.3 Feature binding

At a first pass, the moral I have been drawing from the cases of apparent motion and tracking through occlusion discussed above is that a representation of the light distribution underdetermines the representation of objects carried by the visual system. Consequently, if there are additional represented features that depend on visual objecthood, then we should be unsurprised to find that they, too, are underdetermined by a representation of the light distribution. I claim this is exactly what we find.

To see this, consider the visual representation of binding relations between (other) visually detected features. Binding relations are those relations we represent between two features when we visually represent them as holding of one and the same individual. This situation is unremarkable in visual perception. When we visually represent a red triangle, as it might be, we are not just representing that there is something red and that there is something triangular: we are representing that there is some one thing that exemplifies both *redness* and *triangularity*. As Clark (2000) argues persuasively, the visual system must routinely represent binding relations, or else we would be unable to distinguish visually (as we obviously can) a stimulus consisting of a red triangle and a blue square from a stimulus consisting of a red square and a blue triangle. To make this distinction (which amounts to solving the Many Properties Problem of Jackson (1977)), the visual system must represent binding relations between colour and shape properties—it must group one colour with one shape, and the other colour with the other shape. And as Clark goes on to show, the most plausible explanation of visual binding rests on the idea that the visual system represents features as being exemplified by individuals. That is, it groups *redness* with *triangularity* by predicating both of one individual, *a*, and groups *blueness* with *squarehood* by predicating both of a second individual, *b*.

It is plausible, however, the individuals in terms of which binding is implemented are just the visual objects we have been discussing above.[10] But if, as we

[10] I say this view is plausible, but there are two or three alternatives (depending on how you count) in the running that deserve mention. On one such alternative, which Clark (2000) defends eloquently, sensory individuals are locations (/regions) in the space around the perceiver. On another, defended by Brovold and Grush (2012), sensory individuals are 'gobjects', which are 'anything isolated by gestalt criteria' (2012: 11).

Briefly, I doubt the location view can be a correct general account of perceptual individuals, since there exist cases in which the visual system represents multiple individuals at one location (Blaser

have seen, representing the light distribution underdetermines visual objecthood, and if visual objecthood is needed to fix the visual representation of binding relations between features, then representing the light distribution will also underdetermine the visual representation of binding relations. (In effect, this is just to say that representation of the light distribution is, by itself, unable to distinguish spatiotemporal featural overlap from feature coinstantiation.)

It would seem, then, that interfeatural binding relations are both represented by the visual system and not fixed by the representation of the distribution of light. And this is to say that, as before, we have uncovered an instance of emergent representation in the visual system.

13.2.4 Non-visual objecthood

A final consideration about the relevance of objecthood to our purposes rests in the observation that modalities differ in whether and how they represent objecthood in the first place.

As we have seen, a range of converging considerations support the view that vision parses the distal environment into functional units, or objects, which are then singled out for special treatment by the visual system—e.g. they exist simultaneously, persist in time, serve as loci for the exemplification of visually detected features, and facilitate feature binding, completion, tracking, and figure-ground segmentation in vision. Several authors have argued that there is something similar going on in audition—that the auditory system bundles bits of the environment into simultaneously existing and persisting units that serve analogous functional purposes within audition (Bregman 1990; Kubovy and van Valkenburg 2001; O'Callaghan 2010; Matthen 2010; Nudds 2010). And perhaps, as some have claimed, some similar things can be said in favour of the centrality of objects in touch perception (Klatzky and Lederman 1995, 1999; Pawluk et al. 2011; Fulkerson 2013: ch. 3). On the other hand, it is much less clear that perception is organized in the same ways or to the same extent around objects in olfaction (but see Batty 2010; Gottfried 2010) or gustation.

This sort of variation between modalities raises additional obstacles for the bottom-up strategy for the design of SSDs under consideration: it provides another reason why preserving a representation of the basic distribution of energy is, in general, insufficient by itself to solve the scope problem that the strategy was

et al. 2000), and cases in which the visual system represents one individual at multiple locations (ordinary cases of amodal completion); for further discussion see Cohen (2004) and Clark (2004). I am unconvinced that the gobject view is an alternative to the visual object view, as opposed to an implementation of it. (In any case, the difference between the gobject and perceptual object views won't matter to the present discussion—proponents of gobjects are invited to substitute in their preferred understanding of individuals as needed.)

enlisted to solve. For if the substituted modality represents objects and the substituting modality does not, then any SSD mediating between the two—preserving representations of the distribution of basic energy or not—will (without further supplementation of its representational capacities) inevitably leave out perceptual information about objects that plays important roles in the substituted modality. Fundamentally, if the substituting modality lacks the capacity to bundle the basic energy into object representations as the substituted modality does, then preservation of representations of that basic energy will not, by itself, confer upon the substituting modality the ability to represent the world in the way that the substituted modality can.

Moreover, there may be representational mismatches even for SSDs mediating between substituted and substituting modalities that are both object-representing. For it may turn out that the cues to objecthood in the substituted modality are unrelated to—or at any rate come extensionally apart from—the cues to objecthood in the substituting modality. If so, then preserving representations of objecthood would require bridge principles to trigger object representations in the substituting modality on the basis of appropriate cues in the substituted modality. Again, this is not something that we can assume will fall out simply by ensuring that the SSD preserves a representation of the distribution of basic energy in the substituted modality.

All of this is to say that perceptual objecthood is emergent in our sense.

13.3 Emergent Endogenous Contributions

The examples of emergence discussed in section 13.2 all concerned, in one way or another, objecthood in vision. It is not too hard to come up with a high-level diagnosis of why phenomena involving visual objecthood reveal emergence: objecthood appears to be a (partly) endogenous component of the total representational package generated by perception. It is not the world by itself, but (at least partly) the collective operation of perceptual mechanisms that is responsible for chunking the world into the units that perception cares about and represents. In contrast, the total array of basic energy is exogenous. The constraint we have been examining—viz., the constraint of preserving the representation of the basic energy distribution—is a constraint on preserving the representation of something exogenously fixed. On reflection, it is unsurprising that a device that respects that constraint, and so represents what is exogenously fixed, can fall short of fixing the (not exogenously fixed) representation of objects.

Viewing the problem in these terms suggests that we might find other cases of emergence by looking for other cases of endogenous contributions to perceptual representation. In this section, I will carry out this search by considering two other families of cases where we have reason to think perception makes use of such endogenous contributions: the first involves classic visual illusions, while the second involves what have come to be called 'natural constraints' discussed in computational theories of various sorts.

13.3.1 Emergence in falsidical perception: evidence from illusion

Consider what goes on in a standard instance of a visual illusion, such as results from the interaction of the perceptual system with the Müller-Lyer configuration. Here there is a basic distribution of light energy; and, as usual, that energy causally affects visual transducers, which in turn initiate further causal transactions within the visual system; and the end result is that, again as usual, the visual system represents a range of features of the distal stimulus.

But what makes the case interesting—what makes it a case of illusory perception—is that the visual system ends up in a state that represents (falsidically) *more* than what is fixed by the properties of the mind-independent, distal stimulus. The testimony of perception to the contrary notwithstanding, the lines in the Müller-Lyer configuration are the same in length. But this means that what the energy distribution resulting from the Müller-Lyer configuration provides as an exogenous contribution to the eventual perceptual state cannot possibly include the information that the lines are of different lengths. On the contrary, the perceptual representation of a difference in length must be endogenous in origin—it is, as it were, something added by the perceptual system as a downstream result of its interaction with the impinging energy array.[11] As such, we should not expect that an SSD that preserves under substitution the representation of the exogenously fixed distribution of basic energy will, *ipso facto*, preserve the endogenously generated representation of a difference in line length in the Müller-Lyer configuration.[12] And what I have just said about the Müller-Lyer configuration obtains, *mutatis mutandis*, for many other cases of illusion.[13] If so, then such illusions can plausibly be thought of as giving rise to further instances of perceptual emergence, hence as reasons to doubt the sufficiency of the bottom-up strategy for the design of SSDs.

[11] This way of thinking about illusion echoes (albeit schematically) familiar Kantian themes.

[12] I am not claiming that the representation of a difference in line length (or, more generally, that illusory representations) cannot be preserved under sensory substitution. I am claiming, rather, that preserving a representation of the basic energy distribution alone is insufficient to guarantee this. See below for further discussion.

[13] Though not all. The famously illusory representation of the shape of a half-immersed oar, for example, plausibly *is* fixed by the distribution of basic energy that strikes the retina. That is because this illusion is the result of a refraction of light that occurs prior to its impinging on perceptual systems at all. That said, I take it that very many classical illusions (such as the Müller-Lyer) are unlike this case in that, as claimed in the main text, they depend crucially on endogenously determined aspects of the operation of the perceptual system. In the discussion of illusion that follows I mean to be focusing only on instances that are in this respect like the Müller-Lyer case rather than the half-immersed oar case. (Thanks to Fiona Macpherson for raising this qualification.)

(Something closely analogous to what I have said about illusory perception can be said as well about perception of bi- or multi-stable configurations, which is not obviously correctly described as illusory. In perceiving a Necker cube or a more complex configuration such as that depicted in Figure 13.1, the perceptual system (at a time) 'chooses' from between one of multiple interpretations left open by the stimulus configuration. In so doing, what it represents goes beyond what is fixed by the representation of the basic energy array. For on the one hand, to say that the figure is multiply stable is just to say that the representation of the basic energy distribution, as such, is compatible with multiple available representational disambiguations. And on the other hand, in favouring one of the available disambiguations, the perceptual system is representing something that is incompatible with the others. Once again, therefore, we should not expect that an SSD that preserves under substitution just the representation of the exogenously fixed basic energy distribution will preserve the endogenously generated representation that corresponds to one disambiguation of the configuration over the others.)

Now, the latter prediction is *prima facie* at odds with at least some of the claims about illusion under SSD that have appeared in the literature. Unfortunately, however, the evidence is less straightforward than it might initially appear.[14]

One of the first reports on this matter comes from the personal reflections of Gerard Guarniero (1977b), a congenitally blind PhD student in philosophy who served as a subject for Paul Bach-y-Rita's work with the TVSS, and who went on to

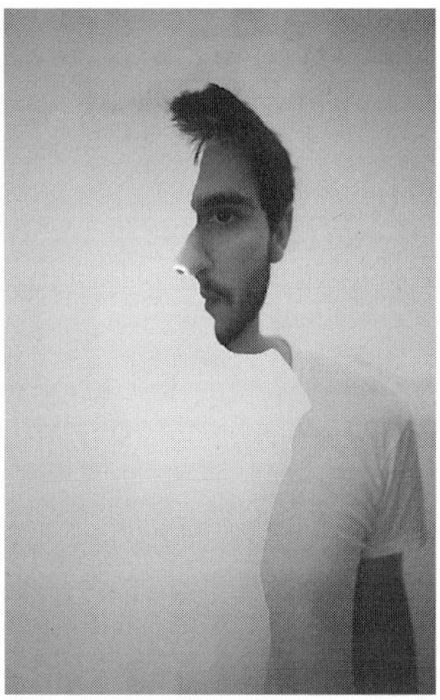

Figure 13.1 In representing a bistable figure in one rather than another of the ways left open by the distal configuration, what the perceptual system represents goes beyond what is fixed by the distribution of light intensity available to its receptors. Image © Mike Edmonds Photography, used by permission. (Q 4740).

[14] One problem about this evidence is that there is surprisingly little of it. Given the thousands of known illusions, one might have expected to find large numbers of published papers investigating whether and under what conditions such effects persist under SSD. That does not seem to be the case.

write a dissertation on space perception (Guarniero 1977a). Guarniero self-reports that some classical illusions are indeed preserved under TVSS (cf. Bach-y-Rita 1984). And these reports are cited approvingly by Noë and O'Regan, who remark that 'TVSS-aided perception is liable to familiar forms of visual distortion and illusion, e.g. distant objects "look" small, objects can occlude each other, etc.' (2002: 19).

Despite such claims, however, it turns out that Guarniero's self-reports do not obviously support the idea that visual illusions (at least in the sense considered above) are preserved under sensory substitution. What Guarniero reports is that, after training and adaptation to the TVSS, he gained fluency at estimating distal properties of objects from proximal representations—that is, he acquired skill at estimating object size from proximal size, estimating parallels from proximal convergence, and correlating distance with proximal elevation. I want to claim that, though these are potentially interesting reports that may bear on important questions about perception (e.g. about just how to understand such so-called proximal representations, and their relations to so-called distal representations; cf. Cohen 2010, 2012), they are not directly relevant to our question about the preservation of illusory representations under sensory substitution.

The first point to make in this connection is that the kinds of cases on which Guarniero reports success do not fit the usual understanding of perceptual illusions—viz., instances in which a subject perceptually represents a feature as qualifying an object that, in fact, it fails to qualify. Indeed, I take it that one main motivation for introducing proximal representations (*qua* alternative to distal/object representations) in the first place is to *avoid* the attribution of perceptual illusion: in so doing, we can say that the proximal representation of convergence while looking at the train tracks recede into the distance is not erroneous, even though a distal representation of convergence would be an illusion in the same circumstance. But if they are not cases of illusion, then they do not speak to our question.

The second point to make is that the abilities Guarniero reports acquiring (namely, the abilities to extract distal representations from proximal representations) are plausibly understood as involving representations formed by inference rather than perception. That is, it is plausible that what Guarniero reports gaining by adaptation to the TVSS is not a capacity to form new perceptual representations, but rather a capacity to form new representations by inferring from the same set of perceptual representations initially present. Thus, relying on standard (if controversial) criteria for the perception/inference distinction, we would expect to find that the new representations Guarniero reports coming to form are cognitively penetrable and selectively impaired with the capacity for general inference. In contrast, the representation resulting from a classic illusion configuration, such as the representation of the difference in line length in the Müller-Lyer configuration, is a parade case of a perceptual representation: it is cognitively impenetrable and spared by lesions that impair the capacity for general inference.

What all this suggests, then, is that Guarniero's reports are plausibly consistent with my claim that illusory representations, such as those present in classic visual illusions, need not be preserved under SSDs that are designed to preserve the representation of the distribution of basic energy in the substituted modality.

In a more recent pair of studies that address our question, Laurent Renier and his colleagues investigated susceptibility to the Ponzo illusion (depicted in Figure 13.2) and the vertical-horizontal illusion (depicted in Figure 13.3) in subjects using a prosthesis for substitution of vision with audition (PSVA) (Renier et al. 2005, 2006). These investigators were able to induce both the Ponzo and vertical-horizontal illusion (in some subjects) under PSVA. But, again, the situation is more complicated than this lets on.

To begin, Renier et al. (2005) report that, initially, their subjects were not susceptible to the Ponzo illusion under PSVA at all, because they were able to perform the line-length estimation task under PSVA without attending to representations of the converging oblique lines crucial to the visual version of the illusion. They found that, by requiring subjects using PSVA to consider the two oblique lines of the stimuli before comparing the length of the two horizontal bars, they could make the illusion re-emerge. But even under this condition, the effect remained weak: they found the effect present in sighted subjects (but still smaller in magnitude than among sighted control subjects not using PSVA), but not at all in their 'early blind' subjects (subjects blind before their twentieth month of age). And Renier et al. (2006) report a similar pattern for the vertical-horizontal illusion: the effect was strongest in sighted control subjects not using PSVA, somewhat weaker in blindfolded sighted subjects using PSVA, and completely absent in early blind subjects using PSVA.

I want to stress three lessons about these results.

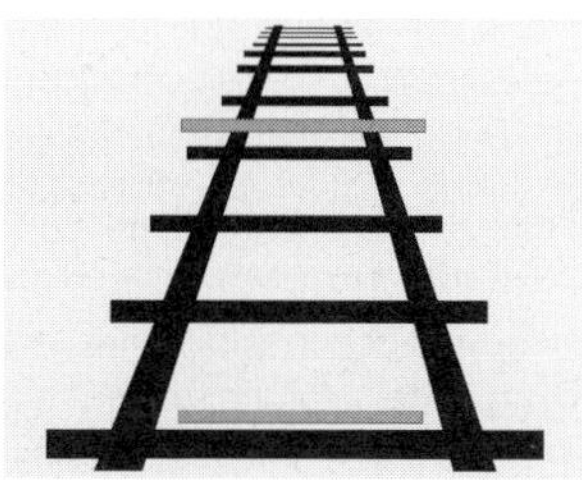

Figure 13.2 The Ponzo illusion is a visual illusion that occurs when parallel horizontal lines of equal length are displayed over a pair of oblique lines that converge toward the top of the display; the classic result is that subjects overestimate the relative length of horizontal lines as these are placed higher in the display.

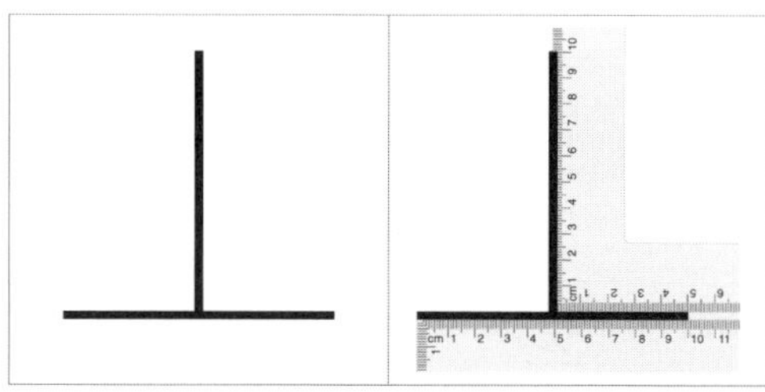

Figure 13.3 In the vertical-horizontal illusion, subjects systematically overestimate the length of vertical lines relative to horizontal lines of equal size.

A first lesson, which emerges from the finding that the investigators failed to replicate the Ponzo illusion under substitution before modifying the task to fix attention on the oblique line elements of the stimulus configuration, is that a substitution that preserves the representation of the distribution of basic energy does not, *ipso facto*, preserve the distribution of perceptual attention. The second lesson is that, since there are aspects of the perceptual representation (here, but plausibly ubiquitously in perception) that depend crucially on which bits of the stimulus are attended, the non-preservation of the distribution of attention means that preserving the representation of the distribution of basic energy is not guaranteed to fix every aspect of the eventual perceptual representation. Specifically, it appears in the case of the Ponzo configuration that attending to the oblique lines crucially interacts with subjects' representation of the length of the horizontal lines. Hence, if a subject confronts an analogue of that configuration in another modality, but fails to attend to just the elements she would have attended to in a visual presentation, she may not go on to represent the configuration as she would have in a visual presentation. Third, and finally, the results with both the Ponzo and the vertical-horizontal configurations show that even if both the representation of the energy distribution and the distribution of attention are preserved, the illusory representation can *still* fail to show up at all (as here with the early blind subjects), or may show up in a weakened form (as here with the sighted subjects). And this is just to say that, as predicted above, preservation of the representation of the basic energy distribution under substitution does not *ipso facto* preserve the illusory feature representations: the latter are perceptually emergent in the sense described.

It seems to me, then, that (advertising to the contrary notwithstanding) the relevant extant evidence concerning classical illusions provides further support for treating the latter as involving perceptual emergence. Of course, the claim I am making is not that no illusory representations of the sort revealed in classical illusions could be preserved under substitution. Rather, I am claiming (i) that not all such illusory representations will be preserved under substitution, (ii) that apparent preservation of such illusory representations may, on further inspection, turn out to be the result of inference, so not instances of preservation of perceptual representation after all, and (iii) that where such illusory representations are preserved, the mere preservation of the representation of the basic energy distribution is insufficient to guarantee this outcome. If these claims are correct, then cases of illusion give us further evidence that the bottom-up strategy for SSDs cannot succeed by itself.

13.3.2 Emergence in veridical perception: evidence from computational theory

Although perceptual illusions provide evidence of endogenous contributions to perceptual representation (and, consequently, evidence of perceptually emergent feature representations), it would be a mistake to assume that such contributions are limited to cases of falsidical perception. One way to see this is by consideration of the sorts of strategies that underlie many of the computational theories of perception that have emerged over the last several decades, which indicate that endogenous contributions play indispensable, and utterly routine, roles in veridical perception as well.

Computational theories are, of course, devoted to describing the computational processes by which perception derives and represents distal features from the initial energy distribution. Theorists in this tradition often characterize the perceptual processes they describe as solving 'inverse problems'—problems of recovering rich information about the distal world from relatively sparse input. These inverse problems are challenging because, in general, the perceptual input underdetermines their solutions; hence researchers will say that the problems are 'ill-posed', or provably unsolvable without imposing further constraints.

For a representative example, consider the problem of computing a visual representation of three-dimensional form. It is an elementary fact of projective geometry that a static two-dimensional array of incident light intensity arriving on the retina could have been produced by infinitely many distal three-dimensional forms. Therefore, a form extraction algorithm that restricts itself to computing over input available in the retinal intensity array will be, for reasons of principle, unable to decide between infinitely many alternatives compatible with its evidence. Or, again, consider the problem of computing the description of surface colour (say, represented as a surface spectral reflectance distribution) from the retinal light intensity array. Since the light arriving at the retina is the result of an interaction between both the illumination incident on the distal surface and the properties of the surface itself, it is a result of elementary arithmetic that the retinal evidence, taken by itself, is ambiguous between infinitely many different descriptions of the surface. Consequently, an algorithm for the derivation of surface descriptions that restricts itself to the evidence available in the retinal intensity array will, as a matter of simple arithmetic, be unable to arrive at a determinate answer. And this situation is entirely typical.

Now, of course perception *does* solve these computational problems: it *does* arrive at a determinate description of three-dimensional form, surface colour, etc. But if these problems are both solved by the perceptual system and provably unsolvable without imposing further constraints beyond those provided by the impinging energy, it follows that perception must be imposing further constraints—viz., constraints not available as such in the exogenous basic energy distribution. For exactly this reason, computational theorizing about perception standardly proceeds by appealing to further constraints that are not exogenously fixed by the distribution of basic energy, but that instead take the form of natural, internalized regularities about the distal world.

An early, vivid, and representative illustration of this explanatory strategy arises in the classic structure from motion theorem of Shimon Ullman (1979).[15] Ullman was interested in the question of how the visual system derives representations of three-dimensional object form from a series of static two-dimensional presentations of multiple dots corresponding to locations on object surfaces. He showed that the visual system can derive the three-dimensional form of a moving object from three static two-dimensional views of four non-coplanar points.[16] Crucially, however, Ullman's derivation depends on the further assumption—not encoded in the exogenous input to vision, *a fortiori*, not encoded in the representation of the total light distribution—that the perceived object undergoes only rigid transformations in space (rotations, translations, reflections, and combinations thereof).

The assumption that moving surfaces are transformed rigidly is an instance of just the sort of 'natural constraint' ('internalized regularity') we have been discussing. That is, it is a generally (though not perfectly) reliable generalization about the perceived world, without reliance on which the input to the perceptual system would underdetermine the solution to the perceptual problem of reconstructing relevant features of the distal world, but with which the exogenous input does permit a solution. Ullman proposed that we should understand the ability of the perceptual system to solve the problems under study as resulting from its having internalized these constraints, presumably as a result of natural selective pressures imposed in an adaptive environment in which they are generally true.

Importantly, treating this and other such constraints as internalized in this sense should not be understood as claiming that they are explicitly represented in closed form in the perceptual system (Pylyshyn 2003: ch. 3). Rather, the idea is that the perceptual system acts (i.e. carries out its characteristic computations from its input) by default in accord with these constraints in something like the way that the planets act by default in accord with Kepler's Laws.[17]

[15] For further classic articulations of the role of natural constraints in computational accounts of perception (particularly in vision), see Marr (1982), Richards (1988) and Shepard (1987, 1994, 2001). In hindsight, it is also possible (if anachronistic) to view Gestalt contraints such as 'good figure' and 'simplicity' (Koffka 1935) as natural constraints in this sense.

[16] The computation assumes that the visual system has already solved the 'correspondence problem'—that it has some method of associating each dot in the *i*th display with a particular dot in the *j*th display, and so treating one as an update of the very same position on the surface of the object whose form it is computing.

[17] There are, of course, theorists who posit much more by way of explicitly represented endogenous contribution in perception. Perhaps a limit case is the view of Purves and Lotto (2003), on which (roughly) perception ordinarily disambiguates the underconstrained exogenous input by appeal to an endogenously supplied and explicitly represented probability distribution over alternative hypotheses about the world. If some such view is right, then there are two distinguishable forms of emergent information in perception. First, there are the endogenous and explicit representational elements themselves. And second, there are the representations of distal features that perception derives from both the latter endogenous elements and the exogenous basic energy distribution. On the view under consideration, perception represents both of these, but neither is fixed by the representation of the basic energy distribution; therefore, both are perceptually emergent.

But if perception does make use of such natural constraints in the way suggested by this family of computational theories, then this gives us further reason for believing in perceptually represented emergent features, so for rejecting the bottom-up design strategy for SSDs. For, if so, then distal features such as form, colour, shape, and the like are represented by perception, although the representation of the basic energy distribution is an insufficient computational basis for their extraction. Hence, such features of the distal world are perceptually emergent in our sense.

13.4 Emergent High-Level Features

In sections 13.2–13.3 we reviewed two families of motivations for believing that perception represents emergent features. In this section I want to consider a third family of cases that support the same conclusion, here involving the representation of what I will call 'high-level' features. While I don't have any principled way of demarcating such features, what I have in mind are features that play a special role in perception, that are categorical, that may have particular adaptive significance, and that typically mediate other perceptual representations, e.g. by automatically attracting perceptual attention (in a way that is unlikely to be preserved under substitution). Moreover, representations of the features I have in mind lack the standard earmarks of having been derived via inference: they persist despite changes in belief, they arise effortlessly, automatically and involuntarily, and universally—viz., in perceivers from different cultures and ages (importantly including infants), and independently of their performance on standard measures of general intelligence. Consequently, we have reason for treating the representations in question as perceptual. I claim that there are several high-level features of this sort that are plausibly perceptually represented, but whose perceptual representation is not fixed by the representation of the complete distribution of basic energy available to perception—including facehood, biological motion, animacy, and perhaps causation. If I am right, then these features, too, are perceptually emergent.[18]

[18] Three concessive qualifications are in order.

The first concessive qualification is that the cases of perceptually emergent properties considered below are intended to be illustrative but not exhaustive. Since I am only trying to argue that there are some such cases, I am happy to allow that there may be many more such examples.

The second concessive qualification concerns the relation between the arguments that follow and related arguments of Susanna Siegel. In a series of important works, Siegel (2006, 2009, 2010) has argued for the related view that several high-level features (her label is 'K-properties')—including *pine tree-hood* and other natural kind properties, mind-independence, and causation, *inter alia*—are represented in visual/perceptual experience. She argues for this conclusion principally by applying her 'method of phenomenal contrast', which involves identifying pairs of perceptual experiences that she claims are phenomenally different from one another, and then arguing that the best explanation of this difference is that one of the perceptual experiences in the pair does and the other does not represent

13.4.1 Facehood

A first example of the kind of high-level feature I have in mind is the categorical feature of being the face of a conspecific.

The recognition of faces is widely believed to be treated specially by perceptual systems in a number of ways that lend credence to the idea that facehood is perceptually represented. Faces receive special visual processing not allocated to visual perception of other body parts or objects (Kanwisher 2010; Sinha et al. 2006; Sugita 2009), and this special processing is carried out by specialized areas (Liu et al. 2010; McCarthy et al. 1997). Perceptual face recognition is susceptible to a characteristic overgeneration error: we (mis-) recognize a face in a cloud or a mountain far more readily than other objects. And face recognition can be selectively impaired in injuries that spare other aspects of perceptual and cognitive processing (this condition is known as prosopagnosia).

But if these considerations suggest that faces are perceptually represented, there is reason to think that the representations in question are also emergent. One way to see this point is by consideration of the so-called Thatcher effect—the finding that local anomalies in the geometric organization of faces are dramatically harder to detect in inverted than in non-inverted faces (Thompson 2010; see Figure 13.4). Now, the standard explanation of our capacity to distinguish easily between the normal and anomalous images when presented right side up but not upside down rests on a representational difference. Namely, the idea is that the visual system represents the specialized high-level property of facehood in one of the right-side-up images (viz., the normal one) but not the other, whereas it does not represent any feature that cleanly distinguishes between the two upside-down images. However, if we restrict ourselves to considering the representation of the complete distribution of basic energy available to vision, then we will be unable to distinguish between the inverted images and the non-inverted images: visual perception represents the same array of lightness intensities in the inverted and non-inverted images (modulo the global inversion that distinguishes the inverted

the target K-properties. I won't rely on Siegel's arguments in what follows, in part because I worry that even if we accept, with Siegel, that K-properties are represented in perceptual experience, we would need further arguments to secure the claims, for which I am arguing, that the relevant high-level properties are both (i) represented in the perceptual system itself (as opposed to non-perceptual elements that contribute to the representational content of perceptual experience) and (ii) not fixed by the representation of the basic energy distribution. On the other hand, if Siegel's arguments are persuasive, and if there is a successful method of extending her conclusions to the view that K-properties are perceptually emergent, then I am happy to take the former on board as yet further reasons to believe in perceptual emergence.

The third concessive qualification is just to remark that the evidence I appeal to below is not knockdown, and certainly not deductive. Notwithstanding this remark, I take these considerations to add up, collectively, to a strong case for perceptual emergence. For better or worse, non-deductive evidence is the only kind of evidence we are going to get in such broadly empirical enquiry.

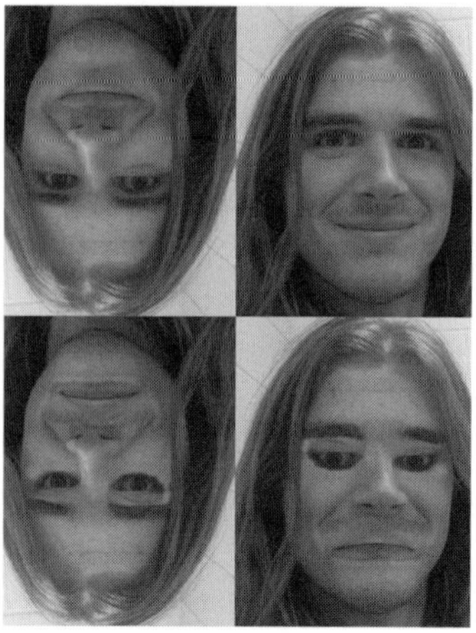

Figure 13.4 Local anomalies in the geometric organization of faces are dramatically harder to detect in inverted than in non-inverted faces.

from the non-inverted images). If this is right, then (i) there is a visual representation of the categorical feature of facehood; and (ii) that representation is not fixed by the visual system's representation of the complete basic energy distribution.

13.4.2 Biological motion

A second example of the kind of high-level feature in perception I have in mind, and about which many of the same things can be said, is the perceptually represented feature of being a 'biological' motion. The classic finding in this area is that subjects can classify—automatically, quickly, and easily—certain but not other, equally complex, patterns of a few moving points of light as reflecting the motion of key joints in a moving organism (Johansson 1973, see Figure 5).

Once again, there are reasons for believing that this categorical feature enjoys a specialized (and possibly adaptively advantageous) role in human perceptual processing. Perception of biological motion appears to involve specialized processing (Lu 2010), to be carried out in specialized areas (Allison et al. 2000; Grossman et al. 2000), and can be spared in injuries that damage gross motor and other spatial abilities (Jordan et al. 2002; Kim et al. 2008).

But there are also reasons for believing that the categorical, perceptually represented feature of being a biological motion is perceptually emergent. The first arises from the mere fact that perception singles out this particular feature for quick and easy classification, while it does not appear to distinguish other, equally complex, dynamic features in moving dots displays. Obviously there are differences in the representation of the total distribution of light carried by perception in biological and non-biological motion cases. But what is highly unobvious is that there is any systematic difference that results from the representation of the total light distribution that distinguishes the two classes of cases neatly, as perception does.

A second clue to the emergence of the feature in question is that there is a Thatcher effect for biological motion as well: it is significantly easier to detect local anomalies (anomalies that perturb the visual classification of the motion as biological) in displays that are right side up than in displays that are inverted (Mirenzi and Hiris 2011). Once again, the explanation of this difference is presumably that the visual system represents the specialized, high-level feature of being a biological motion only about the right-side-up and non-anomalous point light display, which is to say that there is a systematic difference between the visual representation of anomalous and non-anomalous displays when right side up, but not when inverted. But, once again, the representation of the complete distribution of basic energy available to vision doesn't provide for this kind of classificatory distinction: visual perception represents the same total array of lightness intensities in the inverted and non-inverted point light displays (even though there is a global inversion that distinguishes them). Hence, as in the case of face perception, the existence of a Thatcher effect for biological motion suggests that vision represents that high-level feature even though the latter is not fixed by its representation of the complete distribution of basic energy.

13.4.3 Animacy/chasing

A third example of such a high-level feature in perception comes out of recent work on the perception of animacy, and particularly involving the phenomenon of perceived chasing—cases in which subjects perceptually represent a first moving shape as 'chasing' a second (Gao et al. 2009, 2010). This research suggests that representations of chasing behaviour turn on a cluster of dynamic and configural relations between the two shapes, including the 'persistence' of the chaser, overall similarity in the trajectories traced out by both shapes, and whether or not they 'face' in the direction in which they move.

As Gao and Scholl (2011; Scholl and Gao 2013) argue, these representations of chasing/animacy display many of the earmarks classically associated with being perceptual. Thus, such representations are effortlessly and automatically generated, are expressed in infants as young as 9 months old (Csibra et al. 1999; Gergely et al. 1995) and across widely differing cultures, and persist despite subjects' explicit contrary (and correct) belief that the shapes they perceive are not animate. Moreover, they are controlled by subtle visual properties of the stimulus (Scholl and Gao 2013), can be impaired in conditions that otherwise spare motion perception (Heberlein and Adolphs 2004; Rutherford et al. 2006), and appear to implicate activity in specialized brain regions (Gao et al. 2013). But, as with the other high-level features we have considered, the very ease and automaticity with which the visual system recognizes chasing configurations as opposed to other, equally complex, dynamic configurations represented by perception suggests that the high-level perceptual representation of chasing is not fixed by perceptual representation of the complete distribution of light alone.

13.4.4 Causation

A final example of a high-level and possibly emergent categorical perceived feature is causation.[19] Famously, Michotte (1963) showed that certain configurations are spontaneously (and nearly inevitably) described by perceivers in causal terms. Thus, one class of examples Michotte discusses consists of 'launching' events, in which a moving object, *a*, moves across a screen and comes to a halt when it makes contact with a second object, *b*, whereupon *b* begins to move in the same direction in which *a* had been moving. As noted, observers find it extremely tempting to describe the situation in explicitly or implicitly causal terms, perhaps saying that *a* pushed *b* or that *a* caused *b* to move.

Such representations of causation have been studied extensively in the intervening years, and the basic phenomenon—viz., that representations of causation arise in Michotte-type configurations—is now widely accepted. What is less clear is whether these representations should be regarded as perceptual. They do appear to satisfy many of the earmarks of the perceptual. Thus, Michotte himself points out that they are produced quickly, automatically, and mandatorily. Like representations of animacy, representations of causation also seem to persist across manipulations in background beliefs about causal relationships between the items (Schlottmann and Shanks 1992). These representations of causation occur quite generally in response to Michotte-type configurations, e.g. in infants as young as 6 months old (Leslie, 1982, 1984; Leslie and Keeble 1987; Oakes 1994; Oakes and Cohen 1990) and across diverse cultures (Morris and Peng 1994). Moreover, they appear to be under the control of specific visual features of the displays (Scholl and Tremoulet 2000; Scholl and Nakayama 2002). However, such representations do not have all of the classic marks of perceptual status that we have been drawing upon. Thus, some investigators report stable (and possibly parameterized) individual variation in expression (Schlottmann and Anderson 1993). Moreover, it is controversial whether there is a specific neuroanatomical locus for causal perception as opposed to spatial and temporal components (Blakemore et al. 2001). And, finally, so far there are no clear instances of selective impairment for this sort of causal representation (Rips 2011).

In sum, it appears that the types of evidence we have been considering, though suggestive, fail to establish conclusively either that these representations of causation are perceptual or that they are not. However, it does seem plausible that such representations are not fixed by the perceptual representation of the light

[19] See Danks (2009) for an excellent overview of research on these topics.

distribution alone. For the recognition of Michotte-type configurations as causal proceeds more quickly and effortlessly than recognition of other perceptually represented dynamic configurations that seem no less complex in respect of the properties of their light distributions.[20] Given these points, it seems that the right thing to say about the representation of causation is conditional: if causation is perceptually represented, then it is another instance of a perceptually emergent feature.

13.5 Lessons

I have appealed to a range of considerations to argue for the conclusion that perception represents emergent features—that is, features whose representation is not fixed by the representation of the total distribution of basic energy. If I am right about this, then SSDs designed so as to preserve representation of the total distribution of basic energy will not, *ipso facto*, preserve all perceptually represented features. And this means that SSDs designed in this way may nonetheless fail to solve the scope problem, and so leave out elements we may want successful SSDs to capture.

Some authors (e.g. Noë and O'Regan 2002: 19) have had a much more optimistic view about the prospects for SSDs. They have urged that the limitations of extant prototypes are merely *pro tanto*—that they are artefacts of the crude spatial resolution and processing speed of current technology, but in principle superable with sufficient grant money and time. If the arguments of this essay are correct, however, then this optimism is misplaced, for the limitations on SSDs are more fundamental.

However, and without retracting anything of the foregoing, I want to offer several qualifications to the pessimistic assessment just offered.

First, I am in no way denying that sensory substitution is a potentially useful set of technologies. It is consistent with everything I have said that extant or future SSDs may significantly improve lives.

Second, in saying that perception represents emergent features, I do not mean to be mongering mystery about perception or perceptual processing. These representations are obviously the causal/computational outputs of various sorts of perceptual processing. The conclusion I mean to be urging is not an irrealism about all lunches, but only about lunches that are free. It is that preserving in the substituting modality the representation of the basic energy distribution in the substituted modality doesn't capture these (apparently perceptually significant) feature representations or replace the causal/computational processes leading up to them.

[20] This is perhaps one (anachronistic) way of expressing Hume's claim that the impressions delivered to the mind by perception fail to include anything that could amount to a source for the idea of causal efficacy.

Third, and significantly, note that nothing in what I have said implies that SSDs *will* inevitably fail to represent what sensory modalities normally represent. It only implies that if we want them to represent what sensory modalities normally represent, then we will have to do more than preserve the representation of basic energy to which the substituted modalities are sensitive.[21] Hence, if one wants to build a system of perceptual representations that includes representation of such features, then the latter will have to be built in by some other means.

Finally, I want to emphasize that it is intended as a serious, and not merely rhetorical, possibility that one might not insist on including the representation of such emergent features in one's system. For it may suffice for some purposes to allow representation of the latter to be generated by inference (or some other extraperceptual mechanism), or even to do without these representations entirely. But if one does want to include such representations within the scope of perception one is attempting to capture by means of an SSD, then the considerations adduced here suggest that mere preservation of the representation of the basic energy distribution won't suffice for that purpose. To the extent, then, that existing SSDs are constructed to serve the aim of preserving this information, their label as devices for sensory *substitution* may amount to something of an exaggeration.[22]

[21] It is perhaps worth emphasizing that this claim allows that whatever further is required (beyond preservation of the representation of the basic energy) may be something already present in our normal psychological endowment. It may be, for all that I have said, that at least some of the burden of representing perceptually emergent features is borne by amodal capacities that wouldn't need to be rebuilt for the purposes of representing those features under substitution. Thus, for example, it may turn out that the visual representation of causation is subserved partly by amodal (rather than specifically visual) mechanisms that are selectively responsive to causal relations in the world. If so, then an SSD might enlist these very same amodal mechanisms as a way of representing causation. Under the envisaged scenario, then, what it would take to ensure the representation of an ostensibly emergent feature by our SSD would not include the provision of further mechanisms above and beyond what is already present in our psychological architecture.

But this point is not an objection to the point in the main text. For if, as envisaged, the representation of emergent features under substitution is accomplished (partly) by the exploitation of standing amodal capacities that don't need to be reconstructed for use by SSDs, then one thing that such successful representation will require is preservation of those amodal capacities. Because preservation of the latter is not guaranteed by the preservation of the representation of the basic energy to which the substituted modality is sensitive, the envisaged scenario is a way of demonstrating my conclusion, rather than a way of avoiding it.

[22] Many thanks to Robert Briscoe, Daniel Burnston, Alex Byrne, Kevin Connolly, Matthew Fulkerson, Cressida Gaukroger, Güven Güzeldere, Rae Langton, Don MacLeod, Fiona Macpherson, Mohan Matthen, Agustín Rayo, Laurent Renier, Barry Smith, Charles Spence, and members of the philosophy of perception reading group at the University of California, San Diego, for helpful discussions of these issues that much improved the essay. Thanks also to audiences at MIT, the Columbia-Barnard Perception Workshop, the Sensory Substitution and Augmentation Conference at the British Academy, and the SoCal Philosophy Conference, who heard earlier versions of this material and raised all sorts of useful questions.

References

Alexander, S. (1920) *Space, Time, and Deity*. London: Macmillan.

Allison, T., Puce, A. and McCarthy, G. (2000) Social perception from visual cues: role of the STS region. *Trends in Cognitive Sciences* 4: 267–278.

Bach-y-Rita, P. (1984) The relationship between motor processes and cognition in tactile vision substitution. In W. Prinz and A. F. Sanders (eds) *Cognition and Motor Processes*. Berlin: Springer, 150–160.

Bach-y-Rita, P., Collins, C. C., Saunders, F., White, B. and Scadden, L. (1969) Vision substitution by tactile image projection. *Nature* 221: 963–964.

Bahrami, B. (2003) Object property encoding and change blindness in multiple object tracking. *Visual Cognition* 10(8): 949–963.

Batty, C. (2010) A representational account of olfactory experience. *Canadian Journal of Philosophy* 40: 511–538.

Blakemore, S.-J., Fonlupt, P., Pachot-Clouard, M., Darmon, C., Boyer, P., Meltzoff, A. N., Segebarth, C. and Decety, J. (2001) How the brain perceives causality: an event-related fMRI study. *NeuroReport* 12(174): 3741–3746.

Blaser, E., Pylyshyn, Z. W. and Holcombe, A. O. (2000) Tracking an object through feature space. *Nature* 408: 196–199.

Bregman, A. S. (1990) *Auditory Scene Analysis*. Cambridge, MA: MIT Press.

Broad, C. D. (1925) *The Mind and Its Place in Nature*. London: Routledge & Kegan Paul.

Brovold, A. and Grush, R. (2012) Towards an (improved) interdisciplinary investigation of demonstrative reference. In A. Raftopoulos and P. Machamer (eds) *Perception, Realism, and the Problem of Reference*. Cambridge: Cambridge University Press, 11–42.

Burnston, D. and Cohen, J. (2012) Perception of features and perception of objects. *The Croatian Journal of Philosophy* 36: 283–314.

Capelle, C., Trullemans, C., Arno, P. and Veraart, C. (1998) A real-time experimental prototype for enhancement of vision rehabilitation using auditory substitution. *IEEE Transactions Biomedical Engineering* 45: 1279–1293.

Clark, A. (2000) *A Theory of Sentience*. New York: Oxford University Press.

Clark, A. (2004) Feature placing and proto-objects. *Philosophical Psychology* 17(4): 443–469.

Cohen, J. (2004) Objects, places, and perception. *Philosophical Psychology* 17(4): 471–495.

Cohen, J. (2010) Perception and computation. *Philosophical Issues* 20(1): 96–124.

Cohen, J. (2012) Computation and the ambiguity of perception. In G. Hatfield and S. Allred (eds) *Visual Experience: Sensation, Cognition and Constancy*. New York: Oxford University Press, 160–176.

Csibra, G., Gergely, G., Bíró, S., Koos, O. and Brockbank, M. (1999) Goal attribution without agency cues: the perception of 'pure reason' in infancy. *Cognition* 72: 237–267.

Danks, D. (2009) The psychology of causal perception and reasoning. In H. Beebee, C. Hitchcock and P. Menzies (eds) *Oxford Handbook of Causation*. Oxford: Oxford University Press, 447–470.

Fulkerson, M. (2013) *The First Sense: A Philosophical Study of Human Touch*. Cambridge, MA: MIT Press.

Gao, T. and Scholl, B. J. (2011) Chasing vs. stalking: interrupting the perception of animacy. *Journal of Experimental Psychology: Human Perception and Performance* 37: 669–684.

Gao, T., Newman, G. E. and Scholl, B. J. (2009) The psychophysics of chasing: a case study in the perception of animacy. *Cognitive Psychology* 59: 154–179.

Gao, T., McCarthy, G. and Scholl, B. J. (2010) The wolfpack effect: perception of animacy irresistibly influences interactive behavior. *Psychological Science* 21: 1845–1853.

Gao, T., Scholl, B. J. and McCarthy, G. (2013) Dissociating the detection of intentionality from animacy in the right posterior superior temporal sulcus. *Journal of Neuroscience* 32(41): 14276–14280.

Gergely, G., Nfidasdy, Z., Csibra, G. and Bíró, S. (1995) Taking the intentional stance at 12 months of age. *Cognition* 56: 165–193.

Gottfried, J. A. (2010) Central mechanisms of odour object perception. *Nature Reviews Neuroscience* 11: 628–641.

Grossman, E., Donnelly, M., Price, R., Pickens, D., Morgan, V., Neighbor, G. and Blake, R. (2000) Brain areas involved in perception of biological motion. *Journal of Cognitive Neuroscience* 12: 711–720.

Guarniero, G. (1977a) The senses and the perception of space. PhD thesis, New York University.

Guarniero, G. (1977b) Tactile vision: a personal view. *Visual Impairment and Blindness* 71(3): 125–130.

Heberlein, A. S. and Adolphs, R. (2004) Impaired spontaneous anthropomorphizing despite intact perception and social knowledge. *Proceedings of the National Academy of Sciences* 101(19): 7487–7491.

Heil, J. (1983) *Perception and Cognition*. Berkeley: University of California Press.

Jackson, F. (1977) *Perception: A Representative Theory*. New York: Cambridge University Press.

Johansson, G. (1973) Visual perception of biological motion and a model for its analysis. *Perception and Psychophysics* 14(2): 201–211.

Jordan, H., Reiss, J. E., Hoffman, J. E. and Landau, B. (2002) Intact perception of biological motion in the face of profound spatial deficits: Williams syndrome. *Psychological Science* 13(2): 162–167.

Kanwisher, N. (2010) Functional specificity in the human brain: a window into the functional architecture of the mind. *Proceedings of the National Academy of Sciences* 107: 11163–11170.

Kardong, K. V. and Mackessy, S. P. (1991) The strike behavior of a congenitally blind rattlesnake. *Journal of Herpetology* 25: 208–211.

Keeley, B. (2002) Making sense of the senses: individuating modalities in humans and other animals. *Journal of Philosophy* 99: 5–28.

Kim, J., Blake, R., Park, S., Shin, Y., Kang, D. and Kwon, J. (2008) Selective impairment in visual perception of biological motion in obsessive-compulsive disorder. *Depression and Anxiety* 25(7): E15–25.

Klatzky, R. L. and Lederman, S. J. (1995) Identifying objects from a haptic glance. *Attention, Perception, and Psychophysics* 57: 1111–1123. 10.3758/BF03208368.

Klatzky, R. L. and Lederman, S. J. (1999) The haptic glance: a route to rapid object identification and manipulation. In D. Gopher and A. Koriat (eds) *Attention and Performance*

XVII. Cognitive Regulation of Performance: Integration of Theory and Application. Mahwah, NJ: Lawrence Erlbaum, 165–196.

Koffka, K. (1935) *Principles of Gestalt Psychology*. New York: Harcourt, Brace & World.

Kolers, P. and Grunau, M. V. (1976) Shape and color in apparent motion. *Vision Research* 16: 329–335.

Kubovy, M. and van Valkenburg, D. (2001) Auditory and visual objects. *Cognition* 80: 97–126.

Leslie, A. M. (1982) The perception of causality in infants. *Perception* 11: 173–186.

Leslie, A. M. (1984) Spatiotemporal continuity and the perception of causality in infants. *Perception* 13: 287–305.

Leslie, A. M. and Keeble, S. (1987) Do six-month-old infants perceive causality? *Cognition* 25: 265–288.

Linvill, J. G. and Bliss, J. C. (1966) A direct translation reading aid for the blind. *Proceedings of the IEEE* 54(1): 40–51.

Liu, J., Harris, A. and Kanwisher, N. (2010) Perception of face parts and face configurations: an fMRI study. *Journal of Cognitive Neuroscience* 1: 203–211.

Lu, H. (2010) Structural processing in biological motion perception. *Journal of Vision* 10(12): 13.

Marr, D. (1982) *Vision: A Computational Investigation into the Human Representation and Processing of Visual Information*. San Francisco: W. H. Freeman.

Matthen, M. (2005) *Seeing, Doing, and Knowing: A Philosophical Theory of Sense Perception*. Oxford: Oxford University Press.

Matthen, M. (2010) On the diversity of auditory objects. *Review of Philosophy and Psychology* 1(1): 63–89.

Mausfeld, R. (2003) No psychology in—no psychology out: Anmerkungen zu den 'Visionen' eines Faches. *Pyschologische Rundschau* 54(3): 185–195. English translation: www.psychologie.uni-kiel.de/psychophysik/mausfeld/No Psychology In engl.pdf.

McCarthy, G., Puce, A., Gore, J. C. and Allison, T. (1997) Face-specific processing in the human fusiform gyrus. *Journal of Cognitive Neuroscience* 9(5): 605–610.

Meijer, P. B. L. (1992) An experimental system for auditory image representations. *IEEE Transactions Biomedical Engineering* 39: 112–121.

Michotte, A. (1963) *The Perception of Causality*. London: Methuen.

Mirenzi, A. and Hiris, E. (2011) The Thatcher effect in biological motion. *Perception* 40(10): 1257–1260.

Morris, M. W. and Peng, K. (1994) Culture and cause: American and Chinese attributions for social and physical events. *Journal of Personality and Social Psychology* 67: 949–971.

Noë, A. and O'Regan, J. K. (2002) On the brain-basis of visual consciousness: a sensorimotor account. In A. Noë and E. Thompson (eds) *Vision and Mind: Selected Readings in the Philosophy of Perception*. Cambridge, MA: MIT Press, 567–598.

Nudds, M. (2010) What are auditory objects? *Review of Philosophy and Psychology* 1(1): 105–122.

Oakes, L. M. (1994) Development of infants' use of continuity cues in their perception of causality. *Developmental Psychology* 30: 869–879.

Oakes, L. M. and Cohen, L. B. (1990) Infant perception of a causal event. *Cognitive Development* 5: 193–207.

O'Callaghan, C. (2010) Constructing a theory of sounds. *Oxford Studies in Metaphysics* 5: 247–270.

Pawluk, D., Kitada, R., Abramowicz, A., Hamilton, C. and Lederman, S. J. (2011) Figure/ground segmentation via a haptic glance: attributing initial finger contacts to objects or their supporting surfaces. *IEEE Transactions on Haptics* 4(1): 2–13.

Proulx, M. J. (2010) Synthetic synaesthesia and sensory substitution. *Consciousness and Cognition* 19: 501–503.

Purves, D. and Lotto, R. B. (2003) *Why We See What We Do: A Wholly Empirical Theory of Vision*. Sunderland, MA: Sinauer Associates.

Pylyshyn, Z. W. (2003) *Seeing and Visualizing: It's Not What You Think*. Cambridge, MA: MIT Press.

Pylyshyn, Z. W. (2004) Some puzzling findings in multiple object tracking (MOT): I. tracking without keeping track of object identities. *Visual Cognition* 11: 801–822.

Renier, L., Laloyaux, C., Collignon, O., Tranduy, D., Vanlierde, A., Bruyer, R. and De Volder, A. G. (2005) The Ponzo illusion using auditory substitution of vision in sighted and early blind subjects. *Perception* 34: 857–867.

Renier, L., Bruyer, R. and De Volder, A. G. (2006) Vertical-horizontal illusion present for sighted but not early blind humans using auditory substitution for vision. *Perception and Psychophysics* 68(4): 535–542.

Richards, W. A. (1988) *Natural Computation*. Cambridge, MA: MIT Press.

Rips, L. (2011) Causation from perception. *Perspectives on Psychological Science* 6(1): 77–97.

Rutherford, M. D., Pennington, B. F. and Rogers, S. J. (2006) The perception of animacy in young children with autism. *Journal of Autism and Developmental Disorders* 36: 983–992.

Schlottmann, A. and Anderson, N. H. (1993) An information integration approach to phenomenal causality. *Memory and Cognition* 21(6): 785–801.

Schlottmann, A. and Shanks, D. R. (1992) Evidence for a distinction between judged and perceived causality. *Quarterly Journal of Experimental Psychology* 44A: 321–342.

Scholl, B. J. and Gao, T. (2013) Perceiving animacy and intentionality: visual processing or higher-level judgment? In M. D. Rutherford and V. A. Kuhlmeier (eds) *Social Perception: Detection and Interpretation of Animacy, Agency, and Intention*. Cambridge, MA: MIT Press.

Scholl, B. J. and Nakayama, J. (2002) Causal capture: contextual effects on the perception of collision events. *Psychological Science* 13: 493–498.

Scholl, B. J. and Pylyshyn, Z. W. (1999) Tracking multiple items through occlusion: clues to visual objecthood. *Cognitive Psychology* 38: 259–290.

Scholl, B. J. and Tremoulet, P. D. (2000) Perceptual causality and animacy. *Trends in Cognitive Sciences* 4: 299–309.

Scholl, B. J., Pylyshyn, Z. W. and Franconeri, S. L. (1999) When are featural and spatiotemporal properties encoded as a result of attentional allocation? *Investigative Ophthalmology and Visual Science* 40(4): 4195.

Scholl, B. J., Pylyshyn, Z. and Feldman, J. (2001) What is a visual object? Evidence from target merging in multiple object tracking. *Cognition* 80: 159–177.

Shepard, R. N. (1987) Evolution of a mesh between principles of the mind and regularities of the world. In J. Dupre (ed.) *The Latest on the Best: Essays on Evolution and Optimality*. Cambridge, MA: MIT Press, 251–275.

Shepard, R. N. (1994) Perceptual-cognitive universals as reflections of the world. *Psychonomic Bulletin and Review* 1(1): 2–28.

Shepard, R. N. (2001) Perceptual-cognitive universals as reflections of the world. *Behavioral and Brain Sciences* 24: 581–601.

Siegel, S. (2006) Which properties are represented in perception? In T. G. Szabo and J. Hawthorne (eds) *Perceptual Experience*. Oxford: Oxford University Press, 481–503.

Siegel, S. (2009) The visual experience of causation. *Philosophical Quarterly* 59(236): 519–540.

Siegel, S. (2010) *The Contents of Visual Experience*. New York: Oxford University Press.

Sinha, P., Balas, B., Ostrovsky, Y. and Russell, R. (2006) Face recognition by humans: nineteen results all computer vision researchers should know about. *Proceedings of the IEEE* 94: 1948–1962.

Spelke, E. (1990) Principles of object perception. *Cognitive Science* 14: 29–56.

Sugita, Y. (2009) Innate face processing. *Current Opinion in Neurobiology* 19: 39–44.

Thompson, P. (2010) Margaret Thatcher: a new illusion. *Perception* 9(4): 483–484.

Ullman, S. (1979) *The Interpretation of Visual Motion*. Cambridge, MA: MIT Press.

Ward, J. and Meijer, P. (2010) Visual experiences in the blind induced by an auditory sensory substitution device. *Consciousness and Cognition* 19: 492–500.

14

Sensory Substitution and Perceptual Learning

KEVIN CONNOLLY

Abstract When a user integrates a sensory substitution device into her life, the process involves perceptual learning, that is, 'relatively long-lasting changes to an organism's perceptual system that improve its ability to respond to its environment' (Goldstone 1998: 585). In this chapter, I explore ways in which the extensive literature on perceptual learning can be applied to help improve sensory substitution devices. I then use these findings to answer a philosophical question. Much of the philosophical debate surrounding sensory substitution devices concerns what happens after perceptual learning occurs. In particular, should the resultant perceptual experience be classified in the substituted modality (as vision), in the substituting modality (as auditory or tactile), or in a new sense modality? I propose a novel empirical test to help resolve this philosophical debate.

14.1 Introduction

Sensory substitution devices (SSDs) deliver information about the environment by converting the information normally received through one sense modality into information for another sense modality. Typically SSDs are used by the blind to help them better navigate the world. Such devices consist of a video camera which feeds visual information into a converter that transforms it into auditory or tactile stimuli, which the blind person can perceive. In such a case, audition or touch acts as the 'substituting modality' for vision, the 'substituted modality'.

When a user integrates an SSD into her life, the process involves perceptual learning: 'relatively long-lasting changes to an organism's perceptual system that improve its ability to respond to its environment' (Goldstone 1998: 585). Integrating an SSD involves long-lasting changes to a user's perceptual system (see, for instance, research on sensory substitution and brain plasticity, especially

Proceedings of the British Academy, **219**, 236–250. © The British Academy 2018.

Ptito et al. 2005; and Kupers and Ptito 2004). Furthermore, these long-lasting changes allow the user of an SSD to better respond to stimuli in her environment. A blind person, for instance, can use an SSD to respond to the colour of objects, where without the device she could not.

In this chapter, I pose a challenge for sensory substitution researchers, and offer a positive proposal for how researchers might respond to the challenge. The challenge is that to understand and improve the kind of perceptual learning required for sensory substitution, researchers need to focus as much on the *un*learning required as on the learning. That is, they should start by recognizing the long-lasting changes that have already occurred in a person's perceptual system prior to her first experience with an SSD. I detail three such long-lasting changes in section 14.2: latent inhibition (14.2.1), attentional weighting (14.2.2), and unitization/differentiation (14.2.3). I argue that these three perceptual habits are not adapted for sensory substitution and are difficult to break. My positive proposal, however, is that researchers might circumvent these habits by using SSDs that employ novel stimuli, and I outline an empirical way to determine which stimuli are novel. Researchers might speed up the perceptual learning process by reducing the amount of unlearning that sensory substitution requires.

The argument in section 14.2 is in service of a philosophical point, which I make in section 14.3. Much of the current philosophical debate surrounding SSDs is about the nature of one's perceptual experience once one has fully integrated an SSD. The question is whether one's perceptual experience should be classified in the substituted modality (as vision), in the substituting modality (as auditory or tactile), or in a new modality (see Hurley and Noë 2003; Block 2003; Noë 2004; O'Regan 2011; Kiverstein et al. 2015: 661; Deroy and Auvray 2015). I argue that we can use an empirical test for determining novel stimuli to make progress towards resolving this philosophical debate.

14.2 Perceptual Learning Effects

Perceptual learning involves long-lasting changes to one's perceptual system. In this section, I identify three specific kinds of long-lasting changes that will have already occurred in a person's perceptual system prior to her first experience with an SSD: effects of latent inhibition, attentional weighting, and unitization/differentiation. I show some ways in which each of these effects would need to be undone for sensory substitution learning, but I also show how researchers can circumvent the need to undo them if they program SSDs such that the devices deliver novel stimuli.

14.2.1 Latent inhibition

A prominent model of perceptual learning is Ian McLaren and Nick Mackintosh's associative learning model (see McLaren et al. 1989; McLaren and Mackintosh 2000). McLaren and Mackintosh explain how perceptual learning occurs in cases such as learning to discriminate a Merlot from a Cabernet Franc. Suppose you are presented with two similar perceptual stimuli (X and Y) the same number of times. Being similar stimuli, many features are shared between X and Y. When a feature is shared, you are exposed to it twice as much as you are to a non-shared feature (once when presented with X, and a second time when presented with Y). According to the McLaren and Mackintosh model, you become habituated to these shared features, which results in those features becoming less likely to enter into associations (and as such, less likely to be good candidates for use in learning). On the other hand, you are exposed to the non-shared features only half as much as the shared features. So, you become less habituated to the non-shared features. This results in the non-shared features becoming more likely to enter into associations (and so more likely to be good candidates for use in learning).

To take a concrete example, suppose that you drink a Merlot and a Cabernet Franc the same number of times. The features shared in common between them, such as the tannins, are exposed twice as much as the features unique to each of them. You become more habituated to these shared features than to the unique ones, resulting in the shared features becoming less likely to enter into associations. As such, the shared features are poor candidates for use in learning. In contrast, you become less habituated to the features unique to each of the wines. So the unique features, such as the fruitiness of the Merlot, are more likely to enter into associations. As such, the unique features are better candidates for use in learning.

McLaren and Mackintosh's model is strikingly counter-intuitive, despite being well-supported by experimental evidence. On their view, it is easier to learn from unfamiliar stimuli and harder to learn from familiar stimuli. It might seem at first glance that it would be the other way around. And, in fact, for several decades in the history of psychology, that intuitive idea was dogma.

In the late 1950s, psychologists were concerned with the question: Can learning take place without reinforcement?[1] There was evidence for this. One important experiment was conducted by E. C. Tolman and H. C. Honzik in 1930. The experiment involved rats and mazes, and had two stages. In the first stage, rats were allowed to explore a maze without reinforcement (that is, there was no reward at the end of the maze). In the second stage, the rats were rewarded with food at the end of the maze. These rats were more quickly able navigate the maze and receive the reward than a control group that did not take part in the first stage. The idea

[1] My exposition in this section is based largely on Lubow and Weiner 2010.

was that the rats had learned about the routes of the maze during the first stage, even without a reward, and that learning became evident only in the second stage when a reward was offered. These rats experienced what was called 'latent learning', a kind of learning that occurs before reinforcement, but is evident only after reinforcement (Tolman and Honzik 1930: 257).

In 1959, R. E. Lubow and A. U. Moore were attempting a simple demonstration of latent learning, not with rats, but with sheep and goats (see Lubow and Moore 1959). They divided the animals into two groups. In the first stage of the experiment, they presented each member of the first group with a flashing light ten times, and presented each member of the second group with a rotor that turned ten times. None of the ten presentations were reinforced for either group. In the second stage of the experiment, both groups received alternated presentations of the flashing light and the turning rotor. For each presentation, the flash or the turn was followed by a mild shock.

Lubow and Moore were expecting their results to provide an example of latent learning. Specifically, they thought that it would be easier to condition the animals with the stimulus that they were pre-exposed to in stage one—the familiar stimulus. In fact, they found exactly the opposite. Their original hypothesis was that just as the rats in Tolman and Honzik's experiment had learned to navigate the maze even without reinforcement (something that became evident only after reinforcement in stage two), so too would the sheep and goats learn about the stimuli they had been exposed to in stage one, and this learning would become evident after the reinforcement in stage two. So, for instance, if the animal had been presented with a flashing light ten times in stage one, Lubow and Moore predicted that in stage two, the animal would build an association between the flashing light and the shock more quickly than between the turning rotor and the shock.

What Lubow and Moore actually found was the inverse of what they had predicted. If the animal was pre-exposed to the flashing light, then it built an association between the turning rotor and the shock more quickly. If it was pre-exposed to the turning rotor, then it built an association between the flashing light and the shock more quickly. To contrast with latent learning, Lubow and Moore called the effect that they had found 'latent inhibition'. In latent inhibition, pre-exposure to a stimulus type inhibits learning on that stimulus type.[2]

Latent inhibition supports McLaren and Mackintosh's model of perceptual learning. Their model makes the prediction that it is harder to learn from familiar stimuli. As the story of Lubow and Moore's experiment indicates, latent inhibition is a counter-intuitive phenomenon, but it is also a well-established one. While it seems that it would be easier to learn familiar stimuli, in fact the opposite is true.

[2] Fifty years later, Lubow (2010: 4) was surprised that the original experiment worked at all, given that the number of stimulus pre-exposures was so small. Typically latent inhibition requires many more than ten exposures.

Latent inhibition and sensory substitution

HARNESSING LATENT INHIBITION FOR MORE EFFICIENT LEARNING WITH SENSORY SUBSTITUTION DEVICES

What can sensory substitution researchers learn from studies on latent inhibition? One lesson is that effective perceptual learning may be counter-intuitive, and so the way to most effectively train people on SSDs may defy common sense. In particular, since perceptual learning is quicker on novel stimuli due to latent inhibition, researchers might increase the speed of the learning process with SSDs by programming the most novel stimuli into SSDs. To do this, researchers need to be able to test that a stimulus programmed into an SSD is novel to a user, as opposed to familiar. I want to suggest two ways to do this.

One way to determine whether stimuli are novel to a user is by examining their brain responses. Novel stimuli activate networks in the brain that have a signature and are detectable by using electrophysiological recordings of scalp and intracranial 'event-related potentials' (ERPs). These signatures have been specifically shown to exist for novel auditory and tactile stimuli (Knight 1996). ERPs are not the only option, however. For cortically blind research participants at least, another option might be to examine pupil response to determine novel stimuli. Naber and colleagues have provided evidence that the pupil dilates more for novel stimuli (Naber et al. 2013), and there is evidence that pupil dilation measures novelty not just for visual stimuli, but for other modalities as well (see Naber et al. 2013: 2). This could provide a helpful test for sensory substitution researchers. As Naber and colleagues point out, pupil size is 'a simple and outwardly accessible physiological measure' (2013: 2). By measuring pupil dilation or by using ERPs, researchers might determine which stimuli are novel to participants, and program SSDs such that they deliver those stimuli. (Note that this will be important at the end of the chapter, when we engage with the philosophical debate over whether SSD perception should be classified as visual, as auditory or tactile, or as part of a new modality.)

While I think ERPs or pupil dilation measurements are the ultimate standard as to which stimuli are novel and which are not, even without that data, we can make some progress on the question. In ordinary perceptual development, for instance, we can say that the person learns on novel stimuli. The world of an infant is filled with shapes, sounds, colours, tastes, textures, and smells, and for each of those properties, there is a time that they are novel to her. The first experience of green is new, as is the first feel of a block, and the first perception of the sound of a barking dog. Contrast this with sensory substitution. In sensory substitution, the user learns on proximal stimuli[3] to which, in some sense, he has already been exposed.

[3] I take a stimulus to be an objective property or object in the external world. I use 'proximal stimulus' to refer to the property or object in the substituting modality (audition or touch), such as a particular tone delivered by a visual-to-audio SSD. By 'distal stimulus' I mean the property or object in the substituted modality (vision) that the proximal stimulus represents, such as the brightness represented by the tone.

Consider the vOICe, 'a visual-auditory substitution device that works by transforming images from a digital camera embedded in a pair of sunglasses into auditory frequencies ("soundscapes"), which the user hears through headphones' (Kiverstein et al. 2015). The vOICe represents the vertical spatial location of an object by using higher- or lower-pitched tones (the higher the tone, the higher the spatial location of the object). It represents horizontal spatial location by using the left and right headphones. If the spatial location of an object is to the left (or right), the vOICe plays a tone out of the left (or right) headphone. The vOICe represents the brightness of an object with volume (the brighter the object, the louder the volume).

Consider a person using the vOICe. A person using the vOICe has already been exposed to auditory stimuli, prior to her first experience with the SSD. Contrast this with an infant. For an infant, there is a time in which the sounds of birds chirping, voices talking, and fans whirring are all new to him. For the user of the vOICe, on the other hand, she has already heard all of these sounds and many others. Auditory stimuli are not new to her.

SSD users have been pre-exposed not just to auditory or tactile stimuli in general, but also to some of the specific proximal stimuli types delivered by these devices. Consider the EyeMusic device, an SSD that is like the vOICe in converting visual images into sounds, but is unique in also delivering information about colour. EyeMusic represents five colours with notes from five ordinary instruments such as a piano (white) and a marimba (blue) (Levy-Tzedek et al. 2012b: 316). In other words, the device delivers proximal stimuli with which the user is undoubtedly familiar: the notes of a piano and a marimba. Due to latent inhibition, however, prior exposure interferes with new learning. So, new learning might be harder to accomplish with piano and marimba notes. To take a different example, consider 'TVSS', which stands for 'tactile-vision sensory substitution'. TVSS devices convert visual information picked up by a camera into tactile information, which is delivered to the skin (to the tongue or back, in particular). As Bach-y-Rita and Kercel describe it, however, the information delivered by TVSS is 'the usual cutaneous information (pressure, tickle, wetness, etc.)' (2003: 543). But certainly pressure, tickles, and wetness are familiar stimuli, which have been experienced before in a different context. Once again, however, research on latent inhibition shows that prior exposure interferes with new learning. So, it might be harder to train someone with TVSS, given that the device delivers pressure, tickles, and wetness—all familiar stimuli.

It might be objected here that the context of, say, the notes of a marimba surrounded by other SSD stimuli is importantly different from the context of the notes of a marimba surrounded by the notes of other instruments in a band. The worry is that latent inhibition of the marimba notes in one context might not transfer into the SSD context. But latent inhibition does transfer in these contexts, as experiments on latent inhibition for complex stimuli show (for a good summary, see McLaren and Mackintosh 2000: 221). Latent inhibition affects the individual features of a complex stimulus, not the complex stimulus as a whole. If a stimulus, like a marimba note, is presented with one group of stimuli in one context, but with another group of stimuli in another context, latent inhibition affects the marimba, and transfers across contexts.[4]

I have been arguing that prior exposure interferes with new learning. I now want to argue that there are still ways in which sensory substitution researchers can avoid prior exposure. They can start by determining which stimuli are novel to SSD users by using ERPs or by measuring pupil dilation. This might be a complicated process, since a token stimulus can fall under multiple types. An mbira note, for instance, might be novel as an mbira note, but familiar as the note C-sharp. In such a case, a researcher would need to determine carefully which feature is novel in order to construct the most novel stimulus. After researchers have determined such stimuli, they can program SSDs such that the devices deliver them. Since EyeMusic represents colours with notes from familiar instruments like a piano and a marimba, for instance, these could be switched to notes from more unfamiliar types of instruments (the notes of an mbira might be a good substitute for piano notes, for example). Perhaps one reason why a piano and a marimba were chosen is because they are instruments that are familiar to the researchers who selected them. But novelty, not familiarity, facilitates perceptual learning. To speed up the training, more obscure instruments might be a better choice. This is a testable hypothesis.

EyeMusic also uses tones that make up a pentatonic scale (Levy-Tzedek et al. 2012a: 3). This makes sense, because it means that the tones will sound consonant together when heard by someone using the device. However, it is also at odds with efficient perceptual learning. After all, a chord composed from the pentatonic scale will likely be a familiar chord. A scale less familiar to most people, such as the Locrian scale, might deliver more efficient perceptual learning than the pentatonic scale. Of course, it is important to strike a balance between user friendliness and efficient perceptual learning. The pentatonic scale is certainly pleasurable to listen to, and that may be why it was chosen. To balance efficient perceptual learning with user friendliness, however, researchers might use a pleasurable sounding scale that

[4] A second objection based on context is that the environmental context in an SSD training situation is importantly different from the environmental context in which research participants have been previously exposed to piano notes, marimba notes, pressure, tickles, and wetness. The worry is that latent inhibition in the prior context might not transfer into the SSD context. There is indeed quite a bit of evidence for the context sensitivity of the latent inhibition effect (for a good summary, see Hall 1991: 75–78). Roughly, a change in context often attenuates the latent inhibition effect. Crucially, however, context sensitivity is itself attenuated if the person is already familiar with the prior context before she is exposed to the stimuli (McLaren et al. 1994; McLaren and Mackintosh 2000: 224). In other words, if an infant is familiar with her crib context, and is then exposed to pressure and tickles, these stimuli will be latently inhibited, and that effect can transfer into the SSD learning context.

is also unfamiliar to the majority of users. This issue, however, suggests a more general point: researchers will often need to strike a balance between several different desiderata (including efficient engineering), and some of them may be in conflict with efficient perceptual learning.

HARNESSING LATENT INHIBITION FOR EFFICIENT GENERALIZATION

Consider a second way that researchers might use latent inhibition to improve SSD learning. Users of SSDs become able to recognize new token objects of the same type on which they have been trained. So, for instance, if they were trained on a maple leaf with the vOICe, they can become able to recognize new instances of maple leaves using that SSD. This process is called 'generalization' (see Kim and Zatorre 2008; Deroy and Auvray 2015). One thing worth mentioning is that there will be more and less optimal ways to achieve generalization through latent inhibition.

Suppose that the task is to get an SSD user to recognize a novel maple leaf as a maple leaf when she sees it. First, consider the least optimal training scenario for this, given latent inhibition. Suppose that immediately after picking up the sensory substitution device for the first time, the user is exposed just to a maple leaf, but not to other kinds of objects. Given that scenario, each of the maple leaf's features will be equally latently inhibited. This will make it harder to recognize a new token maple leaf as a maple leaf when presented with one. It will be harder to recognize this new maple leaf as such because its prototypical features are unlikely to stand out any more than any other feature. This is because all of its features are equally likely to be latently inhibited, both the prototypical and non-prototypical features alike. To enhance recognition, what we need is for the non-prototypical features to be latently inhibited, so that the prototypical features stand out in contrast.

Suppose, on the other hand, that a user is initially exposed an equal number of times to a wide range of objects different from maple leaves, but sharing some maple leaf features (they might be other kinds of leaves, or non-leaves with pointy edges, etc.). In that case, due to latent inhibition, the user will be less habituated to the features shared between maple leaves and non-maple leaves, resulting in those features becoming less likely to enter into associations, and so less likely to be good candidates for use in learning. In contrast, the user will be less habituated to the features unique to the maple leaf (such as the unique pointy shape of its edges). When introduced to a new token maple leaf, its prototypical features are more likely to enter into associations. As such, those features are better candidates for use in learning.

14.2.2 Attentional weighting

After latent inhibition, a second perceptual learning effect is 'attentional weighting', the idea that the weight of attention can change by 'increasing the attention paid to perceptual dimensions and features that are important, and/or by decreasing attention to irrelevant dimensions and features' (Goldstone 1998: 588).[5] When you learn to recognize a wren, for instance, you might increase attention to the shape of its body, while decreasing attention to the colour of the bird's plumage. If so, you have changed your original attentional weighting. For an expert like a bird-watcher, part of expertise is developing the ability to attend to relevant perceptual dimensions of birds.

Which perceptual dimension the person attends to is often a function of the relevance of the task (see Goldstone and Byrge 2015). For example, when picking the right book to slip into your bag when you are in a hurry, colour and size might be important dimensions to attend to. In contrast, weight might be more important than colour or size for picking out a box of books from other boxes when you are moving. It is important to recognize that attentional weighting has as much to do with what the perceiver chooses to ignore, as it does with what she chooses to attend to (Goldstone 1998: 588–589). When you attend to the weight of the box as you are moving, you are also choosing to ignore many other features of the box, even perhaps its colour and size.

It might be tempting to think of attentional weighting as something that is easy to change. After all, you might just as easily attend to the colour or size of the box of books, rather than the weight. However, there is also evidence that some kinds of attentional weighting become ingrained. As Goldstone points out, 'attentional highlighting of information occurs even if it is to the detriment of the observer' (1998: 589). For instance, letters used first as targets but later used as distractors to be ignored, still grab the attention of research participants (Goldstone cites Shiffrin and Schneider 1977). In such a case, an attentional weighting has become ingrained, and persists even if the person wants to change it.

A second piece of evidence that attentional weighting is not always easy to change is the following. Through experience we develop dispositions to attend in a particular way. For instance, experienced soccer defenders focus longer on the opponent's hips than less experienced players do (Williams and Davids 1998), while experienced goalkeepers fixate longer on the non-kicking leg than less experienced goalkeepers (Savelsbergh et al. 2002). To say that these attentional patterns are easy to change, however, would be to ignore the fact that these are habits developed through years of experience. Experienced soccer players are disposed to attend in a particular way, and that attentional pattern has become deeply ingrained, fortified by years of experience.

[5] My exposition of attentional weighting and unitization/differentiation is largely from Goldstone 1998 and Goldstone and Byrge 2015.

Attentional weighting and sensory substitution

UNWEIGHTING AND REWEIGHTING ATTENTION IN SENSORY SUBSTITUTION

I want to offer a novel proposal for how researchers can weight attention in a way that facilitates SSD learning. First, however, let me say something about the effect of prior attentional habits on SSD learning. Contrast the learning situation for an SSD user with the learning that takes place in ordinary perceptual development. For an infant, the perceptual learning process involves developing an attentional weighting, but does not require breaking any past attentional disposition. By contrast, an SSD user has already developed attentional habits. The learning that takes place in sensory substitution occurs on stimuli with which the user is familiar, either as an auditory or tactile stimulus in general, or as a particular type of stimulus such as the notes of a piano or a marimba with EyeMusic (Levy-Tzedek et al. 2012a, 2012b), or as ordinary tickles, pressure, and wetness to the skin with TVSS (Bach-y-Rita and Kercel 2003: 543). Training a person on an SSD might be difficult since it involves breaking an attentional habit, as opposed to just weighting attention. Once again, novel stimuli become important for training on SSDs. If SSDs were to employ novel stimuli, then a user might simply develop an attentional weighting for the SSD's perceptual array without having to first break their attentional habits.

Now let me suggest the novel way that researchers can weight attention to facilitate SSD learning. In a 2013 study on perceptual learning, participants were trained to classify different kinds of fish locomotion (Jarodzka et al. 2013). Three groups were shown the same four videos, each with a single fish swimming a different locomotion pattern. Each video was accompanied by an audio instruction from a professor of marine zoology explaining the relevant features of each locomotion pattern (Jarodzka et al. 2013: 65). As the professor delivered his instructions, he was also watching each video, and his eye movements were tracked. A control group was shown the four videos with the accompanying audio. A second group was given the four videos with audio, but, in addition, each video had a dot that tracked the spot where the professor's eye movements were focusing. A third group was given the videos and audio, along with a spotlight which both highlighted the spot where the professor's eye movements were focusing and filtered out the other distracting details.

In the testing phase of the experiment, participants were shown four new videos, one for each locomotion pattern, and they were rated for the efficiency at which they fixated on one of the identifying features of the locomotion pattern, as well as the length of time at which they fixated there. Those in the dot group fixated on the identifying features more quickly and focused there longer than the control group. Those in the spotlight group were even quicker, and fixated even longer. Both the dot and the spotlight group were also better than the controls at interpreting what they saw when responding to multiple-choice questions after viewing videos.

The fish locomotion study suggests a novel way to enhance the learning process with sensory substitution devices: attentional cueing might serve a useful function during training. More specifically, cues could shift the weight of attention onto the more task-relevant stimuli delivered by the SSD, and away from less task-relevant stimuli. Suppose you are training users with the vOICe or EyeMusic, and the audio is correlated with a complicated pattern on a computer screen. An attention-grabbing auditory cue such as a beep might be placed just temporally prior to stimuli that researchers want to highlight. This would cause the viewer to focus on the subsequent stimulus. Just as the dot drew the attention of participants in the fish locomotion study, the beep could draw the auditory attention of participants when training on SSDs. Importantly, however, the results of the fish locomotion study suggest that an auditory *spotlight* would be even better. Suppose again that you are training participants with the vOICe or EyeMusic, and the audio is correlated with a complicated pattern on a computer screen. White noise could be played over distracting details to dampen them, but not over important stimuli. Just as the spotlight highlighted important features of fish locomotion, the lack of white noise could highlight important features in a sensory substitution training session.

In short, very recent literature on perceptual learning suggests some novel techniques that researchers might use to teach someone how to use an SSD. These 'sensory substitution training wheels' might give users a better training experience with the device, and make them more proficient with SSDs once the training wheels are removed.

14.2.3 Unitization and differentiation

After latent inhibition and attentional weighting, a third perceptual learning effect is unitization/differentiation. In the process of 'unitization', perceptual features that were once treated by the perceptual system as distinct are later treated by the system as a single unit. A whole host of objects have been shown to be first processed as distinct features, and later processed as a unit. This is the case not just for cats and cars, but also for objects constructed in the lab. For instance, Gauthier and Tarr constructed a set of objects called 'Greebles', which shared a set of spatial features in common. When the participants were exposed to the Greebles for long enough, they would begin to process them as units (Gauthier and Tarr 1997).

In the process of 'differentiation', perceptual features that were once treated by the perceptual system as unified are later treated by the system as distinct. For instance, William James (1890: 509) discusses a case where a man became able to distinguish by taste between the upper and lower half of a bottle for a particular kind of wine. Assuming that the man's perception itself had changed, not just his background belief about what his perception amounted to, James' case is a case of perceptual differentiation. At first, that kind of wine was treated as gustatorily unified by the man's perceptual system, while later the upper and lower half of a bottle were treated as gustatorily distinct.

Unitization and differentiation seem at first glance to be opposites. After all, while in unitization features once treated as distinct are later treated as a single unit, in differentiation, features once treated as a single unit are later treated as distinct (Goldstone 1998: 602). In fact, however, unitization and differentiation are really just performing the same task in two different ways (Goldstone and Byrge 2015). Specifically, both unitization and differentiation create new perceptual units. Goldstone puts the point in the following way: '[U]nitization and differentiation are both processes that build appropriate-sized representations for the tasks at hand' (1998: 604). Both unitization and differentiation give us units to attend to, search for, and build up into more complex percepts (Goldstone and Byrge 2015). It is just that in unitization, these units are composite wholes, while in differentiation the building blocks are parts.

Sensory substitution and unitization/differentiation

RE-UNITIZING AND RE-DIFFERENTIATING

As with latent inhibition and attentional weighting, by the time a person first uses an SSD, her perceptual array will already be arranged in a particular way through the processes of unitization and differentiation. Some features will be arranged together as units, while other features will be differentiated from one another. This means that for some features, unitization or differentiation will need to be undone.

As with latent inhibition and attentional weighting, one way to avert much of the unlearning process for unitization and differentiation is to program SSDs such that they deliver novel stimuli to users. While familiar stimuli may have undergone differentiation and unitization, novel stimuli will not have undergone either of these perceptual processes. As a result, the use of novel stimuli might circumvent much of the unlearning process, making the perceptual learning process more efficient as a whole. After all, novel stimuli will require only unitization and differentiation, without requiring first that these processes are undone from the prior context.

14.3 A Philosophical Conclusion

I want to close with a philosophical upshot. Very recently, the discussion on SSDs has revolved around the nature of one's perceptual experience once one has fully integrated an SSD. In particular, the question is the following: Should that perceptual experience be classified in the substituting modality (as auditory or tactile), in the substituted modality (as visual), or in a new modality? Enactivists such as Noë, Hurley, and O'Regan have argued that the perceptual experience should be classified as visual (Hurley and Noë 2003; Noë 2004; O'Regan 2011). Block (2003) has argued that it should be classified as auditory or tactile. Kiverstein et al. (2015) have argued that the perceptual experience should be classified as part of a new modality. Deroy and Auvray (2015) have argued that these three options are insufficient. Assuming (pace Deroy and Auvray) that the three options are sufficient, my argument suggests a novel way that we can answer this question empirically.

If perceptual experience with an SSD is in the substituted modality (vision), or in a new hybrid modality, then think about the stimuli involved in that experience. Assuming that the SSD user is blind from birth, if the perceptual experience is visual, then the stimuli will be novel to the perceiver. Likewise, if the perceptual experience is in a new hybrid modality, then the stimuli will also be novel to the perceiver. But remember that there are ways to test whether a stimulus is novel or familiar to a person. One option is to examine brain responses. Novel stimuli activate networks in the brain that have a signature and are detectable. This is done by using electrophysiological recordings of scalp and intracranial event-related potentials (ERPs) (see Knight 1996). Another option, for cortically blind participants at least, is to examine their pupil response to determine novel stimuli, since the pupil dilates more for novel stimuli (Naber et al. 2013), and there is evidence that this occurs even for non-visual perceptual stimuli (Naber et al. 2013: 2). By using ERPs or by measuring pupil dilation, researchers might determine whether sensory substitution stimuli are novel to a perceiver. If they are novel, then we have evidence that the perceptual experience with an SSD is best classified either in the substituted modality (as visual), or in a new hybrid modality. If the stimuli are familiar, then we have evidence that the perceptual experience remains in the substituting modality (as auditory or tactile).

There are a lot of remaining questions about perceptual learning and SSDs. First, the learning involved with SSDs has a motor component. Users need to learn how to control the camera with the vOICe, for instance. The motor component of sensory substitution learning is an important topic, which I have not addressed here. Second, although this chapter was about sensory substitution and perceptual learning, it focused predominantly on what perceptual learning can tell us about sensory substitution (see Connolly 2019). A lot can still be said about what sensory substitution can tell us about perceptual learning. Finally, in discussing what perceptual learning can tell us about sensory substitution, the essay focused largely on the proximal stimuli delivered by SSDs, and while it focused a little bit on the distal stimuli, that was not the main focus of the essay. A lot can still be said about what research on perceptual learning can tell us about the distal stimuli that SSDs track.

References

Bach-y-Rita, P. and Kercel, S. W. (2003) Sensory substitution and the human–machine interface. *Trends in Cognitive Sciences* 7(12): 541–546.

Block, N. (2003) Tactile sensation via spatial perception. *Trends in Cognitive Sciences 7*: 285–286.

Connolly, K. (2019) *Perceptual learning: The flexibility of the senses*. New York: Oxford University Press.

Deroy, O. and Auvray, M. (2015) A crossmodal perspective on sensory substitution. In D. Stokes, M. Matthen and S. Biggs (eds) *Perception and its Modalities*. Oxford: Oxford University Press, 327–347.

Gauthier, I. and Tarr, M. J. (1997) Becoming a 'greeble' expert: exploring mechanisms for face recognition. *Vision Research* 37: 1673–1682.

Goldstone, R. L. (1998) Perceptual learning. *Annual Review of Psychology* 49: 585–612.

Goldstone, R. L. and Byrge, L. A. (2015) Perceptual learning. In M. Matthen (ed.) *The Oxford Handbook of the Philosophy of Perception*. Oxford: Oxford University Press, 1001–1016.

Hall, G. (1991) *Perceptual and Associative Learning*. Oxford: Clarendon Press.

Hurley, S. and Noë, A. (2003) Neural plasticity and consciousness. *Biology and Philosophy* 18: 131–168.

James, W. (1890) *Principles of Psychology*. New York: Holt.

Jarodzka, H., van Gog, T., Dorr, M., Scheiter, K. and Gerjets, P. (2013) Learning to see: guiding students' attention via a model's eye movements fosters learning. *Learning and Instruction* 25: 62–70.

Kim, J.-K. and Zatorre, R. J. (2008) Generalized learning of visual-to-auditory substitution in sighted individuals. *Brain Research* 1242: 263–275.

Kiverstein, J., Farina, M. and Clark, A. (2015) Substituting the senses. In M. Matthen (ed.) *The Oxford Handbook of the Philosophy of Perception*. Oxford: Oxford University Press, 659–675.

Knight, R. T. (1996) Contribution of human hippocampal region to novelty detection. *Nature* 383(6597): 256–259.

Kupers, R. and Ptito, M. (2004) 'Seeing' through the tongue: cross-modal plasticity in the congenitally blind. *International Congress Series* 1270: 79–84.

Levy-Tzedek, S., Novick, I., Arbel, R., Abboud, S., Maidenbaum, S., Vaadia, E. and Amedi, A. (2012a) Cross-sensory transfer of sensory-motor information: visuomotor learning affects performance on an audiomotor task, using sensory-substitution. *Scientific Reports*, 2.

Levy-Tzedek, S., Hanassy, S., Abboud, S., Maidenbaum, S. and Amedi, A. (2012b) Fast, accurate reaching movements with a visual-to-auditory sensory substitution device. *Restorative Neurology and Neuroscience* 30: 313–323.

Lubow, R. E. (2010) A short history of latent inhibition research. In Robert Lubow and Ina Weiner (eds) *Latent Inhibition Cognition, Neuroscience and Applications to Schizophrenia*. Cambridge: Cambridge University Press.

Lubow, R. E. and Moore, A. U. (1959) Latent inhibition: the effect of nonreinforced preexposure to the conditional stimulus. *Journal of Comparative and Physiological Psychology* 52: 415–419.

Lubow, R. and Weiner, I. (eds) (2010) *Latent Inhibition Cognition, Neuroscience and Applications to Schizophrenia*. Cambridge: Cambridge University Press.

McLaren, I. P. L. and Mackintosh, N. J. (2000) An elemental model of associative learning: I. Latent inhibition and perceptual learning. *Animal Learning and Behavior* 38(3): 211–246.

McLaren, I. P. L., Kaye, H. and Mackintosh, N. J. (1989) An associative theory of the representation of stimuli: applications to perceptual learning and latent inhibition. In R. G. M. Morris (ed.) *Parallel Distributed Processing – Implications for Psychology and Neurobiology*. Oxford: Oxford University Press.

McLaren, I. P. L., Bennett, C., Plaisted, K., Aitken, M. and Mackintosh, N. J. (1994) Latent inhibition, context specificity, and context familiarity. *Quarterly Journal of Experimental Psychology* 47(4): 387–400.

Naber, M., Frassle, S., Rutishauser, U. and Einhauser, W. (2013) Pupil size signals novelty and predicts later retrieval success for declarative memories of natural scenes. *Journal of Vision* 13(2): 11.

Noë, A. (2004) *Action in Perception*. Cambridge, MA: MIT Press.

O'Regan, J. K. (2011) *Why Red Doesn't Sound Like a Bell: Understanding the Feel of Consciousness*. Oxford: Oxford University Press.

Ptito, M., Moesgaard, S. M., Gjedde, A. and Kupers, R. (2005) Cross-modal plasticity revealed by electrotactile stimulation of the tongue in the congenitally blind. *Brain* 128(3): 606–614.

Savelsbergh, G. J. P., Williams, A. M., Van der Kamp, J. and Ward, P. (2002) Visual search, anticipation and expertise in soccer goalkeepers. *Journal of Sports Sciences* 20: 279–287.

Shiffrin, R. M. and Schneider, W. (1977) Controlled and automatic human information processing: II. Perceptual learning, automatic attending and a general theory. *Psychological Review* 84: 127–190.

Tolman, E. C. and Honzik, H. C. (1930) Introduction and removal of reward, and maze performance of rats. *University of California Publications in Psychology* 4: 257–275.

Williams, A. M. and Davids, K. (1998) Visual search strategy, selective attention, and expertise in soccer. *Research Quarterly for Exercise and Sport* 69: 111–128.

15

Sensory Substitution: Unfulfilled Promises and Fundamental Limitations

CHARLES SPENCE

Abstract Many of the most attention-grabbing claims concerning the uptake of sensory substitution devices in the last 50 years have, noticeably, not come to pass. I highlight a number of the fundamental limitations (some acknowledged, others not) that may have prevented the development and uptake of these devices amongst individuals suffering from sensory loss. First and foremost, it may simply be impossible to fully substitute for the loss of vision (the sense most substituted for) given the imbalance in neural cortical resources given to processing information in the various senses. Second, the inability to substitute for the hedonic attributes of a given modality constitutes an important, if currently under-acknowledged, problem. Most researchers tend to focus their efforts on the substitution of the sensory-discriminative (primarily spatial) aspects of stimulation instead. Third, I highlight the technological limitations associated with providing useful substitution devices for those who have lost their sense of taste or smell, senses which, theoretically, should be far easier to substitute for. Another factor that may have limited the uptake of these devices—aesthetic concerns about the appearance of users wearing them—is, I believe, likely to disappear, as a range of other augmented-perception technologies become more widely accepted.

15.1 Introduction

To my way of thinking, the history of research on the topic of sensory substitution is largely a story of poorly substantiated claims and promises that have gone pretty much unfulfilled. When I look back over the last half-century of research in this field, I am thinking, in particular, of the claims made that the blind would soon

Proceedings of the British Academy, **219**, 251–266. © The British Academy 2018.

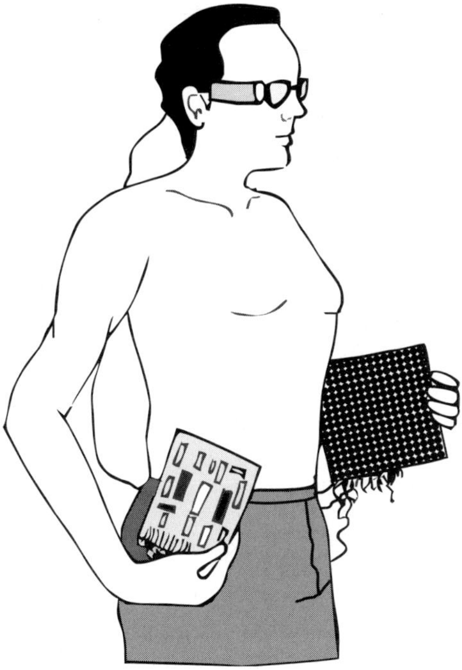

Figure 15.1 Example of early tactile-visual sensory substitution technology introduced by Paul Bach-y-Rita (1972). The large array of tactile stimulators (held in the figure's left hand) would be placed on their stomach or back. Drawing courtesy of Elena Ceriotti, inspired by a photograph that appeared in Bach-y-Rita (1972).

be watching 'tactile television' (Collins 1970), and that traders would be able to keep abreast of the latest stock market figures via vibrating displays presented on their stomachs (Hennessy 1966). These and many other promises built up around research on the development of sensory substitution devices have mostly fallen by the wayside over the intervening decades (see Abrams 2003; Marks 2006; Scadden 1969).

Similarly, more recent attempts to provide a commercially viable sensory substitution device that could provide its users with a sense of magnetic north by means of a vibrating belt (Nagel et al. 2005; cf. Baker 1980) would also seem to have fizzled out, after an initial round of what was undoubtedly intense international media hype (though see Honig 2013, for a recently commercialized version of a vibrating belt). The question therefore has to be asked: Why, given so much promise and given so much scientific, not to mention public, interest in this fundamental area of applied research, have the results thus far obtained (at least in terms of the public uptake of sensory substitution devices amongst those who might have been expected to benefit from such technologies the most) been so very disappointing?

In what follows, I will argue that a number of fundamental, if often little recognized, problems have limited the development of practical sensory substitution devices.

15.2 Cortical 'Real Estate' and the Bandwidth Problem

While the technology associated with delivering tactile stimulation (as needed, for example, for a tactile-to-visual sensory substitution (TVSS) system) has undoubtedly come a long way (Bach-y-Rita and Kercel 2003; Gallace and Spence 2014; Gallace et al. 2007) in the years since the late Paul Bach-y-Rita's exciting early work in this area (e.g. Bach-y-Rita 1972; Bach-y-Rita et al. 1969) (see Figure 15.1), I believe that there may be a more fundamental bandwidth problem that means that systems like the TVSS will never achieve widespread usage amongst those who have lost their sight. For, if one looks at the amount of cortical 'real estate' that is given over to the processing of information from each of the human senses, then I think one of the central problems in this area should immediately come into focus. While it has been estimated that more than half of the brain is given over to the processing of visual information (see Felleman and Van Essen 1991; see also Sereno et al. 1995), the equivalent figure for touch is a little over 10 per cent (see Table 15.1). One therefore has to wonder how the 'tactile brain' could ever hope to substitute for the visual brain given the marked imbalance in terms of the neural resources that are available for the processing of information in the two sensory modalities.[1]

The skin of the stomach and back are particularly insensitive sites relative to other areas of the body surface, such as, for example, the fingertips or tongue.[2] They provide the largest uninterrupted areas of skin surface, and are relatively flat, hence perhaps making the ideal and only solution for the bulky 20 × 20 arrays of tactile stimulators that constituted the earliest TVSS system (see Figure 15.1). However, there are a number of reasons why such a display was unlikely to provide a widely used solution to the problem of sensory substitution. First, it is important to note that, by and large, people are simply not used to directing their attention to their torso (see Van Hulle et al. 2013). What is more, sensitivity is so much lower

[1] Here, it is interesting to note that, when asked, most people will normally say that vision is the sense that they fear losing the most. And, indeed, life insurance policies typically compensate people more financially for a loss of this sense (their most dominant one) than following the loss of any of the others. There may, then, be an argument to be made around the focusing of research development efforts in the field of sensory substitution devices toward the sense, vision, that people apparently value the most.

[2] One interesting question here is why electrical stimulation on the tongue should be experienced in terms of the sensory substitution of, for example, a visual stimulus, rather than as a gustatory stimulus, given that electric taste devices exist (see, for example, Prof. Toko's electric taste (or electric tongue), the Insent TS-5000Z; Lewis 2010; see also Iwata et al. 2003; Ranasinghe et al. 2011, 2012).

Table 15.1 Table summarizing the number of sensors, the number of afferents, information transmission rates/channel capacity (taken from Zimmerman 1989), the estimated percentage of attentional capture (from Heilig 1992), and the percentage of neocortex (e.g. Felleman and Van Essen 1991) involved in the processing of information from each sensory modality. (See Gallace et al. 2012 for some of the limitations affecting the interpretation of these data.)

Sensory system	N. of sensors	N. of afferents	Channel capacity (bits/s)	Psychophysical channel capacity (bits/s)	% Attentional capture	% Neocortex
Vision	$2*10^8$	$2*10^6$	10^7	40	70%	55%
Audition	$3*10^4$	$2*10^4$	10^5	30	20%	3.4%
Touch	10^7	10^6	10^6	5	4%	11.5%
Taste	$3*10^7$	10^3	10^3	1(?)	1%	0.5%
Smell	$7*10^7$	10^5	10^5	1(?)	5%	n.a.

on the back than on the most sensitive skin sites (e.g. Weinsten 1968). To give you some idea of the differences in sensitivity that we are talking about here, note only that two-point discrimination acuity (a standard measure of spatial sensitivity) is less than 1 mm on the fingertips, somewhere around 15 mm on the forehead, 35 mm on the forearm, 39 mm on the back, and 45 mm on the calf (see Gallace and Spence 2014). Or note the following: while the fingertips and tongue have as many as 100 receptors per square centimetre of skin, the back of the hand has fewer than ten.

On top of these location-specific differences in sensitivity, it is worth noting that older participants also lose tactile sensitivity (e.g. Thornbury and Mistretta 1981), as well as having a reduced ability to focus their attention on any tactile stimulation being delivered to their skin while ignoring any other (potentially distracting) information/stimulation that might be being presented to the other senses (Laurienti and Hugenschmidt 2012; Poliakoff et al. 2006). As far as the tongue is concerned, there are a number of advantages associated with using this highly-sensitive part of the body surface (Sampaio et al. 2001). In particular, a device mounted there is obviously protected by the oral cavity, and, what is more, the saliva in the mouth provides a good electrolytic environment requiring just 3 per cent of the voltage needed for stimuli presented on the fingertips (note that electrotactile and not vibrotactile actuators are used with such intra-oral interfaces).

A third issue that may also have limited the uptake of these early sensory substitution systems relates to the viewpoint we take of the world around us. Most people, when asked, localize the 'I' that sees as being somewhere in their head (Bertossa et al. 2008; Limanowski and Hecht 2011; see also Alsmith and Longo 2014). For those who are familiar with it, just think of the front cover of G. A. Miller's classic book on psychology illustrating the way in which it feels for most

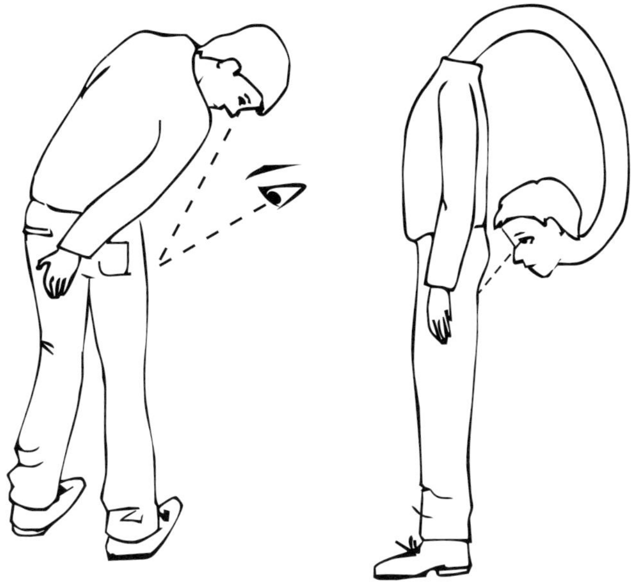

Figure 15.2 Sketches inspired by Corcoran (1977) showing some of the perspectives that an observer might adopt in order to inspect any stimuli that happen to be written on their skin. Drawing courtesy of Elena Ceriotti.

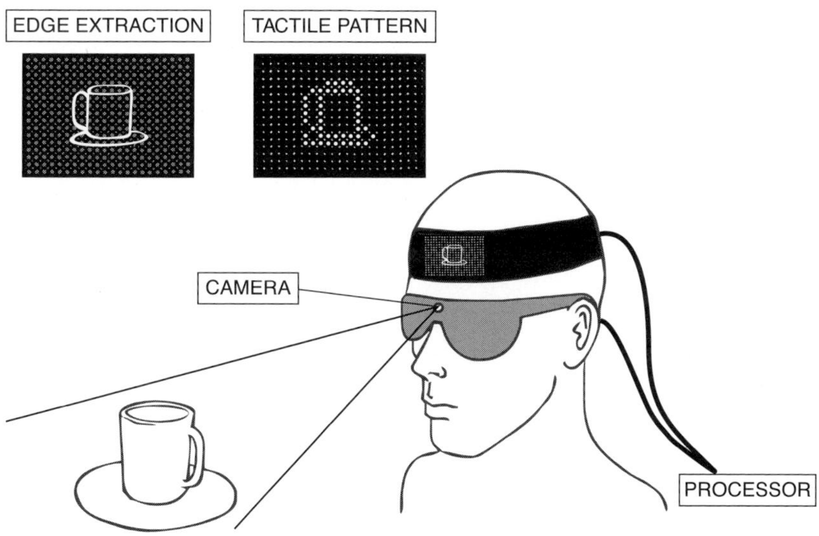

Figure 15.3 Schematic illustration of a forehead-mounted TVSS device, showing the outline impression of a cup and saucer displayed on a user's forehead. Drawing courtesy of Elena Ceriotti, inspired by an original montage that appeared in Marks (2006).

of us when we look out on the world (Miller 1991). Presumably, the torso-based TVSS system implicitly requires something of a shift in the origin of the self in order that any image displayed be correctly interpreted (see Figure 15.2). This may not be a particularly natural thing to do (see Corcoran 1977) and this too may have limited the uptake of such devices relative to, say, one of the more recent forehead-mounted displays (Kajimoto et al. 2006; see Figure 15.3).

Given these limitations, it is perhaps little wonder, then, that the users were unable to gain much information from the early TVSS systems presented on the torso. As the years have gone by, and as the technology and stimulation devices have become ever more compact (not to mention as we have increasingly moved from mechanical to electrical stimulation of the sense of touch), researchers have slowly moved towards TVSS being applied to more sensitive sites on the skin such as, for example, the forehead (Marks 2006) and tongue (Kupers and Ptito 2004; Ptito et al. 2005; Sampaio et al. 2001). While, once again, some of the early results look promising, it remains to be seen whether the unavoidable discomfort associated with having either your forehead or tongue electrocuted on a regular basis makes the information conveyed by such devices worth the effort in the majority of (non-military) applications.

15.3 But What about Neural Plasticity?

Now here one might want to argue that neural plasticity ought to be capable of redressing the neural imbalance somewhat (e.g. Bavelier et al. 2006; Rauschecker 1995; Röder and Rösler 2004; Striem-Amit et al. 2011)—plasticity that might result from the long-term absence of a given sense (e.g. Cohen et al. 1997; Finney et al. 2001; Kujala et al. 1995), or from the long-term practice of a particular perceptual skill (e.g. Münte et al. 2001; Saito et al. 2007). However, that said, I suspect that even in the best-case scenario, neural plasticity will be insufficient to reverse the marked imbalance, especially between vision and any of the other senses (e.g. touch; see also Rönnberg 1995).

15.4 Tactile Information Processing in a Multisensory World

Another important point to note here is that many of the most impressive demonstrations of people's ability to process tactile information, and to interpret patterns of stimulation presented across the skin surface, have been obtained under conditions in which the participants involved were exposed to no other competing sensory stimulation, and likely had no other task to perform than solely to interpret and respond to the pattern of tactile stimulation impinging on their skin surface (see Gallace and Spence (2014) for a review). However, as soon as one starts to look at tactile information processing in a more multisensory context, when multiple sensory inputs compete for an individual's limited attentional resources, then people's tactile information processing abilities suddenly start to look far less impressive. This again provides another reason for doubt when it comes to the implementation of sensory substitution devices that recruit the skin surface for use in real-life situations of essentially ubiquitous multisensory stimulation (Gallace and Spence 2014).

To give an illustrative example here, while most people can accurately discriminate the direction of motion of stimuli across the skin when presented in isolation, their judgements are likely to be biased heavily toward the direction of any dynamic visual, or perhaps even auditory, stimuli that may happen to be presented at more or less the same time (e.g. Soto-Faraco et al. 2004). Similarly, an observer's judgements of how many tactile stimuli have been delivered to a given point on their skin site can be similarly biased by what they happen to see or hear at around the same time (Lee and Spence 2008). Although there has been far less research on the topic to date, reasonably sensory dominance effects have also been reported in blind individuals. Though, that said, the auditory dominance over touch seen in, for example, the two-flash illusion tends to be somewhat weaker than in blindfolded sighted participants (Hötting and Röder 2004).

15.5 Reducing Workload by Means of Correspondences

I certainly believe that the recent move toward using the rules of cross-modal correspondence (Spence 2011) in the design of sensory substitution devices will undoubtedly help in terms of reducing the cognitive workload for users when it comes to interpreting the meaning of the information presented in the substituting modality (Hamilton-Fletcher and Ward 2013; Proulx 2010). Here, though, it may well turn out to be important that a designer's intuitions regarding what counts as corresponding dimensions are tested empirically, given some of the counter-intuitive findings that have emerged from the world of sonification (i.e. auditory interface design; e.g. see Kramer et al. 1999; Walker 2002; Walker and Ehrenstein 2000). Wright and Ward's (2013) intriguing recent work on the development of substitution dimensions based on the use of genetic algorithms may well provide a way forward for researchers in this regard. It should presumably also help to reduce the substantial amount of training that is normally needed in order to interpret the output from such devices. My gut feeling, though, is that even this innovative approach to the design of sensory substitution technologies will simply be insufficient in and of itself to overcome the processing imbalance outlined above, at least in the case of TVSS.

15.6 So What Is the Way Forward?

If one follows the cortical 'real estate' argument through to its logical conclusion, then the most natural way forward in the area of sensory substitution research might be to use a modality such as vision in order to substitute for a loss of gustation or olfaction—that is, for one of the senses that require much less cortical processing (see Table 15.1). At this point, though, several other important points come to the fore: (1) unfortunately, there are currently no systems available for vision-to-gustation/olfaction sensory substitution, or VG/OSS, as one might wish to call it; (2) even if such systems were to be available, they would likely not be very satisfactory (or successful) for the very simple reason that one presumably could never substitute for the reward/hedonic value of gustatory and olfactory stimuli (which is such a critical aspect of the stimulation we receive in these 'lower' senses)[3]—a similar problem also soon raises its head once one starts to think about the practicalities of substitution devices for those who have lost their ability to perceive pain (e.g. those suffering from leprosy; Auvray et al. 2010; Brand and Yancey 1993); and (3) the technology required is simply not available at the present time: while a number of research teams have been working on laboratory-based devices such as electronic noses (e.g. Gent 2013), it would seem likely that we are going to have to wait quite some time before such a device becomes available in a form that is suitably portable for someone who has lost their sense of smell (not to mention being able to more than simply detect cork taint in a wine, or discriminate between the odorous compounds associated with apples and pears—pretty much the limit of the capacity of these devices currently).[4] And even if the technical problems were to be solved, one would, anyway, still be left with the challenge of how to substitute for the multisensory experience of flavour, which itself reflects the

[3] Here I am reminded of the comment by one of the users of the TVSS, who was able to decode the fact that he was 'looking at' a *Playboy* centrefold via the TVSS, but that somehow it just wasn't stimulating (in the way that seeing the very same image would be expected to be). Bach-y-Rita (2002: 509) puts it thus: 'Subjects trained with the tactile visual substitution system have noted the absence of qualia, which in a number of cases has been quite disturbing. Thus, well-trained subjects are deeply disappointed when they explore the face of a wife or girlfriend and discover that, although they can describe details, there is no emotional content to the image. In two cases, blind university students were presented Playboy centrefolds, and although they could describe details of the undressed women, it did not have the affective component that they knew (from conversation with their sighted classmates) that it had for sighted persons. Similar experiences have previously been noted in congenitally blind persons who acquire sight following surgery: colors have no affective qualities, and faces do not transmit emotional messages (e.g., Gregory & Wallace, 1963)' (my thanks to Daniel Yon for bringing this anecdote to my attention). The absence of such an affective response, I presume, means that using such a device isn't really like seeing in a very important sense (cf. Merabet et al. 2004).

[4] That said, if one looks at suicide rates it is the loss of the sense of smell that one really needs to watch out for. Suicide rates are higher following the loss of the sense of smell than following the loss of any other sense, including vision—a statistic that could be used by those wishing to justify the costs associated with developing sensory substitution devices for the lower, non-visual sense.

integration of olfactory with gustatory and oral-somatosensory tactile inputs (ISO 1992, 2008; Iwata 2011; Lewis 2010; Spence 2012; see also Putzar et al. 2007).[5]

Hence, while sensory substitution devices may be very good at capturing and presenting the sensory-discriminative attributes of the stimulation in the substituted modality (at least in the case of those devices substituting for a loss of vision), there is, as yet, no evidence that they can provide the more affective/hedonic attributes of sensory stimulation (cf. Pfaffmann 1960). I would like to suggest that this may be one of the key reasons why such devices have not seen a much greater uptake amongst those suffering from some sort of sensory deficit. Remember that reward is one of the key drivers motivating human behaviour (e.g. Baxter and Murray 2002; Blood and Zatorre 2001; Burke et al. 2008; Theeuwes and Belopolsky 2012). What is more, that inability to substitute for the hedonic qualities in the substituting modality is going to be more salient for what have been termed the 'lower', or more emotional, senses of olfaction, touch, and gustation (than for the higher senses of audition and vision). Note here that researchers have argued that all smells are intrinsically hedonically valent—either pleasant or unpleasant (e.g. see Benderly 1988; Hinton and Henley 1993; Schiffmann 1974).

15.7 Methods of Assessment

Finally, if one looks back over the history of research on the topic of sensory substitution, one cautionary note that comes to the fore is the danger of relying too heavily on the free subjective report that was such an important, not to mention salient, feature of much of the early reporting in this area (e.g. see Guarniero 1974, 1977). With this in mind, it is worrying to see this kind of evidence once again starting to gain prominence in the field (e.g. see Ward and Meijer 2010, for one representative example). I am firmly of the belief that in order to really move forward with research in the field of sensory substitution, scientists and philosophers will need to work on more objective tests of the phenomena that they are most interested in (such as externalization, or 'distal attribution'—that is, the ability to locate a stimulus as occurring away from the receptor surface) (e.g. Bach-y-Rita et al. 1969; Siegle and Warren 2010).

[5]The only people who present to my office suffering from sensory loss are those complaining of a loss of taste. Ironically, however, what these individuals have nearly always lost is their sense of smell instead (Rozin 1982). In fact, those rare individuals who have lost their ability to taste (either because they have had their tongue removed—typically not voluntarily (see Brillat-Savarin 1835)—or as a result of herpes; see Pfaffmann and Bartoshuk 1990) do not report much of a loss of sensation.

15.8 Perspective-Taking on the Skin

One possibility here that we have been working on in our own research (see Auvray et al. 2009; Skatova et al. 2008) involves the use of the ambiguous letters task. In brief, a long history of research has shown how if an ambiguous letter is presented ('written') on the skin (e.g. letter pairs such as b/d and p/q are especially popular), then an observer may either interpret the pattern of stimulation in a way that suggests that they are looking out through their skin (from the inside out, as it were), or else take a perspective suggesting that they had adopted the viewpoint of someone who might have been drawing on their skin (see Krech and Crutchfield 1958, for the initial report of this fascinating phenomenon) (see Figure 15.4). Interestingly, the perspective taken by a participant has been shown to depend on a number of factors, including the skin site stimulated (Natsoulas and Dubanoski 1964), the posture adopted (e.g. Corcoran 1977; Parsons and Shimojo 1987), and whether one

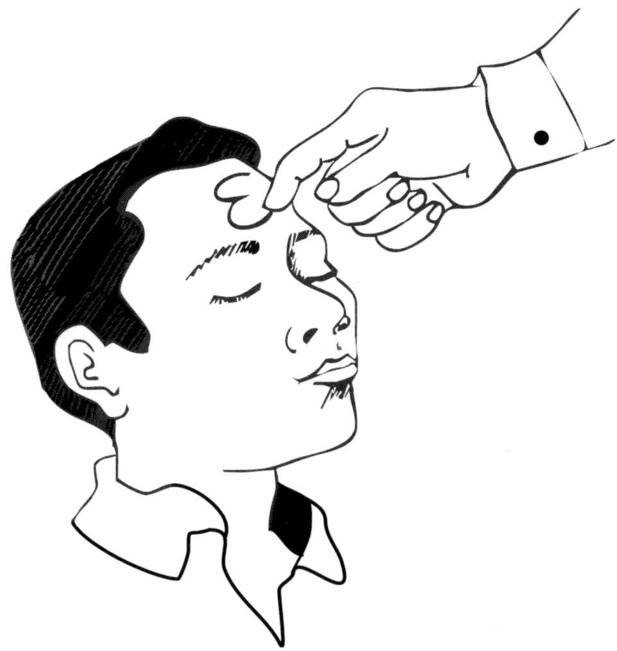

Figure 15.4 Schematic illustration of the ambiguous letter task. Krech and Crutchfield (1958) in their textbook, *Elements of Psychology*, used this task in order to highlight the fact that different perspectives could, and in fact were, taken by participants who had been instructed to discriminate, or else to identify, the identity of the letter that had been drawn on their forehead. Drawing courtesy of Elena Ceriotti, inspired by an original image from Krech and Crutchfield (1958). (As an interesting aside, here, one might wish to consider what effect the presence of the experimenter writing on the participant's skin might have had on the perspective taken by the participant; cf. Galinsky et al. 2006; Natsoulas 1966.)

happens to find oneself in a dominant/powerful or submissive role (cf. Galinsky et al. 2006). This task has also been extended to the congenitally blind (Shimojo et al. 1989). Anyway, one can see how such an indirect measure (simply reporting on the identity of the letter that is perceived) might one day be used as a proxy measure with which to infer whether tactile stimuli presented on the skin, say, have been externalized or not (see Arnold et al. 2016, 2017).

15.9 Aesthetic Concerns

Finally, one of the other factors that may, traditionally, have limited the uptake of such devices, is aesthetic concerns: concerns about what a user might look like while wearing such an ungainly augmentation/substitution technology. Here, though, I believe that such concerns are likely to disappear in the very near future, as a range of other augmented perception technologies become more widely accepted (fashionable even), just think Google glasses,[6] within society at large, even for those who are not suffering from any obvious form of sensory loss.

15.10 Conclusions

In conclusion, despite many confident and optimistic claims having been made over the years regarding the likely future of sensory substitution devices, few of the more spectacular, or attention-grabbing, predictions have actually come to pass. What is more, there are remarkably few people out there suffering from sensory deficits who appear to find the benefits of utilizing such devices to outweigh the associated costs (be those costs aesthetic—see Figure 15.1—or cognitive). What is more, this would not seem to be simply a lack of concern about the loss of one's senses, given the success of (and huge interest in) cochlear implants (House 1976), not to mention glasses (i.e. repairing or enhancing one's abilities from within a given sensory modality).

Instead, I wish to argue that there are a number of more fundamental limitations that have constrained the uptake of sensory substitution devices amongst those suffering from some form of sensory impairment. First and foremost, I do not think that one can ever fully substitute for a loss of vision given the cortical imbalance in the neural processing resources given over to each of the senses. However, a second and seemingly under-acknowledged problem in this area relates to the failure to substitute for the loss of the hedonic attributes of sensory stimulation in the substituted modality. Most researchers would seem a little too happy to focus their

[6] See www.google.com/glass/.

research efforts on substituting for the sensory-discriminative aspects of stimulation (especially the reproduction of spatial information), and seemingly ignore the substitution of the more hedonic aspects of sensory information. Finally, there is also a very real problem here in terms of the extant technology, as highlighted by any attempt to provide a portable sensory substitution device for those who have lost their sense of smell, say. Until these fundamental problems have been resolved, it is hard to see how this field of research will be able to move forward, at least in terms of supporting the more widespread uptake of such sensory substitution devices amongst those who might be expected to benefit from them most.

References

Abrams, M. (2003) Can you see with your tongue? The brain is so adaptable, some researchers now think, that any of the five senses can be rewired. *Discovery Magazine*, 6 January, http://discovermagazine.com/2003/jun/feattongue.

Alsmith, A. J. T. and Longo, M. R. (2014) Where exactly am I? Self-location judgements distribute between head and torso. *Consciousness and Cognition* 24: 70–74.

Arnold, G., Spence, C. and Auvray, M. (2016) Taking someone else's spatial perspective: natural stance or effortful decentring? *Cognition* 148: 27–33.

Arnold, G., Spence, C. and Auvray, M. (2017) A unity of the self or a multiplicity of locations? How the graphesthesia task sheds light on the role of spatial perspectives in bodily self-consciousness. *Consciousness and Cognition* 56: 100–114.

Auvray, M., Gallace, A. and Spence, C. (2009) What perspective do people take when interpreting tactile letters presented on their bodies? Poster given at the 10th International Multisensory Research Forum (IMRF), 29 July–2 August, New York.

Auvray, M., Myin, E. and Spence, C. (2010) The sensory-discriminative and affective-motivational aspects of pain. *Neuroscience and Biobehavioral Reviews* 34: 214–223.

Bach-y-Rita, P. (1972) *Brain Mechanisms in Sensory Substitution*. New York: Academic Press.

Bach-y-Rita, P. (2002) Sensory substitution and qualia. In A. Noë and E. Thompson (eds) *Vision and Mind*. Cambridge, MA: MIT Press, 497–514.

Bach-y-Rita, P. and Kercel, S. W. (2003) Sensory substitution and the human-machine interface. *Trends in Cognitive Sciences* 7: 541–546.

Bach-y-Rita, P., Collins, C. C., Saunders, F., White, B. and Scadden, L. (1969) Vision substitution by tactile image projection. *Nature* 221: 963–964.

Baker, R. R. (1980) Goal orientation by blindfolded humans after long-distance displacement: possible involvement of a magnetic sense. *Science* 210: 555–557.

Bavelier, D., Dye, M. W. and Hauser, P. C. (2006) Do deaf individuals see better? *Trends in Cognitive Sciences* 10: 512–518.

Baxter, M. G. and Murray, E. A. (2002) The amygdala and reward. *Nature Reviews Neuroscience* 3: 563–573.

Benderly, B. L. (1988) Aroma driven: on the trail of our most emotional sense. *Health* 20(December): 62–65, 77.

Bertossa, F., Besa, M., Ferrari, R. and Ferri, F. (2008) Point zero: a phenomenological inquiry into the seat of consciousness. *Perceptual and Motor Skills* 107: 323–335.

Blood, A. J. and Zatorre, R. J. (2001) Intensely pleasurable responses to music correlate with activity in brain regions implicated in reward and emotion. *Proceedings of the National Academy of Sciences of the United States of America* 98: 11818–11823.

Brand, P. and Yancey, P. (1993) *Pain: The Gift Nobody Wants*. New York: HarperCollins.

Brillat-Savarin, J. A. (1835) *Physiologie du goût* [*The Philosopher in the Kitchen / The Physiology of Taste*]. Bruxelles: J. P. Meline. Translated by A. Lalauze (1884) *A Handbook of Gastronomy*. London: Nimmo & Bain.

Burke, K. A., Franz, T. M., Miller, D. N. and Schoenbaum, G. (2008) The role of the orbitofrontal cortex in the pursuit of happiness and more specific rewards. *Nature* 454: 340–345.

Cohen, L. G., Celnik, P., Pascual-Leone, A., Corwell, B., Faiz, L., Dambrosia, J., Honda, M., Sadato, N., Gerloff, C., Catala, M. D. and Hallett, M. (1997) Functional relevance of cross-modal plasticity in blind humans. *Nature* 389: 180–183.

Collins, C. C. (1970) Tactile television—mechanical and electrical image projection. *IEEE Transactions on Man Machine Systems*, MMS-11: 65–71.

Corcoran, D. W. J. (1977) The phenomena of the disembodied eye or is it a matter of personal geography? *Perception* 6: 247–253.

Felleman, D. J. and Van Essen, D. C. (1991) Distributed hierarchical processing in primate cerebral cortex. *Cerebral Cortex* 1: 1–47.

Finney, E. M., Fine, I. and Dobkins, K. R. (2001) Visual stimuli activate auditory cortex in the deaf. *Nature Neuroscience* 4: 1171–1173.

Galinsky, A. D., Magee, J. C., Inesi, M. E. and Gruenfeld, D. H. (2006) Power and perspectives not taken. *Psychological Science* 17: 1068–1074.

Gallace, A. and Spence, C. (2014) *In Touch with the Future: The Sense of Touch from Cognitive Neuroscience to Virtual Reality*. Oxford: Oxford University Press.

Gallace, A., Tan, H. Z. and Spence, C. (2007) The body surface as a communication system: the state of the art after 50 years. *Presence: Teleoperators and Virtual Environments* 16: 655–676.

Gallace, A., Ngo, M. K., Sulaitis, J. and Spence, C. (2012) Multisensory presence in virtual reality: possibilities and limitations. In G. Ghinea, F. Andres and S. Gulliver (eds) *Multiple Sensorial Media Advances and Applications: New Developments in MulSeMedia*. Hershey, PA: IGI Global, 1–40.

Gent, E. (2013) 'Electronic nose' better than human sense of smell. *Engineering and Technology Magazine*, 8 May, http://eandt.theiet.org/news/2013/may/nose-electronic.cfm.

Gregory, R. L. and Wallace, J. G. (1963) Recovery from early blindness: a case study. *Quarterly Journal of Psychology*, Monograph No. 2.

Guarniero, G. (1974) Experience of tactile vision. *Perception* 3: 101–104.

Guarniero, G. (1977) Tactile vision: a personal view. *Journal of Visual Impairment and Blindness* 71: 125–130.

Hamilton-Fletcher, G. and Ward, J. (2013) Representing colour through hearing and touch in sensory substitution. *Multisensory Research* 26(6): 503–532.

Heilig, M. L. (1992) El cine del futuro: the cinema of the future. *Presence: Teleoperators and Virtual Environments* 1: 279–294.

Hennessy, J. R. (1966) Cutaneous sensitivity communications. *Human Factors* 8: 463–469.

Hinton, P. B. and Henley, T. B. (1993) Cognitive and affective components of stimuli presented in three modes. *Bulletin of the Psychonomic Society* 31: 595–598.

Honig, Z. (2013) Triposo Travel Belt vibrates to help you locate attractions (video). www.engadget.com/2013/09/13/triposo-travel-belt/?ncid=rss_semi (accessed 13 September 2013).

Hötting, K. and Röder. B. (2004) Hearing cheats touch, but less in congenitally blind than in sighted individuals. *Psychological Science* 15: 60–64.

House, W. F. (1976) Cochlear implant. *Annals of Otology, Rhinology and Laryngology* 85: 1–93.

ISO (1992) *Standard 5492: Terms Relating to Sensory Analysis*. International Organization for Standardization. Vienna: Austrian Standards Institute.

ISO (2008) *Standard 5492: Terms Relating to Sensory Analysis*. International Organization for Standardization. Vienna: Austrian Standards Institute.

Iwata, H. (2011) VR for food texture. *Foods and Food Ingredients Journal of Japan* 216: 4.

Iwata, H., Yano, H., Uemura, T. and Moriya, T. (2003) Food simulator. ICAT 2003, 3–5 December, Tokyo, Japan.

Kajimoto, H., Kanno, Y. and Tachi, S. (2006) Forehead electro-tactile display for vision substitution. *Proceedings of the Virtual Reality Society of Japan Annual Conference*, 1A4–4.

Kramer, G., Walker, B., Bonebright, T., Cook, P., Flowers, J., Miner, N., et al. (1999) *The Sonification Report: Status of the Field and Research Agenda*. Report prepared for the National Science Foundation by members of the International Community for Auditory Display. Santa Fe, NM: International Community for Auditory Display.

Krech, D. and Crutchfield, R. S. (1958) *Elements of Psychology*. New York: A. A. Knopf.

Kujala, T., Huotilainen, M., Sinkkonen, J., Ahonen, A. I., Alho, K., Hamalainen, M. S., et al. (1995) Visual cortex activation in blind humans during sound discrimination. *Neuroscience Letters* 183: 143–146.

Kupers, R. and Ptito, M. (2004) 'Seeing' through the tongue: cross-modal plasticity in the congenitally blind. *International Congress Series* 1270: 79–84.

Laurienti, P. J. and Hugenschmidt, C. E. (2012) Multisensory processes in old age. In A. Bremner, D. Lewkowicz and C. Spence (eds) *Multisensory Development*. Oxford: Oxford University Press, 251–270.

Lee, J.-H. and Spence, C. (2008) Feeling what you hear: task-irrelevant sounds modulate tactile perception delivered via a touch screen. *Journal of Multisensory User Interfaces* 2: 145–156.

Lewis, L. (2010) Strawberry shortcake? No, it's squid guts and cream. *The Times*, 25 August, 33.

Limanowski, J. and Hecht, H. (2011) Where do we stand on locating the self? *Psychology* 2(4): 312–317.

Marks, P. (2006) Gadgets get the feel of the tactile world. *New Scientist* 2560 (15 July): 27.

Merabet, L., Thut, G., Murray, B., Andrews, J., Hsiao, S. and Pascual-Leone, A. (2004) Feeling by sight or seeing by touch? *Neuron* 42: 173–179.

Miller, G. A. (1991) *Psychology: The Science of Mental Life*. London: Penguin.

Münte, T. F., Kohlmetz, C., Nager, W. and Altenmüller, E. (2001) Superior auditory spatial tuning in conductors. *Nature* 409: 580.

Nagel, S. K., Carl, C., Kringe, T., Märtin, R. and König, P. (2005) Beyond sensory substitution—learning the sixth sense. *Journal of Neural Engineering* 2: R13–R26.

Natsoulas, T. (1966) Locus and orientation of the perceiver (ego) under variable, constant, and no perspective instructions. *Journal of Personality and Social Psychology* 3: 190–196.

Natsoulas, T. and Dubanoski, R. A. (1964) Inferring the locus and orientation of the perceiver from responses to stimulation of the skin. *American Journal of Psychology* 77: 281–285.

Parsons, L. M. and Shimojo, S. (1987) Perceived spatial organization of cutaneous patterns on surfaces of the human body in various positions. *Journal of Experimental Psychology: Human Perception and Performance* 13: 488–505.

Pfaffmann, C. (1960) The pleasure of sensation. *Psychological Review* 67: 253–268.

Pfaffmann, C. and Bartoshuk, L. M. (1990) Taste loss due to herpes zoster oticus: an update after 19 months. *Chemical Senses* 15: 657–658.

Poliakoff, E., Ashworth, S., Lowe, C. and Spence, C. (2006) Vision and touch in ageing: crossmodal selective attention and visuotactile spatial interactions. *Neuropsychologia* 44: 507–517.

Proulx, M. J. (2010) Synthetic synaesthesia and sensory substitution. *Consciousness and Cognition* 19: 501–503.

Ptito, M., Moesgaard, S. M., Gjedde, A. and Kupers, R. (2005) Cross-modal plasticity revealed by electrotactile stimulation of the tongue in the congenitally blind. *Brain* 128: 606–614.

Putzar, L., Goerendt, I., Lange, K., Rösler, F. and Röder, B. (2007) Early visual deprivation impairs multisensory interactions in humans. *Nature Neuroscience* 10: 1243–1245.

Ranasinghe, N., Karunanayaka, K., Cheok, A. D., Fernando, O. N. N., Nii, H. and Gopalakrishnakone, P. (2011) Digital taste and smell communication. *Proceedings of the 6th International Conference on Body Area Networks* (BodyNets 2011), ICST, Brussels, 78–84.

Ranasinghe, N., Cheok, A. D. and Nakatsu, R. (2012) Taste/IP: the sensation of taste for digital communication. *Proceedings of the 14th ACM International Conference on Multimodal Interaction* (ICMI 2012), New York, 409–416.

Rauschecker, J. P. (1995) Compensatory plasticity and sensory substitution in the cerebral cortex. *Trends in Neurosciences* 18: 36–43.

Röder, B. and Rösler, F. (2004) Compensatory plasticity as a consequence of sensory loss. In G. A. Calvert, C. Spence and B. E. Stein (eds) *The Handbook of Multisensory Processes*. Cambridge, MA: MIT Press, 719–747.

Rönnberg, J. (1995) Perceptual compensation in the deaf and blind: myth or reality? In R. A. Dixon and L. Bäckman (eds) *Compensating for Psychological Deficits and Declines: Managing Losses and Promoting Gains*. Mahwah, NJ: Lawrence Erlbaum, 251–274.

Rozin, P. (1982) 'Taste-smell confusions' and the duality of the olfactory sense. *Perception and Psychophysics* 31: 397–401.

Saito, D. N., Okada, T., Honda, M., Yonekura, Y. and Sadato, N. (2007) Practice makes perfect: the neural substrates of tactile discrimination by Mah-Jong experts include the primary visual cortex. *BMC Neuroscience* 7: 79.

Sampaio, E., Maris, S. and Bach-y-Rita, P. (2001) Brain plasticity: 'visual' acuity of blind persons via the tongue. *Brain Research* 908: 204–207.

Scadden, L. (1969) A tactual substitute for sight. *New Scientist* 41: 677–678.

Schiffmann, S. S. (1974) Physiochemical correlates of olfactory quality. *Science* 185: 112–117.
Sereno, M. I., Dale, A. M., Reppas, J. B., Kwong, K. K., Belliveau, J. W., Brady, T. J., Rosen, B. R. and Tootell, R. B. H. (1995) Borders of multiple visual areas in humans revealed by functional magnetic resonance imaging. *Science* 268: 889–893.
Shimojo, S., Sasaki, M., Parsons, L. M. and Torii, S. (1989) Mirror reversals by blind subjects in cutaneous perception and motor production of letters and numbers. *Perception and Psychophysics* 45: 145–152.
Siegle, J. H. and Warren, W. H. (2010) Distal attribution and distance perception in sensory substitution. *Perception* 39: 208–223.
Skatova, A., Spence, C., Auvray, M. and Gallace, A. (2008) On the recognition of letters drawn on the skin. Paper presented at the Third International Conference on Cognitive Science, Moscow, June.
Soto-Faraco, S., Spence, C., Lloyd, D. and Kingstone, A. (2004) Moving multisensory research along: motion perception across sensory modalities. *Current Directions in Psychological Science* 13: 29–32.
Spence, C. (2011) Crossmodal correspondences: a tutorial review. *Attention, Perception, and Psychophysics* 73: 971–995.
Spence, C. (2012) Multi-sensory integration and the psychophysics of flavour perception. In J. Chen and L. Engelen (eds) *Food Oral Processing: Fundamentals of Eating and Sensory Perception*. Oxford: Blackwell Publishing, 203–219.
Striem-Amit, E., Bubic, A. and Amedi, A. (2011) Neurophysiological mechanisms underlying plastic changes and rehabilitation following sensory loss in blindness and deafness. In M. M. Murray and M. Wallace (eds) *Frontiers in the Neural Bases of Multisensory Processes*. Boca Raton, FL: CRC Press, 395–422.
Theeuwes, J. and Belopolsky, A. V. (2012) Reward grabs the eye: oculomotor capture by rewarding stimuli. *Vision Research* 74: 80–85.
Thornbury, J. M. and Mistretta, C. M. (1981) Tactile sensitivity as a function of age. *Journal of Gerontology* 36: 34–39.
Van Hulle, L., Juravle, G., Spence, C., Crombez, G. and Van Damme, S. (2013) Attention modulates sensory suppression during back movements. *Consciousness and Cognition* 22: 420–429.
Walker, B. N. (2002) Magnitude estimation of conceptual data dimensions for use in sonification. *Journal of Experimental Psychology: Applied* 8: 211–221.
Walker, B. N. and Ehrenstein, A. (2000) Pitch and pitch change interact in auditory displays. *Journal of Experimental Psychology: Applied* 6: 15–30.
Ward, J. and Meijer, P. (2010) Visual experiences in the blind induced by an auditory sensory substitution device. *Consciousness and Cognition* 19: 492–500.
Weinstein, S. (1968) Intensive and extensive aspects of tactile sensitivity as a function of body part, sex, and laterality. In D. R. Kenshalo (ed.) *The Skin Senses*. Springfield, IL: Thomas, 195–222.
Wright, T. and Ward, J. (2013) The evolution of a visual-to-auditory sensory substitution device using interactive genetic algorithms. *Quarterly Journal of Experimental Psychology* 66: 1620–1638.
Zimmerman, M. (1989) The nervous system in the context of information theory. In R. F. Schmidt and G. Thews, *Human Physiology*, 2nd complete edn. Berlin: Springer-Verlag, 166–173.

16

Sensory Substitution and Non-Sensory Feelings

DAVID SUAREZ, DIANA ACOSTA-NAVAS,
UMUT BAYSAN AND KEVIN CONNOLLY

Abstract One limitation of sensory substitution devices (SSDs) is their inability to reproduce the non-sensory feelings that are normally associated with visual experiences, especially hedonic responses. This is sometimes reported to cause SSD users frustration and it is unclear that improvements in acuity, bandwidth, or training will resolve the issue. We offer a novel solution. Researchers can produce hedonic responses by eliciting these feelings artificially, pairing distal objects that should be pleasurable to pleasurable outputs from the SSD. We outline two strategies for accomplishing this: first, by means of a prefixed, hardwired association of distal objects to SSD outputs; and second, by means of a flexible, feedback-based association created by subject-directed matching of distal objects to SSD outputs. We evaluate both strategies, and argue that the feedback-based strategy is more promising. Researchers could use this strategy to help the blind, allowing them to take pleasure in objects they perceive using SSDs.

16.1 Introduction

Perception provides us with sensory contents such as shapes, colours, flavours, and smells. In ordinary perception, these contents are accompanied by a variety of non-sensory feelings. Perception arouses *noetic feelings* concerning the presence or familiarity of what one is perceiving, *emotions* such as love and hate, *hedonic responses* such as pleasure and pain, and *aesthetic feelings* of beauty and ugliness. Although some non-sensory feelings seem to be naturally associated with specific sensory contents, non-sensory feelings do not seem to be supervenient on the sensory contents they accompany, since non-sensory feelings can vary while sensory contents remain the same. In Capgras syndrome, for instance, patients perceive

Proceedings of the British Academy, **219**, 267–277. © The British Academy 2018.

the face of a close relative, yet do not have a feeling of familiarity. Such patients consider their relatives to be impostors, since they have no feeling of familiarity when seeing them (Christodoulou 1977).

The failure of supervenience of non-sensory feelings on sensory contents seems also to be supported by the cases in which sensory substitution devices (SSDs)[1] are used. SSD users very often report an absence of hedonic, emotional and aesthetic feelings, despite being capable of identifying the visual scenes that would typically elicit those feelings. Hedonic responses are generated by some stimuli in the substituting modality,[2] but these responses are not associated to the visual scenes that would normally generate them. Therefore, even though many users of SSDs are eventually able to attribute stimuli in substituting modalities to distal objects, it takes training—and, in many cases, explicit instruction in the mapping between substituting and substituted modalities—to generate the right non-sensory feelings from the appropriate distal objects. Ordinary distal attribution occurs 'when the sensations felt on the skin or in the ears are projected onto a distant perceived object, which should correspond to the one captured by the camera' (Deroy and Auvray 2015: 333). After a period of training, subjects come to attribute their sensory contents to distal objects rather than to the proximal stimuli delivered by the SSD, but this is not usually the case with non-sensory feelings.

This raises the question whether an analogous phenomenon to distal attribution can occur with non-sensory feelings, given enough training of the appropriate sort. So, for example, will subjects project their hedonic responses onto the distal objects perceived by means of the SSD, rather than attributing them to the outputs of the SSD itself? The degree to which this will occur is an empirical question, to be answered by future research, but here we should note two things. First, distal attribution of non-sensory contents is part of normal experience. When we see a beautiful painting, we project the pleasure we feel onto the painting; it is not just our immediate visual sensations that we take to be pleasing, but the painting itself which is pleasurable to see. Second, for this very reason, distal attribution of non-sensory contents is both expected and desired by SSD users.

[1] A sensory substitution device (SSD) delivers information about the environment, normally perceived through stimulation in one sensory modality (the 'substituted modality'), through the production of stimulation in another sensory modality (the 'substituting modality'). Most SSDs aim to substitute for vision, and consist of a video camera that feeds information into a conversion unit which converts that information into auditory or tactile stimuli. Such devices can be used by the blind to assist in their autonomous navigation of the world.

[2] We take a stimulus to be an objective property or object in the external world. We use 'proximal stimulus' to refer to the property or object directly delivered to the substituting modality, such as a particular tone delivered by a visual-to-audio SSD. By 'distal stimulus' we mean the property or object in the substituted modality that the proximal stimulus is used to represent, such as the brightness represented by the tone.

One might wonder why SSDs *should* duplicate normal non-sensory feelings. After all, if sensory substitution aims only at providing alternative means for delivering sensory contents, then the duplication of *non*-sensory feelings would be irrelevant to that goal. However, the duplication of non-sensory feelings can plausibly be included amongst the *therapeutic* goals of sensory substitution. Beyond enabling practical capacities dependent on sensory contents such as object recognition and autonomous navigation, sensory substitution also has the potential to provide patients with pleasure, emotional connection, aesthetic experience, and a sense of being grounded in a shared reality. As Bach-y-Rita and his colleagues report (Bach-y-Rita 2002; Bach-y-Rita et al. 2003), users of TVSS devices[3] found the 'absence of qualia' (i.e. the absence of affective responses) rather disappointing, if not disturbing. This suggests that users of SSDs hope for more than just enhancements to their practical capacities, but also for experiences that enrich their lives in other ways. Similarly, Spence (2013) has argued that flavour and olfactory substitution devices would be far less appealing if they failed to produce the pleasures associated with tasty or fragrant stimuli. In the absence of such pleasures, it seems unlikely that patients with impairments of taste or olfaction would have much of a desire for hedonically-neutral, purely informational substitutes. So, while sensory substitution does aim at enabling practical capacities, it seems plausible to think that the provision of other life-enriching experiences constitutes a worthwhile therapeutic goal.

The goal of this essay is to explore whether or not sensory substitution devices can capture the non-sensory feelings that typically accompany perception. In the next section, we present evidence that SSDs do not currently capture such feelings. Next, we explore whether this failure is fully explicable by the fact that the acuity and bandwidth of the SSDs are poor. Finally, we offer a suggestion: by using a feedback mechanism, subjects might pair pleasurable objects in their environment with pleasurable sounds (or pleasurable patterns of touch) delivered by SSDs. This will enable them to experience hedonic responses when they perceive those objects through the SSDs.

16.2 Current SSDs Fail to Generate Normal Non-Sensory Feelings

Since the early days of research on sensory substitution, it has been reported that SSDs do not always preserve the non-sensory feelings that are associated with

[3] Tactile-vision sensory substitution (TVSS) devices are SSDs that convert patterns of luminance picked up by a camera into isomorphically-organized tactile stimuli which are delivered to the skin through a matrix of solenoids usually mounted on the back, or through a matrix of electrodes held on the tongue.

normal perceptual experiences. In particular, SSDs fail to generate normal emotional and hedonic responses (Bach-y-Rita 2002) or to convey to the subject the 'values and the quality of lived experience associated with perceived entities' (Lenay et al. 2003). Researchers call these absent features, *qualia*. Evidence about the absence of (normal) qualia and subsequent frustration in SSD usage includes a case where two (presumably heterosexual) male subjects using a TVSS apparatus were shown pictures of nude women, and another case where subjects were shown pictures of their partners. In these cases, as Bach-y-Rita reports, although subjects were able to recognize what they were being shown, they were surprised and disappointed to discover that they did not find these stimuli pleasing (2002: 509). Bach-y-Rita also reports a few cases in which qualia were developed, but he emphasizes their scarcity (2002: 510). Concerning the reports about the absence of (normal) qualia in SSD usage, Lenay et al. (2003) suggest that the subsequent frustration could result from the fact that blind subjects typically use sensory substitution devices alone rather than in groups. Lenay et al. argue that qualia are 'closely linked to the existence of a shared history and collective memory, a memory which can only emerge in the course of interactions between several subjects in a common environment' (2003: 285).

The disappointment experienced by SSD users is akin to the frustration experienced by people with early blindness who regain their vision after sight recovery operations. It should be noted that such cases are very rare (Ostrovsky et al. 2006), so it is difficult to draw strong conclusions from the available reports. Moreover, only a small number of these reports treat issues related to the experience of qualia. Nevertheless, one exception is the case of SB (Gregory and Wallace 1963; Gregory 1990). SB lost his sight when he was 10 months old, and regained it through a surgical intervention when he was 52 years old. Although he learned to recognize objects very successfully thereafter (he was even able to read the time from a clock a few days after the surgery), his perceptual experiences remained qualitatively different from those of a normally-sighted subject. Facial expressions that he was able to recognize did not carry emotional messages; he did not dislike any colours; he was not very enthusiastic about vivid and colourful scenes (he preferred to sit in the dark); and he was bored on sightseeing tours. While these examples do suggest that there were some non-sensory feelings associated with his visual experiences, his experiences were, nevertheless, clearly quite different from those of the normally-sighted. In particular, the difference between SB's postoperative visual experience and a normally-sighted person's visual experience could be interpreted as primarily a difference in his profile of hedonic responses. The difficulty of generating normal profiles of hedonic responses after sight recovery operations resembles the difficulty of transferring hedonic aspects from one sensory modality to another. With respect to SSDs in particular, Deroy and Auvray note that 'shapes perceived in one sensory modality are not directly associated to pleasures or pains felt while perceiving the same shape in another sensory modality' (2012: 4).

Bach-y-Rita (2002), however, is rather optimistic about the possibility of conferring such hedonic messages to the substituting modalities. He thinks that the case is analogous to the acquisition of a second language:

> The emotional aspects of the new language are often lacking, especially with emotionally charged words and expressions, such as curse words. It appears that both spoken language and other sensory messages require long experience within the context of other aspects of cultural and emotional development to be able to contain qualia.
>
> (Bach-y-Rita 2002: 510)

So, with sufficient training, Bach-y-Rita suggests that SSD usage would generate normal hedonic responses. He also speculates that if such SSD 'systems are used from infancy, the qualia will develop, even if the system is not continuously in use' (Bach-y-Rita 2002: 510). In fact, data seem to support this hypothesis, as '[s]ystems for blind babies . . . have already provided some suggestive evidence for the development of qualia, such as the infant's smile upon perceiving the mother's approach' (Bach-y-Rita 2002: 510).

Regardless of whether Bach-y-Rita's optimism about capturing the normal qualitative aspects of experience through longer exposure to SSDs is justified or not, it can be fairly stated that, currently, SSDs fail to generate normal non-sensory feelings. In the following sections, we will consider the possible sources of the problem and discuss solutions to it.

16.3 Is the Problem Just Bandwidth or Acuity?

In a 2001 study, Sampaio, Maris and Bach-y-Rita took subjects who had received some training with TVSS, and tested them with a standard ophthalmological test. The 'visual' acuity of these subjects measured on average only 20/430. Without training, their acuity with TVSS was even worse, averaging only 20/860 (Sampaio et al. 2001: 205). Given these results, perhaps the reason why SSDs do not generate affective characteristics is because the acuity of a subject is so poor when using an SSD. That would explain why Bach-y-Rita's male SSD subjects did not respond in the expected way when presented with the pictures of the nude women. The 'picture' was not clear enough.

Vision and audition may present a bandwidth problem for SSDs, but it is not clear that the same would be true with respect to touch, smell, or taste. According to Charles Spence, we can transduce 40 bits per second through vision and 30 through hearing. In contrast, we transduce just 5 bits per second through the skin, and just 1 bit per second through taste and smell (Spence 2013). If the bandwidth of vision and audition is so high that it cannot be fully captured by SSDs making use of the remaining modalities, then this would explain why users of visual or auditory SSDs would have poor acuity while using them, and hence lack the expected non-sensory responses. By contrast, the bandwidths of touch, smell, and taste do not present a comparable problem. This is because the bandwidths of these senses are low enough to be captured by an SSD using vision or audition as the substituting modality. But take a sense like smell. Even though smell does not present the bandwidth problem that vision presents, it seems plausible that an SSD designed to substitute for olfaction would still not capture the non-sensory feelings associated with smell. For example, suppose we were able to deliver all of the information relevant to olfactory perception through vision instead, with the same informational bandwidth, and the same acuity as normal olfaction. Nevertheless, it seems plausible to think that delivering this information would still be insufficient, on its own, to generate the pleasure many of us associate with the smell of a rose. Given this plausible assumption, it can be suggested that receiving the information normally provided by a given sensory modality may not be sufficient (even with the appropriate SSD acuity, bandwidth, and training) for the duplication of the substituted modality's normal profile of non-sensory feelings.

16.4 Natural vs. Artificial Associations

Even if SSDs are currently incapable of reproducing accurate profiles of non-sensory feelings, it is worth considering whether it would be possible to create artificial associations between the distal stimuli that SSDs are tracking, and the natural hedonic responses SSDs produce with proximal stimuli. For example, users of the FeelSpace belt[4] report having pleasurable sensations when using the device (Konig 2013), and users of the vOICe[5] describe some of the sounds they hear as beautiful. Researchers might take these natural responses and artificially associate them with pleasant or unpleasant distal visual scenes. The problem is that these natural responses are not associated to the distal stimuli that SSDs are tracking, but rather to the proximal auditory or tactile stimuli produced by the SSDs. As a result, when using SSDs, subjects' natural responses to perceived objects rarely correspond to their expectations about what those responses should be. When subjects 'see' objects that they expect to elicit hedonic responses, but do not experience what they expect, they often feel frustrated. One question, then, is whether it is possible to create artificial associations between objects that normally elicit positive hedonic responses in sighted subjects, and proximal stimuli that SSD users find naturally pleasurable. For example, can researchers produce SSDs that would

[4] The FeelSpace belt is designed to help subjects orient themselves in space by indicating the direction of magnetic north through vibrations around subjects' waists.

[5] As Kiverstein et al. describe it, 'The vOICe is a visual-auditory substitution device that works by transforming images from a digital camera embedded in a pair of sunglasses into auditory frequencies ("soundscapes"), which the user hears through headphones' (2015: 661).

associate a pleasant-looking lilac with a naturally pleasant sound or pattern of touch? Would this enable researchers to reproduce normal profiles of non-sensory feelings?

Furthermore, supposing all of this were successful, another issue remains unsettled: whether subjects will attribute these non-sensory feelings to the objects perceived. So, for example, assume that an SSD is successful in associating the presentation of a pleasant-looking lilac with a naturally pleasant sound. If we are aiming to duplicate *all* the aspects of a normal visual experience then something more than a congruence of a pleasant object with a pleasant proximal stimulus may be required—namely, that the subject experiences the pleasure associated with their perception as deriving *from the lilac itself*, rather than from the sound produced by the SSD. In what follows, we hope to show a way in which it is possible to create artificial associations, but we leave it as an open empirical question whether distal attribution of non-sensory feelings will occur.

With regard to whether it is possible to create artificial associations, there seems to be a relevant difference between devices that deliver visual information by means of sound and those that use touch. Unlike auditory stimuli, tactile stimuli can only vary along two dimensions: intensity and location. This makes it harder to devise patterns of touch that are more pleasurable than others, in a way that resembles the wide spectrum of hedonic responses that visual images are capable of eliciting. On the other hand, it is known that some sound patterns are more pleasant than others. Both musical theory and psychological research about emotional responses to sounds could be consulted so as to find typically pleasing sounds. Assuming that such reliable information about the hedonic qualities of sounds is available, would it also be possible to use the sounds that we know to be pleasant or emotionally evocative to convey pleasant or emotionally evocative visual stimuli to blind subjects?

There are two possible ways to do this: either by means of a prefixed, hardwired, association of pleasant distal objects to pleasant proximal stimuli, or by means of a flexible, feedback-based mechanism, which creates associations based on subjects' matching of the hedonic properties of distal objects to patterns of proximal stimuli that SSD users take to have the corresponding hedonic properties.

The first option would involve using the current code used by the vOICe to 'translate' images into sounds, and using the available knowledge of natural cross-modal correspondences to complement this code. This would involve figuring out which sounds are naturally associated to the distal objects that produce certain hedonic responses, and adding those sounds to the sound patterns that represent those distal objects. Another, perhaps simpler, way to do this would be to select sounds that typically cause hedonic responses (regardless of the objects to which they are typically associated), and add these sounds to the system. This would involve programming the device in such a way that it is capable of discriminating certain visual patterns as being, for example, either a face or a landscape. With this ability for categorization, the device could associate types of pleasant sounds to categories of visual scenes, and play those sounds, in addition to the original code, when the subject is confronted with one of those scenes. This association would be programmed onto the device, just like the basic code.

Hardwiring pleasant acoustic patterns into an SSD is a way to secure that seeing a pleasant object will elicit the expected hedonic response. This option, however, seems artificial, distorting the normal phenomenology of pleasure. That is, this strategy would impose fixed hedonic responses onto the subject, while failing to account for the fact that, in the normal case, hedonic responses are flexible and dynamic. For instance, many hedonic responses are acquired only after several exposures to, say, a painting or a person's face. Also, the same visual scene does not always elicit the same hedonic response. This variation is dependent on a wide variety of factors. Some, like lighting conditions, which a device could detect, could in principle be taken into account in the programming. Others, like mood changes, are more arbitrary and highly subjective, and would be very difficult, if not impossible, to build into the device's architecture.[6]

Perhaps a more appropriate way of building these hedonic features into the SSD is through a more flexible mapping between pleasant sounds and pleasant images, which is responsive to the subject's preferences. This task would require a feedback-based mechanism, through which the subject is able to set and alter associations between images and sounds. Consider how such a mechanism might have worked when Bach-y-Rita's male subjects using TVSS were shown pictures of nude women. First, the subject 'sees' the woman. Then he notes the absence of a hedonic response. Next, he uses the feedback mechanism to indicate that the image should be pleasurable. The next time he 'sees' that image, the device will use that feedback to deliver pleasurable proximal stimuli. The mechanism could include a 'scale of pleasantness' for subjects to qualify visual scenes; or even allow the subject to classify visual scenes according to which kind of hedonic response they expect them to elicit.

The possibility of building such a mechanism raises two related issues. In the first place, building in a feedback mechanism could imply an elimination of the fixed mapping of visual-to-auditory properties, which is the very basis of the system, and the feature in virtue of which subjects can learn to use SSDs to recognize, discriminate, and perform other perceptual tasks. It is important to note that building in a feedback mechanism would change the nature of training with the device in a crucial way. Specifically, training would run in two directions, since both the subject and the device would learn from one another: subjects would learn the translation code of the device, in order to discriminate sensory contents, and

[6]This becomes even more complicated if we consider not only the variations in hedonic responses to images, but also the variations in hedonic responses to sounds. Since these two responses need not vary coherently, the interactions between them would become hard to deal with when programming such a device.

through their feedback, devices would also 'learn' to associate pleasant acoustic stimuli to what the subject considers to be pleasant scenes. Whether this flexibility would hinder the learning process, or perhaps facilitate it, is an empirical question. The success of this mechanism, however, would depend on the possibility of maintaining a fixed code for the translation of visual information into auditory information, while having some flexibility for pleasant sounds to be assigned to the visual scenes that the subject considers pleasant.

On the other hand, introducing this flexibility may be a good strategy to address the problems of artificiality and rigidness that would appear if we had hardwired associations between pleasant sounds and pleasant sights. Yet, it is not entirely clear whether it would be a good strategy to reproduce the way in which visual images produce hedonic responses. Having such feedback allows for the possibility of having hedonic responses that are not imposed on the subject, but it might cause the opposite problem: the hedonic response would appear more like a choice on the part of the subject, rather than a response to a pleasant image.

Nevertheless, it could be the case that, after a period of training, the visual images themselves start to be perceived as pleasant. As mentioned above, Bach-y-Rita thought that hedonic qualities may appear in sensory substitution in the same way that they appear for the non-native speakers of a language: after a long exposure to the context and cultural aspects of the language (Bach-y-Rita 2002: 510). This analogy also suggests that it is the use of the device which creates associations of visual scenes with hedonic responses, just as it is the use of the language that furthers the creation of such associations.

It may be thought that, when people learn to use a second language, the emotional aspects of the language are learned by two different means: first, by perceiving the way in which native speakers use emotionally charged words in particular situations, and second, by using the words in the appropriate contexts. If this analogy is correct, then it would seem that the development of hedonic and emotional responses for users of SSDs would not only depend on the amount of training, but also on their active involvement in the training process. Non-native speakers learn to associate emotional contents to words, not just by hearing the words, but also by actively using them in emotionally charged situations. Initially, the emotional content may seem dissociated from the word; it may seem to the subject as if he is choosing to pair a neutral word with an emotionally charged situation. Nonetheless, after a period of training, the emotional content may be associated to the word itself, and not merely to the context in which it is used. Likewise, providing feedback to the SSD may constitute an active involvement of the user, in virtue of which he is able to couple hedonic responses with visual scenes that initially seem hedonically neutral. This active involvement might have a similar effect: after a while, the visual scenes themselves may come to seem pleasant. At some point, it may happen that subjects attribute the hedonic properties to the distal visual scenes, and not to proximal auditory stimuli.

This discussion opens a set of related philosophical questions: Is it possible for SSD users to associate pleasant auditory stimuli to pleasant visual scenes by giving feedback to the devices? Would such associations lead to the attribution of pleasant properties to distal visual scenes rather than the proximal auditory stimuli, or would the pleasantness be attributed to the subject's choice of stimuli instead of being attributed to the scene? Would the active involvement of the subject in the process of association make a difference to the way that pleasantness is experienced? More generally, would a feedback mechanism facilitate training with SSDs, or would it hinder the learning process? These questions, and related ones, are open both to philosophical debate and to empirical research.

The main advantage of the feedback mechanism is that it could contribute to making the experience of SSD users more pleasurable. If the frustration reported by SSD users is not due to the absence of hedonic responses to the stimuli given to them (since there are hedonic responses to some sounds), but rather to the lack of consistency between their expectations of what should cause a hedonic response (e.g. seeing their wife's face) and what actually causes such a response (e.g. a meaningless pattern of sounds), this proposal should be helpful in addressing that problem. By building a feedback mechanism into the system, subjects would be given the possibility of pairing pleasant auditory stimuli to visual stimuli that they expect to be pleasant, thereby increasing the consistency of their expectations with their actual experiences. This way, their experiences would be more fluent, and this would, in turn, increase the likelihood of generating the expected non-sensory feelings by means of SSDs. We hope that the implementation of feedback mechanisms in SSDs will turn out to be an avenue of research that is worth pursuing.[7]

References

Bach-y-Rita, P. (2002) Sensory substitution and qualia. In A. Noë and E. Thompson (eds) *Vision and Mind: Selected Readings in the Philosophy of Perception*. Cambridge, MA: MIT Press, 497–514.

Bach-y-Rita, P., Tyler, M. E. and Kaczmarek, K. A. (2003) Seeing with the brain. *International Journal of Human-Computer Interaction* 15(2): 285–295.

Christodoulou, G. N. (1977) The syndrome of Capgras. *British Journal of Psychiatry* 130: 556–564.

Deroy, O. and Auvray, M. (2012) Reading the world through the skin and ears: a new perspective on sensory substitution. *Frontiers in Psychology* 3(457): 1–13.

Deroy, O. and Auvray, M. (2015) A crossmodal perspective on sensory substitution. In D. Stokes, M. Matthen and S. Biggs (eds) *Perception and its Modalities*. Oxford: Oxford University Press, 327–347.

[7] We thank Susanna Siegel for her helpful comments on an earlier draft of the essay.

Gregory, R. L. (1990) *Eye and Brain: The Psychology of Seeing*. Oxford: Oxford University Press.

Gregory, R. L. and Wallace, J. G. (1963) Recovery from early blindness: a case study. *Quarterly Journal of Experimental Psychology*, Monograph 2.

Kiverstein, J., Farina, M. and Clark, A. (2015) Substituting the senses. In M. Matthen (ed.) *The Oxford Handbook of the Philosophy of Perception*. Oxford: Oxford University Press, 659–675.

Konig, P. (2013) Properties and mechanisms of sensory augmentation. Paper delivered at the Sensory Substitution and Augmentation Conference, British Academy, London.

Lenay, C., Gapenne, O., Hanneton, S., Marque, C. and Genouelle, C. (2003) Sensory substitution: limits and perspectives. In Y. Hatwell, A. Streri and E. Gentaz (eds) *Touching for Knowing*. Amsterdam: John Benjamins, 275–292.

Ostrovsky, Y., Andalman, A. and Sinha, P. (2006) Vision following extended congenital blindness. *Psychological Science* 17: 1009–1014.

Sampaio E., Maris S. and Bach-y-Rita, P. (2001) Brain plasticity: 'visual' acuity of blind persons via the tongue. *Brain Research* 908: 204–207.

Spence, C. (2013) Commentary on Jonathan Cohen's 'On Some Limitations of Sensory Substitution'. Paper delivered 26 March at the Sensory Substitution and Augmentation Conference, British Academy, London.

17

The Role of Noetic Feelings in Sensory Substitution[1]

JÉRÔME DOKIC

Abstract A central issue in the study of sensory substitution devices is whether and to what extent the original source of knowledge about the world that they seem to enable substitutes for ordinary perception. I argue that this issue divides into two sub-issues, which concern respectively the sensory and the affective aspects of the phenomenology of perception. The sensory aspect determines the representational contents of experience, while the affective aspect is constituted by noetic feelings such as familiarity and presence. A pessimistic view may be formulated according to which neither familiarity nor presence can be reproduced in sensory substitution. There are important phenomenological differences between ordinary perception and sensory substitution due to the massively parallel architecture of the former. However, drawing on a discussion of Capgras syndrome and derealization disorder, I show that we also enjoy higher-level, post-perceptual feelings of familiarity and presence. In the last part of the essay, I draw on the psychological literature on metacognition and sketch a fluency-based account of both these feelings, which leads to a more optimistic view about whether they can be enjoyed by trained users of sensory substitution devices.

17.1 Introduction

A CENTRAL ISSUE IN THE study of sensory substitution devices (henceforth, SSDs) is whether and to what extent the original source of knowledge about the external world that they seem to enable substitutes for ordinary perception. This issue has both

[1] I would like to thank David Bain for his detailed and most helpful comments on a distant ancestor of this essay. Thanks also to Jean-Rémy Martin for fruitful ongoing discussion and collaboration on the topic of noetic feelings.

theoretical and practical implications. On the theoretical side, the hope is to attain a better understanding of the nature of perception itself. On the practical side, one might be interested in making the use of these devices as comfortable as possible by trying to match relevant aspects of the phenomenology of ordinary perception.

It should be relatively uncontroversial that expert use of SSDs can yield original *non-inferential knowledge* about the world.[2] For instance, trained subjects using the TVSS or the vOICe do not have to start from explicit considerations about the contents of their tactile or auditory experiences to conclude that there is a cube in front of them.[3] Rather, they spontaneously judge that there is a cube in front of them, without having to pay attention to their tactile or auditory experiences. Moreover, their judgement can even aspire to the status of *perceptual* knowledge, at least if 'perceptual knowledge' is interpreted in a broad sense, as referring to non-inferential knowledge causally based on sensory stimulations.

However, as Millar (2000: 74) has plausibly argued, 'perceptual knowledge can embrace more than the perceptually manifest'. This means that the contents of perceptual knowledge can go beyond what is perceptually presented, i.e. the contents of the underlying perceptual experience. We often move spontaneously from a sensory experience with a certain content (for instance, 'This is a bird') to a judgement with a richer content (for instance, 'This is a cardinal'), thanks to purely cognitive, or at least post-perceptual, habits or recognition heuristics.[4]

A more specific question then arises, namely whether SSDs yield genuine perceptual *experience* of the world over and above the contents directly provided by the substituting modality (e.g. touch in the case of the TVSS and audition in the case of the vOICe). In other words, the question is whether SSDs are sources of original perceptual contents. If this question is answered positively, further sub-questions arise, such as whether SSDs produce modality-specific or amodal contents and, if the former is the case, whether the relevant sensory modality is the substituting modality (Dominance interpretation) or the substituted one (Deference interpretation), or perhaps both at the same time (see, for example, Auvray and Myin 2009; Auvray and Deroy 2012; Ward and Wright 2012).

As I shall argue in this essay, even if the foregoing set of questions is clearly important, it addresses only one aspect of the phenomenology of using SSDs,

[2] Here I use 'non-inferential' in the philosopher's sense, meaning that it does not seem to the subject that she explicitly reasons to the relevant conclusion. This is compatible with there being implicit inferences in the psychologist's sense.

[3] The TVSS or tactile-vision sensory substitution device was created by Paul Bach-y-Rita (1972) and maps visual information extracted by a camera onto a two-dimensional array of vibrating points. The vOICEe converts the same visual information into auditory events, encoding space by means of time and qualitative dimensions of sounds (Meijer 1992).

[4] This example comes from McDowell (2008), who acknowledges that the acquisition of non-inferential knowledge that a perceived bird is a cardinal does not entail that the concept of a cardinal must be involved in a canonical specification of perceptual content.

namely the intentional or representational *contents* that these devices can enact. Another aspect has to do with the varieties of *non-sensory or trans-sensory feelings* that usually accompany ordinary perception, such as feelings of presence and absence, feelings of familiarity and unfamiliarity, feelings of certainty and uncertainty.[5] Correspondingly, there is a different set of questions that we can ask about the phenomenology of using SSDs, which concern the kinds of feeling that they are able to generate and their relationship to the feelings usually involved in ordinary perception.

I shall contend that these two sets of questions are relatively independent from each other. That is, claims to the effect that SSDs generate, or do not generate, the same kinds of feeling as ordinary perception may not much depend on whether the expert use of these devices is considered to result from a mere cognitive habit or, more ambitiously, from a genuine extension (or essential modification) of the subject's perceptual competences.

The essay is structured as follows. The next section introduces the claim that the phenomenology of ordinary perception is dual, in the sense that it involves both sensory and affective aspects. This claim is discussed with reference to two pathological cases, namely derealization disorder and Capgras syndrome, which concern respectively feelings of presence and feelings of familiarity. The third section offers preliminary considerations about whether these feelings are in fact involved in the expert use of SSDs. In the fourth section, a pessimistic view is formulated according to which neither kind of feeling can be reproduced in SSDs, because the relevant affective states are realized by low-level stimulus-driven systems present only in ordinary perception. However, the fifth section introduces a different, higher-level sense of presence, which could in principle be reproduced in SSDs. Finally, in the sixth section I sketch a fluency-based account of both experienced presence and familiarity, which leads to a slightly more optimistic view about whether these feelings can be enjoyed by trained users of SSDs.

17.2 The Dual Phenomenology of Perception[6]

An essential and pervasive aspect of the phenomenology of ordinary perception is provided by the sensory contents of our experiences. However, this does not exhaust perceptual phenomenology. When you are observing the pigeon just there perched on the branch, you may have visual experiences of greyish shades, of shapes, of movements and so on. Now, together with these sensory experiences

[5] I borrow the term 'trans-sensory' from Mangan (2001). The idea is that the same feeling, for instance a feeling of familiarity, can be bound to contents from different sensory modalities. The feeling that a familiar person is present, for instance, can be elicited by a given face or a given voice, or both.
[6] This section is adapted from Dokic and Martin (2015).

you also feel that you are looking at a *real* pigeon and not, for instance, a mere figment of your imagination. This feeling of reality or presence, which Husserl called '*Leibhaftigkeit*' (Husserl 1907), constitutes the experiential basis of spontaneous judgements of reality, such as 'There is a pigeon perched on the branch'. Were someone to lose this kind of feeling, she would be prevented from forming such judgements owing to the absence of the relevant experiential basis. What it is like to have a perceptual experience would be different in the absence of feelings of presence. Along with other kinds of feeling which can be bound to sensory contents, such as the feeling of familiarity (or unfamiliarity) and the feeling of certainty (or uncertainty), the feeling of presence contributes to the overall phenomenology of perception.

In order to understand how perceptual feelings work, it is worth making a detour through the psychological theory of metacognition. We can draw a distinction between two sources of metacognitive judgement, specifically *theory-based* judgements on the one hand and *experience-based* judgements on the other hand (Koriat 2000, 2006). Theory-based judgements are conclusions of explicit inferences from our encyclopaedic background knowledge or independent knowledge that we have about our own cognitive skills. In contrast, experience-based judgements result from affective experiences, namely what is referred to as *noetic feelings*. As an illustration, my belief that I know who was the forty-third President of the USA can be based either on reasoning (from the premises that I have learnt the names of all the USA Presidents at school and/or that I have an excellent memory) or on the gut feeling that I know the answer. Feelings of knowing are examples of noetic feelings among others, including feelings of not knowing, feelings of forgetting, and feelings of confidence. These specific affective experiences constitute the output of a monitoring process, which involves implicit inferences from a variety of internal cues, such as availability of partial information or fluency. In this respect, the level of availability of partial information or the level of fluency will modulate the phenomenological profile of the corresponding feeling. In particular, if the information to recall has been fluently encoded, the subject's feeling of knowing will be stronger than if the information has been encoded with difficulty. It appears that feelings are not sensitive to the specific memory contents at stake, but only to the quality of the on-line memory processes (Koriat 2006). Feelings are process- or quality-based rather than content-based (see also Dokic 2012).

In a previous co-authored work, I hypothesized that the distinction between theory-based and experience-based judgements can be applied to metaperceptual judgements (Dokic and Martin 2012). For example, the feelings of certainty or uncertainty present in metamemory are present in metaperception too. The judgement that I am unsure if the particular bird I am looking at is a blackbird or a raven can be based on either theory (for instance, I explicitly try to categorize the bird on the basis of its features, and I eventually fail to determine whether it is a blackbird or a raven) or experience (I have a feeling of uncertainty about the kind of bird perceived, perhaps because it is too dark or there is a mist). Other feelings such as the feeling of familiarity are more peculiar to metaperception. The judgement that I have seen this place before can be based on either theory (for instance, I explicitly remember that it is not the first time that I have visited this town) or experience (the place just feels familiar). Finally, as described above, our ordinary perceptual experiences are usually accompanied by feelings of presence. The judgement that there is a real as opposed to an imagined pigeon there on the branch can be based on either theory (for instance, I realize that there is no reason to imagine a pigeon and that I have never imagined anything like that in the past) or experience (the pigeon feels real to me). Normally, of course, when we look at things around us, we have the feeling of being related to actual and present things rather than mere representations, imaginings or memories. Feelings of presence are the result of a reality monitoring process, whose function is to determine whether an informational state has been internally or externally generated (Frith 1992). So, like feelings in memory, feelings in perception are not sensitive to presented contents as such but only to the quality of perceptual (and probably also cognitive) processes.

To the extent that perceptual phenomenology is dual, potential dissociations between the sensory and the affective dimensions of perceptual experiences can be predicted. Such dissociations show up in specific pathological cases, including derealization disorder (DD) and Capgras syndrome (CS), which I now briefly present.

17.2.1 Derealization disorder

Patients presenting DD (also called 'depersonalization') experience a kind of affective detachment from the external world, which appears strange, inconsistent and unreal (Sacco 2009): '[their perception is not] lived but is more like a mechanical, purely receptive sensory process, unaccompanied by its affective tone' (Parnas and Sass 2001: 105). Patients report that it is as if they were watching a movie or a picture of the world, instead of the real things around them: 'In fact, the people and things around you seem as unreal to you as if you were only dreaming about them' (Shorvon et al. 1946: 784). Shorvon et al. report another patient's description: 'Through the eyes I look out at a world that might be a picture of the world' (1946: 784). It is as if patients were confronted with a mere representation of the world. The causes of DD are multiple, including cognitive, neurological and psychiatric disturbances. However, the crucial point to highlight is that the contents of the patients' experiences should motivate the presence of an affective phenomenology which is in fact absent. The patients do not have the feeling of being directly presented with the actual sensory contents that they are nevertheless consciously experiencing. In other words, their perceptual states are not accompanied by feelings of presence any more; as Shorvon et al. already noted, '[their] perceptions do not awaken a feeling of reality [. . .]' (1946: 780).

DD suggests that the sensory and the affective aspects of perceptual phenomenology can be dissociated. In addition, subjective reports of patients support the thesis that affective phenomenology is necessary for the ordinary relational phenomenology to be instantiated. To the extent that the sensory aspect of their perceptual experiences is intact, patients can produce judgements about properties of objects with a high degree of confidence (e.g. 'This pigeon is grey (as opposed to red)'). In contrast, since the affective aspect of their perceptual experiences is deeply affected, they cannot produce judgements to the effect that they are acquainted with actual states of affairs (e.g. 'There is a real pigeon there in front of me (as opposed to a figment of my imagination'), at least with a high degree of confidence.

17.2.2 Capgras syndrome

Patients with CS hold the belief that one of their relatives (e.g. their spouse) has been replaced by an impostor. The formation of this delusional belief results from the fact that the affective component that normally accompanies our perceptual experiences of familiar persons, namely the feeling of familiarity, is absent. In fact, some models propose the existence of two information-processing pathways of face recognition (e.g. Bauer 1986).[7] A first pathway (the ventral visuo-semantic stream) encodes semantic information about facial features in order to construct a visual image of face and constitutes the medium of overt recognition. A second pathway (the dorsal visuo-affective stream) processes the affective response to familiar faces and is responsible for both the feeling of familiarity and covert automatic recognition. Some data in favour of the dissociation between an overt and a covert mechanism of face recognition show that normal subjects produce larger automatic arousal, as measured by skin conductance responses, when they are shown familiar faces than when they are shown unfamiliar faces (e.g. Quayle et al. 1999). This automatic response to familiar faces has precisely been interpreted as a kind of covert recognition. Furthermore, patients with prosopagnosia produce larger skin conductance responses for familiar faces than for unfamiliar faces, while at the same time being unable to overtly recognize any of the (familiar or unfamiliar) presented faces (Bauer 1986). In the light of these results, it has been suggested that CS is the mirror image of prosopagnosia. More precisely, in CS the visuo-semantic stream would be intact while the visuo-affective stream would be impaired. This hypothesis is supported by empirical results showing that the skin conductance responses of Capgras patients are not stronger for familiar

[7] The neuroanatomical validity of the original two-route model has been questioned and refined (see, for example, Ellis and Lewis 2001). Nonetheless, the hypothesis of a dissociation between overt and covert recognition is much less controversial.

faces than for unfamiliar faces (Ellis and Lewis 2001). Patients lack the affective reaction normally accompanying familiar faces; they do not experience familiarity. This abnormal and incongruous affective reaction constitutes the experiential basis from which the impostor delusion will be constructed.

Therefore, in CS, as in DD, the sensory phenomenology of subjects should motivate the presence of an affective phenomenology which is in fact absent. The person the subject is facing looks (perhaps exactly) like one of her relatives, but the subject lacks the feeling of familiarity associated with ordinary perception of a familiar person. The relative 'looks right' but 'feels wrong'. Conversely, some studies with healthy people show that it is possible to have a feeling of familiarity for a stimulus that is not, however, semantically recognized (Young et al. 1985). These data suggest that the feeling of familiarity can be dissociated from conscious identification of the source of familiarity.

17.3 Feelings of Presence and Familiarity in SSDs: Preliminary Considerations

Assuming that the phenomenology of ordinary perception is dual, let us move to the question of whether SSDs generate the feelings characteristically involved in ordinary perception. In this and the following sections, I would like to focus on two kinds of feeling, having to do with presence and familiarity.

17.3.1 The case of presence

Trained users of SSDs, including congenitally blind people, often say that they have a sense of the presence of distal objects experienced with the help of the device. For instance, in the case of the TVSS, objects can seem to be really 'out there' in the world (see Bach-y-Rita 2004; O'Regan 2011: 137). It is natural to interpret the phrase 'out there', in this context, as indicating not merely that objects are experienced as having some location in objective space (i.e. the subjects' experiences have spatial contents), but also that the subjects feel 'en rapport' with them, or have the feeling that the experienced objects are really there in front of them.

On this interpretation, the experiences of trained users of SSDs are very unlike those of derealized patients. Consider the following description by the French psychiatrist Jean-Étienne-Dominique Esquirol:

> An abyss, they say, separates them from the external world, I hear, I see, I touch, say many lypemaniacs [i.e. depressed people, given that depression can lead to derealization], but I am not as I formerly was. Objects do not come to me, they do not identify themselves with my being; a thick cloud, a veil changes the hue and aspect of objects.
> (Esquirol 1838: 414)

As suggested above, derealized patients do not enjoy the relational phenomenology involved in ordinary perception. Thus, they do not have the feeling that the objects of their experiences are 'out there', in the relevant sense of that phrase.

The natural interpretation is plausible, but a theoretical worry must be answered before it can be fully endorsed. The worry is that the sense of presence reported by trained users of SSDs is not a genuine feeling. At least some subjects who have not been told that they are using a device which converts distal information into bodily experience fail to have a sense of presence of distal things (Auvray et al. 2005). This might suggest that the sense of presence in the *other* cases of using SSDs rests on an independent *judgement* of presence. The subjects eventually experience a spatial object which they independently know to be 'out there' in their immediate environment. Their judgements of presence are based on a background theory rather than a primitive feeling.

In contrast, genuine feelings of presence seem to be *belief-independent*, which means that we can coherently have the feeling that a perceived object is present and judge or believe that it is not actually present. Perhaps this is what happens in some cases of virtual reality: the subject has a convincing perceptual experience of an object which feels present, but she independently knows that she is not facing anything real. The relational aspect of the phenomenology of one's experiences seems to be constituted at a level more fundamental than that of either belief or judgement.

As a consequence, the possibility has not yet been excluded that even a trained user of the TVSS or the vOICe has experiences which are in some respects *analogous* to the experiences of derealized patients. Such a user would be able to entertain new representational contents about distal objects, but she would not have the feeling that these objects are 'out there', or 'come to her'. In contrast to some derealized patients, she need not be delusional, and may independently judge or believe that her experience is about external objects really there in front of her. Still, she would not enjoy the relational phenomenology involved in ordinary perception. If this is a genuine possibility, then even the expert use of SSDs is not sufficient to generate genuine, belief-independent feelings of presence.

17.3.2 The case of familiarity

On the face of it, the case of familiarity is less favourable than that of presence. Anecdotal evidence suggests that experiences enabled by SSDs seem to lack the 'affective tone' characteristic of ordinary perception. For instance, some users of the TVSS have reported that they do not have the emotions that they should or expect to have when 'perceiving' the face of a familiar person:

> Thus, exploring the face of one's loved-one can be very disappointing, since the emotional messages that the long experience with vision has provided have not been perceived with our TVSS.
>
> (Bach-y-Rita 2002: 500)

Bach-y-Rita describes experiences enabled by the TVSS as lacking *qualia*, which presumably include affective states such as the feeling of familiarity. For instance:

> Subjects trained with the tactile vision substitution system have noted the absence of qualia, which in a number of cases has been quite disturbing. Thus, well-trained subjects are deeply disappointed when they explore the face of a wife or girlfriend and discover that, although they can describe details, there is no emotional content to the image.
>
> (Bach-y-Rita 2002: 509)

It is very tempting to describe the experiences reported in these passages as being Capgras-like. Of course, the patients are not deluded about what they experience. They know that they are facing a familiar person. Otherwise, they would have different expectations, and would not be disappointed by their experiences. Still, their experiences lack the feeling of familiarity that normally accompanies the perception of a loved one, whatever sensory modality is involved.

In what follows, I shall contrast two views about the involvement of noetic feelings in the use of SSDs. According to the pessimistic view, feelings of presence and familiarity cannot be part of the phenomenology of using a device such as the TVSS or the vOICe. On a more optimistic view, there can indeed be significant overlap between the phenomenology of using SSDs and the phenomenology of ordinary perception, at least as far as feelings of presence and familiarity are concerned.

17.4 A Pessimistic View

On the pessimistic view, SSDs cannot reproduce the feeling of presence and the feeling of familiarity involved in ordinary perception. The argument is that these feelings are generated from low-level stimulus-driven processes which are simply lacking in the experiences enabled by SSDs. The complex cognitive architecture of ordinary perception cannot be reproduced by these devices, at least as we know them.

Consider the feeling of presence. Matthen (2005, 2010) argues that it is generated by the brain outside the visuo-semantic system, namely in the dorsal stream. More precisely, on his account, the feeling of presence is a conscious emanation of the largely unconscious workings of the visuo-motor system.[8]

Of course Matthen's account cannot be that the activity of the visuo-motor system is *necessary* for there being a feeling of presence. One can have a feeling of presence bound to non-visual (for instance auditory) contents. In both cases,

[8] See Milner and Goodale (2006) for a classical formulation of the two-visual-systems hypothesis.

though, the feeling of presence is caused by low-level stimulus-driven systems. On the pessimistic view, these systems, which operate in parallel with the systems in the ventral stream that produce the sensory contents of one's experience, are precisely lacking in SSDs. As a consequence, there are no analogues of belief-independent feelings of presence in the experiences enabled by these devices.[9] In this respect, the case of sensory substitution is quite different from that of virtual reality, where the ordinary visuo-motor system can be exploited (indeed, fooled) and contribute to the feeling of being acquainted with a real world.

One might object to this diagnosis and insist that there is an analogue of the visuo-motor system in SSDs. Expert users of these devices can spontaneously reach to and grasp distal objects without having to think of their movements. One user of the TVSS is reported to have quickly stepped back when the experimenter increased the magnification on a zoom lens (Bach-y-Rita 1972), reproducing the characteristic looming response caused by the visuo-motor system in ordinary perception.

The defender of the pessimistic view might object that the 'quasi' visuo-motor system realized by SSDs is very different from our biological visuo-motor system. Given the parallel architecture of the human visual system, the spatial ability to reach to and grasp objects is not grounded on the spatial contents of conscious experience. In contrast, the ability of expert users of the TVSS or the vOICe to reach to and grasp objects *must* be a post-perceptual ability, since it feeds from the conscious tactile or auditory contents provided by these devices. This architectural difference, so the defender of the pessimistic view argues, makes an important phenomenological difference.

It has also been suggested that the visuo-motor system contributes to the phenomenological distinction between the background and the foreground of visual space (a position that Block (2005) attributes to Sean Kelly). This in turn may underlie the feeling that visual space is a part of larger space easily accessible through appropriate bodily movements. Again, it is doubtful that these phenomenological aspects can be involved in the experiences enabled by the TVSS or the vOICe, to the extent that peripheral vision does not seem to have any analogue in them.

Now consider the case of familiarity. One might justify the claim that the experiences enabled by SSDs are Capgras-like, in the sense that they lack the affective tone characteristic of the ordinary perception of familiar objects, by reference to the empirical hypothesis about CS described in section 17.2 above. According to this hypothesis, Capgras patients have a deficit pertaining to their visuo-affective system, which links (through the dorsal stream) visual stimulations with relevant activity in the limbic system. As a consequence of this deficit, the visual perception

[9] Note that I am not ascribing the pessimistic view to Matthen. I am just describing this view as a possible extension of Matthen's conception of the architecture of feelings of presence.

of a familiar person does not generate the feeling of familiarity that should normally be experienced. On this view, the feeling of familiarity is generated *in parallel* with the production by the visuo-semantic system of an experience with a specific sensory content. This is precisely what is lacking in SSDs. There is no analogue of the visuo-affective system in the TVSS or the vOICe. In other words, there is no analogue of a rapid, largely unconscious process of appraisal of visual stimulations.

The fact that feelings of presence and familiarity in ordinary perception can be generated by para-perceptual processes makes other experiences possible that do not seem available in SSDs. Feelings of presence and familiarity are usually bound to specific sensory contents. We feel the presence of a particular object, which may or may not seem familiar. These feelings, though, can also be experienced independently of their being manifestly bound to specific sensory contents. This is obvious enough in the case of familiarity. For instance, we can have a feeling of 'déjà vu' without knowing which aspect of the visual scene is in fact familiar (Brown 2003). It also appears that dorsal stream processes enable us to 'sense' the presence of something in the visual field even before we can actually visually identify it (Rensink 2004). These phenomena, which are part and parcel of the phenomenology of ordinary perception, can barely be reproduced in SSDs.

In a nutshell, the defender of the pessimistic view points out that the highly parallel neural architecture of human perception is responsible for phenomenological aspects of our ordinary experience, including affective aspects, which seem to be absent from the experiences enabled by currently available SSDs.

However, even if the phenomenology of using SSDs cannot indeed match all of the phenomenological subtleties of ordinary perception, at least as far as certain kinds of feeling are concerned, broader notions of presence and familiarity may be available to be reproduced in SSDs. So a more optimistic view can eventually be envisaged, as I shall argue in the following sections.

17.5 A Different Sense of Presence

Derealized patients seem to lack a feeling of presence but it is plausible that they have an intact visuo-motor system. They have peripheral vision, and are capable of visual sensing without seeing. As a consequence, they should share at least part of the phenomenology of ordinary perception. Still, something is missing, which concerns a different sense of presence.[10]

[10] Of course one might argue that the visuo-motor system of derealized patients is intact but for some other reason does not generate the feeling of presence that it generates in normal perception. I find this line of argument implausible, given that other phenomenological aspects of ordinary perception due to the activity of the visuo-motor system (such as peripheral vision and automatic obstacle-avoidance behaviour) seem to be preserved in derealization.

What clearly emerges from the reports of derealized patients is that they lack the feeling of being directly related to the perceived world as opposed to a mere picture-like representation. Interestingly, Matthen (2005) introduced the notion of felt presence by reference to a contrast between seeing an F face-to-face and seeing an F in a picture. The same visuo-recognitional abilities can be involved in both cases, but the presence of an F is felt only in the former case. Now if derealized patients have an intact visuo-motor system, their experience cannot be exactly like that of watching a picture or even a movie. They know, at least tacitly, that the laws of sensorimotor contingencies provided by their experience are not the same as the laws of sensorimotor contingencies provided by the experience of watching a movie. For instance, they are aware that unlike real visual perspectives, the perspective internal to an actual movie cannot be made to vary at will. In this respect, the phenomenology of their experience is closer to the phenomenology of direct perception than to the phenomenology of perceiving things in (static or dynamic) representations.

There is nevertheless a shared component between the experience of derealized patients and the ordinary experience of watching a movie, which may explain why they are attracted by the movie or picture metaphor. The spectator typically does not self-ascribe any experience involving the visual perspective internal to the movie. For instance, I watch a scene in which a man is walking, but I am not inclined to say that I am visually related to the walking man. The only experience I am inclined to self-ascribe is that of seeing a screen which represents a walking man.

An important enabling condition of perception is that there should be an appropriate spatial relationship between the subject and the perceived object.[11] Assuming that I, as an ordinary perceiver, have at least tacit knowledge of this enabling condition, I may refrain from self-ascribing the experience of seeing a walking man because it does not seem to me that I occupy the visual perspective internal to the movie. I do not feel spatially related to the man. In contrast, when I see a real man, it does seem to me that I occupy the visual perspective internal to my experience.

One might try to explain the relevant contrast as follows. The contents of perception are egocentric, in the sense that I *see* that I am spatially related to an object. For instance, I see a man walking toward *me*, or a tree to *my* left. The experience of seeing a scene in a movie is different. Unless I am fully immersed in the movie, it does not seem to me as if I am a constituent of the depicted scene. I do not see or seem to see that a man is walking toward *me*, or a tree to *my* left. However, this explanation is wanting. Several authors have argued that the contents of perception are *selfless*. The occupant of the perspective internal to our visual experiences need not, and perhaps cannot, be visually represented as such (Perry 1993; Campbell

[11] For a detailed discussion of this claim, see Cassam (2007). What counts as an appropriate spatial relationship depends on the sensory modality at stake.

1994; Brewer 1999; Dokic 2015). When egocentric terms like 'left', 'right', 'up', 'down', 'in front' and 'bchind' are used to specify the contents of our perceptual experiences, they should be used *non-relationally*, as explained by Brewer in the following passage:[12]

> There is a primitive use of [sentences involving egocentric terms] in which this is effectively tied to the thinker himself, in his actual location at just that time, in such a way that he has no comprehension of what it would be for the object or place represented as standing in that 'relation' to him then to be differently spatially related to *something else at some other time*. So he is not really *thinking relationally* at all. Although it is *a*'s spatial relations *with him then* which determine its truth or falsity, his thought is more properly regimented as '*R′a*': '*a* is to the right and a little in front', say, as opposed to '*a* is to the right and a little in front *of me now*'.
>
> (Brewer 1999: 193)

Now if the contents of ordinary perception are selfless, we should be entitled to claim that the very same contents can be seen in a movie. For instance, both ordinary vision and the experience of watching a movie can involve the representation of a man walking *closer*, or a tree *to the left*, while the occupant of the relevant visual perspective is not represented.

One might object to this last claim on the grounds that only the visuo-motor system is able to assign relative egocentric coordinates to visible objects (see Matthen 2012). Assuming that this system is not fooled when the subject is knowingly watching a movie, the contents depicted by a movie cannot match the egocentric contents of ordinary perception. However, this objection would miss the point of the claim, which is about the explicit contents of the relevant experiences, rather than the practical ability to locate objects in one's egocentric space. Even if Matthen is right and watching a movie does not involve the assignment of egocentric coordinates to depicted objects, we can see selfless egocentric directions in the movie. There is a difference between depicting a vase to the left of a cup, and depicting the former to the right of the latter. Perhaps our ability to see such a difference in a movie or in a photograph is somehow inherited from our visuo-motor ability to locate objects in real space, but it does not follow that actual egocentric coordinates in Matthen's sense are assigned to the depicted vase or cup.

If spatial perception is selfless, the content of my visual judgement that there is a tree to my left must be richer than the content of the grounding visual experience. It does not follow that my judgement involves an explicit identification of the origin of my visual frame of reference as myself. On the contrary, my judgement

[12] The point under discussion does not depend on the claim that the spatial contents of our experiences *must* be specified by means of egocentric terms (as Evans (1982) famously argued: see for instance p. 157). Perhaps one can hear a sound without knowing where it comes from in egocentric space. Still, our auditory experience has some perspective internal to it, which in the normal case is felt as our perspective.

is normally immune to error through misidentification. If I do not know that there is a tree to my left on the basis of my visual experience, I do not know that there is a tree to someone else's left either.[13] However, the view under consideration does entail that my inclination to judge or believe that the tree is to my left is at least partly independent of the sensory contents of my experience.

My suggestion is that derealized patients do not feel that they occupy the perspective internal to their perceptual experiences and thus are at best weakly inclined to self-ascribe them. Of course, they do in fact occupy such a perspective. This is why they can use their visuo-motor system to reach to and grasp objects around them. However, they have difficulties in making this fact explicit at the level of thought. The transition from the visual experience of a tree to the left to the judgement that there is a tree to their own left is not as obvious to them as it is to us. Even if they know that if they decided to initiate a movement, characteristic sensory changes would be experienced, they lack the motivation to *judge* that some of these changes concern their bodily self. The patients do not feel themselves *in* the world which their sensory experiences are about.

In the ordinary case of watching a movie, immersed subjects may temporarily feel themselves to be occupying the visual perspective internal to the movie, but most often subjects will feel themselves to be occupying the visual perspective internal to their visual experience of the screen itself. In contrast, derealized patients do not feel themselves to be occupying *any* experiential visual perspective.

On the present suggestion, the problem in DD does not lie in perception per se. Derealized patients do not suffer from an unusual form of perceptual illusion. Rather, it concerns post-perceptual stages, and more precisely the interface between perception and belief.

As a consequence, we should draw a distinction between two kinds of feeling of presence. One kind of feeling of presence is involved in both ordinary perception and DD, thanks to the operations of the visuo-motor system, but not in optic ataxia, which involves an impairment of this system. It is a low-level feeling, generated by stimulus-driven, para-perceptual processes in the dorsal stream. As the feeling of being able to move one's body around and use it to grasp objects, we might also call it the *feeling of bodily accessibility*. Objects can be felt to be accessible in this sense even for derealized patients, who seem to lack a full sense of embodiment or ownership of their body. Another kind of feeling of presence constitutes

[13]The term 'immunity to error through misidentification' comes from Shoemaker (1968) but the phenomenon is discussed in Wittgenstein's *Blue Book*. Here I rely on a fairly standard, epistemological reading of the term. Succinctly, the epistemic ground of a judgement which is immune to error through misidentification must be such that 'in the event that the statement in question is somehow defeated, it cannot survive as a ground for the corresponding existential generalization' (Wright 1998: 19). The connection between a judgement being immune to error through misidentification relative to the first person and the fact that the explicit content of the epistemic ground does not involve the self is emphasized by Recanati (2012).

the relational phenomenology of ordinary perception but is missing in DD. It is a high-level feeling, generated by post-perceptual processes, having to do with one's spontaneous self-ascriptions. As the feeling of being entitled to make judgements about one's experiential and spatial relation to the perceived world—what I shall call 'self-locating judgements'—we might also call it the *feeling of acquaintance*.

Now if we accept that because of their serial architecture, present-form SSDs cannot involve low-level feelings of presence, the question remains as to whether they can involve high-level feelings of presence, namely feelings of acquaintance. In order to answer this question, we must enquire further into the mechanisms at stake in the generation of the latter kind of feeling in ordinary perception.

17.6 A Fluency-Based Account

A widely accepted conclusion of the psychological study of metacognition is that many noetic feelings have to do with the *fluency* of perceptual and/or cognitive processes. For instance, the feeling of knowing can be due to the fluency of processing the question itself or attempting to answer it (Koriat 2006), i.e. the 'subjective ease' with which these mental operations are performed.[14]

The feeling of acquaintance (i.e. the kind of feeling of presence lacking in DD) might reflect processing fluency too. More precisely, if the view sketched in the previous section is on the right track, this feeling can be conceived as tracking the fluency of post-perceptual self-locating processes, or whatever sub-personal processes cause the subject's inclinations to make self-locating judgements such as 'This is a cube there in front of me' or 'I am actually seeing a cube rather than a representation of a cube'.

On the fluency-based account of the feeling of acquaintance, the fact that derealized patients lack the inclinations to form self-locating judgements is not caused by the absence of the feeling of acquaintance. The explanation goes the other way around; patients do not feel acquainted with the perceived world because they lack the relevant cognitive inclinations. In other words, the feeling of acquaintance manifests a cognitive habit rather than a perceptual achievement. Derealized patients might lack such a habit or, more probably, the motivation to activate it.[15]

To the extent that they are tied to post-perceptual doxastic inclinations, feelings of acquaintance are in an important sense *cognitive* (in contrast to feelings

[14] See for instance Wurtz et al. (2007), and Oppenheimer (2008).

[15] In the case of DD, the absence of the relevant cognitive motivations seems to be caused by a mere brain dysfunction, which causes a general lack of motivation. This contrasts with the case of unconvincing virtual reality, where subjects fail to feel immersed in the presented world because of constitutive features of the setup (lack of interactivity, uncanny valley effects, etc.). See Casati and Pasquinelli (2005) for a discussion of realism in virtual reality which in some respects is congenial to the present account.

of accessibility). They can still be said to be belief-independent to the extent that they can survive the rational formation of contrary judgements. For instance, the subject may feel inclined to judge that there is a cube in front of her, but refrain from actually forming this judgement because she independently knows that she is using a virtual reality device.[16]

In the case of SSDs, the real issue is thus whether the initial post-perceptual processes leading from sensory experience to self-locating judgements can be as fluent as in ordinary perception. If the subjective ease with which these processes are carried out matches the subjective ease with which they are carried out in ordinary perception, the same feeling of acquaintance will be generated.

Note that the mere fact that the subject forms self-locating judgements such as 'There is a cube in front of me' is not enough to generate the relevant feeling. An additional constraint is that these judgements should result from cognitive habits rather than explicit reasoning from independent background beliefs (for instance, about how a given SSD works). Only cognitive habits will be able to produce feelings of acquaintance independently of the judgements that the subject will eventually form all things considered. Indeed, the subject may either follow (as in ordinary perception) or resist (as in some cases of virtual reality) her felt inclinations to form self-locating judgements on the basis of her experience.

There is no reason why *in principle* trained users of SSDs cannot acquire the habit of forming self-locating judgements on the basis of their (tactile or auditory) experiences. Since the acquisition of such a habit should depend only on post-perceptual processes, the simple architecture of present-form SSDs should not be an obstacle. Even if the processes underlying the formation of spontaneous self-locating judgements may not be the same as in ordinary perception, the crucial point is that the subjects should be able to feel acquainted with the original spatial contents that they have learned to extract from their experiences.

The psychological literature on metacognition suggests that the feeling of familiarity too is a function of processing fluency. In general, familiar objects are easier to process, either perceptually or conceptually. This can generate the feeling that one knows these objects from previous experience. Now, lack of familiarity in SSDs might be explained by the complexity of the objects being processed. Human faces are clearly complex objects, which in ordinary perception are processed within a sub-module of the visual system (see, for example, Farah 2000). In contrast, in SSDs they are processed just as any other simpler object, say a cube. This might explain why even expert users of these devices do not experience feelings of familiarity while processing familiar faces. Moreover, since high fluency typically generates a positive affect (i.e. it 'feels good'; see Reber et al. 2004), the

[16] The extent to which feelings of acquaintance are belief-independent is an interesting issue. Intuitively they are more liable to be cognitively penetrated than sensory contents. For further discussion about the belief-independence and cognitive penetrability of noetic feelings, see Dokic and Martin (2015).

absence of qualia in the identification of familiar faces through the use of SSDs is not so surprising after all.

However, there might be a more general explanation of the apparent lack of feelings of familiarity in SSDs. There is an empirical model of feelings of familiarity according to which they are a function of both observed and expected processing fluency (Whittlesea and Williams 2001a, 2001b). Feelings of familiarity do not simply reflect fluency; they reflect the discrepancy between actual fluency and fluency as expected by the brain in the relevant context. We can now speculate that in SSDs, the expected fluency of processing simple objects such as a cube is generally higher than observed fluency. As a consequence, no feeling of familiarity should be experienced.[17] The reason is simple: processing 'visual' information about a cube on the basis of conscious tactile experiences, as in the TVSS, is bound to be less fluent than either seeing or touching a cube ordinarily.

17.7 Conclusion

The general question tackled in this essay is whether trained users of SSDs can enjoy the same kind of phenomenology as that of ordinary perception. I have argued that since perceptual phenomenology is dual, i.e. has both sensory and affective dimensions, this question should be divided into two sub-issues. The foregoing discussion has focused on one sub-issue, which concerns the possible involvement of feelings of presence and familiarity in the perceptual or perceptual-like experiences enjoyed by trained users of SSDs. Some reasons to be optimistic in this respect have been adduced: the relevant experiences can in principle generate cognitive feelings of presence and, perhaps to a lesser extent, feelings of familiarity.

An important lemma of the discussion is that the generation of noetic feelings in SSDs (at least those having to do with presence and familiarity) may *not* depend on the fact that these devices deliver genuine sensory contents. In principle noetic feelings can be bound to sensory contents, but also to contents produced by post-perceptual, cognitive habits. This is another illustration of the relative independence of the two dimensions—sensory and affective—of ordinary perceptual phenomenology.

In fact, for some purposes, the question of whether trained users of SSDs can have belief-independent noetic feelings may be more important, on the phenomenological level, than the question of whether they enjoy original and genuine sensory contents. Just as in virtual reality, the solution may not lie in increasing

[17] Of course here we have to suppose that processing fluency can be evaluated across sensory modalities, since a blind user of the TVSS, for instance, can expect fluency relative to the processing of a cube mainly on the basis of her previous tactile experience.

resolution or seeking sensory hyper-realism, but in other factors having to do with the implicit metacognitive monitoring of the perceptual and cognitive processes occurring in the use of SSDs.

References

Auvray, M. and Deroy, O. (2012) Reading the world through the skin and ears: a new perspective on sensory substitution. *Frontiers in Psychology* 3: 457. doi: 10.3389/fpsyg.2012.00457.

Auvray, M. and Myin, E. (2009) Perception with compensatory devices: from sensory substitution to sensorimotor extension. *Cognitive Science* 33: 1036–1058.

Auvray, M., Hanneton, S., Lenay, C. and O'Regan, K. (2005) There is something out there: distal attribution in sensory substitution, twenty years later. *Journal of Integrative* Neuroscience 4: 505–521.

Bach-y-Rita, P. (1972) *Brain Mechanisms in Sensory Substitution*. New York: Academic Press.

Bach-y-Rita, P. (2002) Sensory substitution and qualia. In A. Noë and E. Thompson (eds) *Vision and Mind: Selected Readings in the Philosophy of Perception*. Cambridge, MA: MIT Press, 497–514. Translated from J. Proust (ed.) (1996) *Perception et intermodalité*. Paris: Presses Universitaires de France, 81–100.

Bach-y-Rita, P. (2004) Tactile sensory substitution studies. *Annals of the New York Academy of Sciences* 1013: 83–91.

Bauer, R. M. (1986) The cognitive neuropsychology of prosopagnosia. In H. D. Ellis, M. A. Jeeves, F. Newcombe and A. Young (eds) *Aspects of Face Processing*. Dordrecht: Martinus Nijhoff, 253–267.

Block, N. (2005) Review of Alva Noë's *Action in Perception*. *Journal of Philosophy* 102: 259–272.

Brewer, B. (1999) *Perception and Reason*. Oxford: Oxford University Press.

Brown, A. S. (2003) A review of the déjà vu experience. *Psychological Bulletin* 129: 394–413.

Campbell, J. (1994) *Past, Space and Self*. Cambridge, MA: MIT Press.

Casati, R. and Pasquinelli, E. (2005) Is the subjective feel of 'presence' an uninteresting goal? *Journal of Visual Languages and Computing* 16: 428–441.

Cassam, Q. (2007) *The Possibility of Knowledge*. Oxford: Clarendon Press.

Dokic, J. (2012) Seeds of knowledge: noetic feelings and metacognition. In M. Beran, J. L. Brandl, J. Perner and J. Proust (eds) *Foundations of Metacognition*. Oxford: Oxford University Press, 302–320.

Dokic, J. (2015) Perception and space. In M. Matthen (ed.) *The Oxford Handbook of the Philosophy of Perception*. Oxford: Oxford University Press, 441–458.

Dokic, J. and Martin, J.-R. (2012) Disjunctivism, hallucinations, and metacognition. *WIREs Cognitive Science* 3: 533–543. doi: 10.1002/wcs.1190.

Dokic, J. and Martin, J.-R. (2015) That looks the same but feels different: a metacognitive approach of cognitive penetrability. In A. Raftopoulos and J. Zeimbekis (eds) *Cognitive Penetrability of Perception: New Philosophical Perspectives*. Oxford: Oxford University Press, 241–267.

Ellis, H. D. and Lewis, M. B. (2001) Capgras delusion: a window on face recognition. *Trends in Cognitive Sciences* 5: 149–156.

Esquirol, J. E. (1838) *Des Maladies Mentales*, vol. I. Paris: Baillière.

Evans, G. (1982) *The Varieties of Reference*. Oxford: Oxford University Press.

Farah, M. J. (2000) *The Cognitive Neuroscience of Vision*. Oxford: Blackwell.

Frith, C. D. (1992) *The Cognitive Neuropsychology of Schizophrenia*. Hillsdale, NJ: Erlbaum.

Husserl, E. (1907) *Ding und Raum* (*Thing and Space*), ed. U. Claesges. *Husserliana*, vol. 16. The Hague: Martinus Nijhoff.

Koriat, A. (2000) The feeling of knowing: some metatheoretical implications for consciousness and control. *Consciousness and Cognition* 9: 149–171.

Koriat, A. (2006) Metacognition and consciousness. In P. D. Zelazo, M. Moscovitch and E. Thompson (eds) *Cambridge Handbook of Consciousness*. New York: Cambridge University Press, 289–325.

Mangan, B. (2001) Sensation's ghost. *Psyche* 7(18).

Matthen, M. (2005) *Seeing, Doing, and Knowing*. Oxford: Oxford University Press.

Matthen, M. (2010) Two visual systems and the feeling of presence. In N. Gangopadhyay, M. Madary and F. Spicer (eds) *Perception, Action, and Consciousness: Sensorimotor Dynamics and Two Visual Systems*. Oxford: Oxford University Press, 107–124.

Matthen, M. (2012) Visual demonstratives. In A. Raftopoulos and P. Machamer (eds) *Perception, Realism, and the Problem of Reference*. Cambridge: Cambridge University Press, 43–67.

McDowell, J. (2008) Avoiding the myth of the given. In J. Lindgaard (ed.) *John McDowell: Experience, Norm, and Nature*. Oxford: Blackwell, 1–14.

Meijer, P. B. L. (1992) An experimental system for auditory image representations. *IEEE Transactions on Biomedical Engineering* 39: 112–121.

Millar, A. (2000) The scope of perceptual knowledge. *Philosophy* 291: 73–88.

Milner, D. and Goodale, M. (2006) *The Visual Brain in Action*, 2nd edn. Oxford: Oxford University Press.

Oppenheimer, D. M. (2008) The secret life of fluency. *Trends in Cognitive Sciences* 12(6): 237–241.

O'Regan, J. K. (2011) *Why Red Doesn't Sound Like a Bell: Understanding the Feel of Consciousness*. Oxford: Oxford University Press.

Parnas, J. and Sass, L. A. (2001) Self, solipsism, and schizophrenic delusions. *Philosophy, Psychiatry, and Psychology* 8(2): 101–120.

Perry, J. (1993) Thought without representation. In *The Problem of the Essential Indexical: And Other Essays*. Oxford: Oxford University Press, 205–226.

Quayle, A. H., Ellis, H. D. and Young, A. W. (1999) The emotional impact of faces (but not names): face specific changes in skin conductance responses to familiar and unfamiliar people. *Current Psychology* 18(1): 88–97.

Reber, R., Schwarz, N. and Winkielman P. (2004) Processing fluency and aesthetic pleasure: is beauty in the perceiver's processing experience? *Personality and Social Psychology Review* 8(4): 364–382.

Recanati, F. (2012) Immunity to error through misidentification. what it is and where it comes from. In S. Prosser and F. Recanati (eds) *Immunity to Error through Misidentification. New Essays*. Cambridge: Cambridge University Press, 181–201.

Rensink, R. A. (2004) Visual sensing without seeing. *Psychological Science* 15(1): 27–32.

Sacco, R. G. (2009) The circumplex structure of depersonalization/derealization. *International Journal of Psychological Studies* 2: 26–40.

Shoemaker, S. (1968) Self-reference and self-awareness. *Journal of Philosophy* 65(19): 555–567.

Shorvon, J. H., Hill, J. D. N., Burkitt, E. and Halstead H. (1946) The depersonalization syndrome. *Proceedings of the Royal Society of Medicine* 39: 779–792.

Ward, J. and Wright, T. (2012) Sensory substitution as an artificially acquired synaesthesia. *Neuroscience and Biobehavioral Reviews*, http://dx.doi.org/10.1016/j.neubiorev.2012.07.007.

Whittlesea, B. W. A. and Williams, L. D. (2001a) The discrepancy-attribution hypothesis: I. The heuristic basis of feelings of familiarity. *Journal of Experimental Psychology: Learning, Memory, and Cognition* 27(1): 3–13.

Whittlesea, B. W. A. and Williams, L. D. (2001b) The discrepancy-attribution hypothesis: II. Expectation, uncertainty, surprise, and feelings of familiarity. *Journal of Experimental Psychology: Learning, Memory, and Cognition* 27(1): 14–33.

Wright, C. (1998) Self-knowledge: the Wittgensteinian legacy. In C. Wright, B. C. Smith and C. Macdonald (eds) *Knowing Our Own Minds*. Oxford: Clarendon Press, 13–45.

Wurtz, P., Reber, R. and Zimmermann, T. D. (2007) The feeling of fluent perception: a single experience from multiple asynchronous sources. *Consciousness and Cognition* 17: 171–184.

Young, A. W., Hay, D. C. and Ellis, A. W. (1985) The faces that launched a thousand slips: everyday difficulties and errors in recognizing people. *British Journal of Psychology* 76: 495–523.

Index

Page numbers in **bold** refer to tables and in *italics* refer to figures.